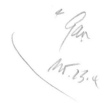

Better Breastfeeding

A mother's guide to feeding and nutrition

Daina Kalnins, MSc, RD,
with Debbie Stone, RN, IBCLC, RLC, and
Joyce Touw, RN, BScN, PNC (C), IBCLC, RLC

The Hospital for Sick Children

Robert
ROSE

For complete cataloguing information, see page 311.

Disclaimer
This book is a general guide only and should never be a substitute for the skill, knowledge, and
experience of a qualified medical professional dealing with the facts, circumstances, and symptoms
of a particular case.

The nutritional, medical, and health information presented in this book is based on the research,
training, and professional experience of the authors, and is true and complete to the best of their
knowledge. However, this book is intended only as an informative guide for those wishing to know
more about health, nutrition, and medicine; it is not intended to replace or countermand the advice
given by the reader's personal physician. Because each person and situation is unique, the authors and
the publisher urge the reader to check with a qualified health-care professional before using any
procedure where there is a question as to its appropriateness. A physician should be consulted before
beginning any exercise program. The authors and the publisher are not responsible for any adverse
effects or consequences resulting from the use of the information in this book. It is the responsibility
of the reader to consult a physician or other qualified health-care professional regarding his or her
personal care.

Editors: Bob Hilderley, Senior Editor, Health; and Sue Sumeraj, Editor, Recipes
Copyeditor: Fina Scroppo
Indexer: Gillian Watts
Design & Production: Daniella Zanchetta/PageWave Graphics Inc.
Illustrations: Kveta (Three in a Box)
Cover photo: Larry Williams (Corbis)

The publisher acknowledges the financial support of the Government of Canada through the
Book Publishing Industry Development Program.

Published by Robert Rose Inc.,
120 Eglinton Ave. E., Suite 800,
Toronto, Ontario, Canada M4P 1E2
Tel: (416) 322-6552 Fax: (416) 322-6936

Printed and bound in Canada

1 2 3 4 5 6 7 8 9 CP 15 14 13 12 11 10 09 08 07

Contents

✳ Preface

FOR YEARS, HUMAN INFANTS have survived from generation to generation nurtured by their mother's milk, and after years of scientific investigation into the growth and development of children, the evidence is clear. Human breast milk is the optimal way of feeding human infants to ensure their well-being. Increasingly, health-care providers are promoting natural breastfeeding rather than artificial formula-feeding for babies in their first year of life and beyond. The World Health Organization (WHO) recommends that infants be breastfed exclusively for the first 6 months of their lives, and that breastfeeding continue thereafter as solid foods are introduced into their diet. This recommendation has been endorsed by the American Academy of Pediatrics, the Canadian Paediatric Society, the American Dietetic Association and the Dietitians of Canada. Human breast milk provides all of the energy and nutrients that a full-term infant requires for normal growth and development (preterm infants may require vitamin and mineral supplements).

While breastfeeding is a most enjoyable experience for most women, the mention of breastfeeding to new mothers raises a variety of emotions, ranging from "Of course, I'm going to breastfeed," to "I'll give it a try," to "There's no way I'm going to breastfeed." In making the decision to breastfeed or formula-feed their babies, many new mothers can't look to their mothers or female relatives for advice because most of these women, caught up in an era that advocated artificial feeding and lacked the experience of breastfeeding, formula-fed their babies. Advances in nutrition science and the changing needs of working mothers over the past century have led to the promotion of a manufactured infant-food "formula" to replace human milk, which enables any caregiver to feed the infant with a bottle. Other women feel embarrassed if they breastfeed. We have no difficulty watching horses, cows, dogs, or cats nurse their newborns, yet today people still express a vast range of emotions when it comes to watching a human infant nursing at a mother's breast.

For breastfeeding to be successful, education of the mother during pregnancy, as well as support from health-care workers with breastfeeding expertise, is needed. With the appropriate support from trained health-care workers, in most cases, breastfeeding issues can be resolved.

Better Breastfeeding aims to resolve these issues. This book was written for women who are making the decision to breastfeed and desire more information during lactation. It should serve as a convenient and authoritative resource for new mothers and fathers, and others who are part of the woman's supportive circle, in understanding the value of breastfeeding and in the practice of breastfeeding.

Specifically, this book presents the scientific evidence for the benefits of breastfeeding for mother and child, expert advice on healthy eating during breastfeeding, and an understanding of breastfeeding physiology and breast milk composition. The book features a full set of practical strategies for breastfeeding successfully, including many how-to guides and troubleshooting tips. Uniquely, 150 recipes are provided to improve the mother's and, through her breast milk, the baby's health. There is something for everyone, whether you're a meat or fish lover, or someone following a vegetarian diet. The recipes provided are simple to prepare and are designed to be included in the family's meal plans for years to come.

Written by a registered dietitian and two registered nurse lactation consultants at the world-renowned Hospital for Sick Children in Toronto, this book offers expert advice on managing the most common complications experienced by women during breastfeeding. By being prepared to deal with these complications and knowing that there are proven solutions, it will be possible for women to breastfeed successfully. The outcome of this beautiful experience is the improved well-being of mother and child. If we can help you achieve this outcome by helping you to breastfeed successfully, we will have done our job.

✳ Top 10 Tips for Better Breastfeeding

1. Become informed about the benefits of breastfeeding. Before your baby arrives, get ready to provide this most important start to your baby's life.

2. Commit yourself to breastfeeding. It can take up to about 4 to 6 weeks for you to establish a feeding routine and feel comfortable with this new skill. Your baby and you need time to get to know each other.

3. Take care of yourself. Follow a well-balanced diet and enjoy the benefits of regular activity. Try to get plenty of rest, especially in the first few weeks after delivery.

4. Include a variety of foods in your diet. Eat a variety of fruits and vegetables, healthy grains and fiber, and foods that are high in iron. You may require a vitamin D and iron supplement. Eat when you are hungry and drink when you are thirsty.

5. Watch your baby's hunger cues and signs of fullness to know when and how much to feed. (We'll help you figure this one out.) If your baby's output (wet and soiled diapers) is normal, then the amount of breast milk she is taking in is enough.

6. Monitor your baby's weight gain. In the first few weeks of breastfeeding, it is important that your family physician or pediatrician track your baby's weight.

7. If you cannot be with your baby, supply your breast milk by expressing and storing it. Breast milk is the best nutrition, whether it is straight from the breast or expressed and delivered by bottle, cup or spoon.

8. Satisfy your baby's demand. Breastfeeding is a supply and demand system. During growth spurts, babies want to feed more often (which will increase your milk volume) before settling back to the previous routine.

9. Accept help from others in order to feel less alone in the early days of motherhood. If you have any questions or concerns during breastfeeding, get professional help. Gratefully accept the offer of family and friends to help with meals, housework and errands while you establish breastfeeding with your baby.

10. Understand that every baby is an individual.

PART 1

Better Nutrition and Techniques for Breastfeeding

CHAPTER 1

Benefits of Breastfeeding

DECIDING TO BREASTFEED your baby is a decision you will likely make during your pregnancy. In doing so, remember that, without a doubt, breastfeeding is the best form of nutrition for a newborn baby. Breast milk is nature's perfect food, meeting 100% of a healthy infant's nutritional requirements, with the possible exception of vitamin D, until a baby is 6 months old.

Most health-care providers recommend breast milk rather than formula, not only because breast milk is highly nutritious, but also because it offers immunity against many childhood and adult diseases. The list of associated health benefits provided to the infant by breastfeeding includes protection against gastrointestinal illness, diabetes, high blood pressure, heart disease and some cancers; prevention of allergies, obesity, respiratory illness and celiac disease; and improved blood pressure, bone health, cognitive function and iron status. Breastfeeding may also reduce anxiety later in childhood.

Studies of the possible benefits of breastfeeding have shown associations with positive effects not only for the child, but also for the mother. Breastfeeding has been linked to prevention of diseases including premenopausal breast cancer, ovarian cancer and osteoporosis in the mother later in life. There are also significant psychological benefits to the mother and child in the bonding experience breastfeeding provides.

Benefits for Mothers

Psychological Bonding and Well-Being

Perhaps one of the most important benefits for mothers is the immediate attachment that occurs with her baby during breastfeeding. The psychological benefit of this close bonding builds a trusting relationship. A mother may also experience an improvement in her self-esteem, derived from the assurance of knowing she is providing the best possible nutrition for her baby. Hormones (such as oxytocin and prolactin) released during breastfeeding can also result in a reduced level of anxiety, providing a calming effect during this initial adjustment to the mother's new role.

✳ Value-Added Benefits

Beyond direct health benefits for mother and baby, breastfeeding offers several associated added values.

Ecological: Breast milk is delivered without the additional packaging or processing involved in the making of infant formula. The reduction of waste from leftover cans and containers of formula, as well as the reduction of the waste involved in processing infant formula, contributes to the health of our planet.

Economic: The costs of breastfeeding are significantly less than the cost of formula-feeding when you take into account the cost of infant formula, bottles, caps, and nipples. Specialty allergy formulas can be at least double the cost of regular infant formula.

Convenience: Breastfeeding is very convenient. It is possible to breastfeed anytime, anywhere. Breast milk is always fresh and at the perfect temperature. There is no worrying about where you will heat up a bottle in the shopping mall or at the park.

Cleanliness: Breast milk does not require preparation or sterilization techniques that are dependent on a clean water supply.

Disease Prevention

Diabetes and Heart Disease
By having an effect on carbohydrate and fat metabolism in the mother, breastfeeding may provide protection against the development of diabetes and heart disease.

Osteoporosis
Women who breastfeed also benefit by reducing their risk of developing osteoporosis later in life.

Cancer
Breastfeeding also helps to protect a woman from breast cancer. The longer the mother breastfeeds, the more protection she has against developing breast, ovarian and endometrial cancers in later years.

Weight Loss

Weight loss accompanies breastfeeding because fat stores that were deposited during pregnancy are used to provide energy for the mother to feed her baby and food for the infant. Weight loss may not happen immediately, but within

Did You Know ...

Childhood Anxiety Reduction

Researchers recently reported that 10-year-old children who had been breastfed had less anxiety than their formula-fed peers. The close physical contact early on between a baby and a mother during breastfeeding may be one explanation for the findings. Another may be that breast milk affects the metabolic processes associated with the stress response.

A combination of studies reveals that the longer the total time of breastfeeding, the more protection from developing breast cancer the mother receives. A woman breastfeeding for a total of 1 year reduces her chances of developing breast cancer by 6%, while a woman breastfeeding for a total of 2 years reduces her chances by 11%. Longer periods of total breastfeeding time provide even further protection. The earlier that breastfeeding occurs in a woman's reproductive years, the stronger this protective effect may be.

6 months to 1 year from the baby's birth, a breastfeeding mother, on average, will more readily lose weight than a mother who formula-feeds her child. However, if a mother takes in an excess of calories through her diet, she may not achieve any weight loss.

Afterpains

Breastfeeding helps to stimulate the production of the hormone oxytocin, which causes the uterus to contract and helps the uterus return more quickly to its prepregnancy size. Because the uterus is contracted more quickly post-delivery, bleeding is reduced, preventing the loss of iron, which can be a factor in lower milk production. In the first few weeks of breastfeeding, these contractions, called afterpains, can be painful, but this should not discourage mothers from breastfeeding. Your health-care provider may be able to prescribe medication to ease the pain of these contractions.

Contraception

The absence of a menstrual period during breastfeeding, called lactational amenorrhea, can also prevent additional unwanted pregnancies in the first 6 months for mothers who are exclusively breastfeeding. Breastfeeding can act as a contraceptive because it affects luteinizing hormone (LH) release, decreasing these levels and preventing ovulation. However, breastfeeding cannot be relied upon to provide complete protection against pregnancy. Much depends on the breastfeeding pattern and the health of the mother. As the frequency of breastfeeding decreases, the chance of ovulation — and thus a woman's fertility — increases. Mothers who do not want to become pregnant again should discuss other methods of contraception with their doctor.

Benefits for Babies

Enhanced Immunity

During breastfeeding, the mother continues to protect her newborn infant from outside the womb much as she did inside the womb during pregnancy. Breast milk provides an infant's immune system with specific factors that help the

Is there anyone who should not breastfeed?

Some women should not breastfeed, for the following reasons:

- Women with HIV or HTVL 1 infection living in developed countries. There is potential to transmit the virus to the baby.
- Women with active, untreated tuberculosis. These women need to be separated from their child for the first 2 weeks of treatment, but they may express their breast milk for the baby.
- Women with active herpes lesions on the breast.
- Women who develop chicken pox shortly before or after childbirth. These women need to be separated from their babies until the mother is no longer contagious, but expressed breast milk can be given to the baby.
- Women with cancer. Drugs that fight cancer (antineoplastics) are harmful to babies. If these drugs are used in the treatment of the mother, the baby should not receive breast milk.
- Women who need to take certain other drugs, such as amiodarone and chloramphenicol or some radioactive agents (this list is not all-inclusive). These women should not breastfeed. Consult your health-care provider before taking any drugs while breastfeeding.
- Women who use drugs of abuse.
- In addition, babies with galactosemia need to be on a lactose-free diet, and thus cannot receive breast milk.

baby's body fight off common infections and diseases, such as diarrhea, ear infections, respiratory infections and urinary tract infections.

The immune factors that breast milk provides are specific proteins and fats, including enzymes, immunoglobulins, growth factors, antigens, cytokines, chemokines, eosinophils-derived granular proteins, polyamines and polyunsaturated fatty acids, as well as leukocytes (white blood cells). These protective factors help to prevent the growth of harmful microorganisms and also promote the growth of the small intestines, which helps decrease the chances of other problematic proteins making their way through the intestinal wall and into the bloodstream. In turn, the protective effect can stave off an allergy to that protein. Stimulating the growth of the small intestine also helps to create a barrier against the entrance of unwanted organisms.

How long should I breastfeed to enhance my baby's immunity against disease?

The longer a baby breastfeeds, the greater the protective effect against illness, not only as a baby, but also later as a child and adult. Although we do not know exactly how early nutrition influences disease development later in life, the fact that breastfeeding has a protective effect on preventing illness in newborns, especially when compared to formula-feeding, means that it likely plays a role in future disease prevention as well.

Did You Know ...

Probiotics and Prebiotics

Probiotics are the beneficial microorganisms that make up the healthy microflora in the small intestines. They include *Lactobacillus* and *Bifidobacteria.* Prebiotics help these beneficial bacteria to grow. Probiotics help babies defend against other more harmful microorganisms.

Gastrointestinal Health

In early pregnancy, the umbilical cord provides nutrition directly to the baby's blood system, not to the intestinal tract. By 20 weeks of age, the fetus is swallowing the amniotic fluid, which provides the growing intestines with nutrients, allowing for the stimulation and development of immune function. This combination of nutrition from the umbilical cord and the ingestion of the amniotic fluid provides all the nutrition the fetus needs to grow and develop normally.

At birth, when the umbilical cord is severed, the gastrointestinal (GI) tract continues to grow, adapting to the food provided to the newborn. Many changes occur when that intestinal tract is fully exposed to nutrients after birth. Through breast milk, protective proteins and microorganisms that are introduced play a very important role in the further development of the GI tract. Some substances found in breast milk work as prebiotics, which help to encourage growth of the probiotics, the beneficial bacteria and microflora in the intestine necessary for healthy digestion of food and absorption of nutrients.

Disease Protection

The primary reasons for hospital admission of infants are diarrhea and respiratory infections. Breastfeeding helps the baby defend against these common infections, as well as other specific diseases, and this protection continues on later in life.

Diarrhea

Many studies have demonstrated that infants who are Breastfed are less likely to have diarrheal illnesses than infants who were not breastfed. By enhancing immunity, breast milk prevents overgrowth of harmful microorganisms that cause diarrhea. These microorganisms cannot survive or survive for very short periods. Recent studies show that breastfeeding reduced the number of days diarrhea lasted when compared to formula-fed infants.

 If my child develops an illness that causes diarrhea, should I still continue to breastfeed? What if I become ill as well?

Yes, you will continue to pass on protective factors that may help your baby's gastrointestinal tract heal. However, babies who are receiving formula must stop taking the feeding for about 24 hours and switch to a solution of electrolytes and water until their digestive system is able to handle the formula again. This is yet another good example of how much better tolerated breast milk is compared to formula, especially in illness.

And yes, if you develop an illness, you can continue to breastfeed after consulting with your health-care provider. Your own immune system provides protection for you and immediate protection for your baby through the breast milk — an accelerated and rapid response form of protection.

Respiratory Illness

There is strong evidence to suggest that breastfeeding offers protection against the development of respiratory syncytial virus (RSV) infection, which is a common and potentially life-threatening infection. Infants are particularly susceptible to RSV. Breastfed babies have fewer days of illness and a lower number of episodes of respiratory illness. A recent study found that infants less than 1 year of age who were breastfed were hospitalized less than infants who were formula-fed.

Several studies also show that breastfeeding protects an infant against respiratory disease later on in childhood. Both prolonged breastfeeding (for at least 4 months) and the delayed introduction of solid foods (until 6 months) have a protective effect against respiratory illness, and this lasts into later childhood. In one large study of more than 2,200 children, breastfeeding for at least 6 months resulted in those children having fewer respiratory tract infections, as well as fewer ear infections, than those who were breastfed for 4 months. This provides further encouragement for mothers to continue to breastfeed exclusively for 6 months and beyond.

How breast milk protects against respiratory illness is not completely understood, but researchers suggest it may be oligosaccharides (specific types of sugars) that prevent certain bacteria from attaching to the respiratory cells. Lactoferrin found in breast milk prevents the use of iron by some bacteria that need it to grow, therefore reducing the possibility that they can cause infection.

Urinary Tract Infections

Protective factors in breast milk can help prevent urinary tract infections in infants. The oligosaccharides bind to bacteria in the urinary tract, preventing infection from occurring.

Asthma

Breastfeeding for longer than 4 months seems to protect infants from developing asthma. Breast milk helps to decrease wheezing and respiratory tract infections, which can lead to asthma later on. In one study, this protective effect continued until children were 6 years of age. Other factors, such as the environment (pollution, dust mites in the home, smoking), also have an affect on the development of asthma. By decreasing the incidence of wheezing and reducing the number of respiratory infections through exclusive breastfeeding, the incidence of asthma can be reduced.

Celiac Disease

Several studies have now shown that early feeding practices can play a role in the development of celiac disease. If infants were breastfeeding at the time of the introduction of solid foods, they were better protected against developing celiac disease. The longer the infants were breastfed, the more protection they received, or at least the onset of celiac disease was put off until the infant was older. The longer duration of breastfeeding results in the delayed introduction of foods that contain gluten (such as cereals).

In celiac disease, the protein gluten found in wheat, rye and barley flour is not tolerated by the immune system. Intake of this protein causes damage to the lining of the small intestine, or mucosa. Genetic factors also play a role in developing celiac disease, but the exact mechanism is not known. Once the gluten is eliminated from the diet, the mucosa repairs and the effects of celiac disease are no longer present. Symptoms of celiac disease include diarrhea and irritability. These symptoms are not specific to celiac disease, so sometimes diagnosis is delayed.

Cardiovascular Disease

Infants who are breastfed have lower blood pressure and a healthier blood fat profile than infants who are formula-fed. The better lipid profile may help prevent heart disease in adulthood. These factors may also help prevent obesity.

Childhood Cancers

Some studies show that children who were breastfed as infants are less likely to develop childhood cancers, including Wilms' tumor, acute leukemia and neuroblastoma (a cancer of the nervous system). One study found that children who were never breastfed or who were breastfed on a short-term basis had an increased risk of developing Hodgkin's disease versus children who were breastfed for at least 6 months. Although the protection of breastfeeding is not overly dramatic, there is an association that cannot be ignored.

Osteoporosis

Bone health is influenced by the type of feeding an infant receives. In one study, breastfed infants were more likely to have a greater bone mass by 8 years of age than infants who were not breastfed.

Inflammatory Bowel Disease

Recent studies indicate that breastfeeding, through the positive effect on the immune system and protection of the intestinal mucosa, may prevent infants from developing inflammatory bowel disease.

Other Associated Benefits

Other health benefits, although less direct or immediate, have been associated with breastfeeding.

Atopic Dermatitis

In atopic dermatitis (eczema), the skin becomes inflamed and red, causing itchiness and discomfort. Maintaining breastfeeding and delaying the introduction of solid foods until at least 6 months can help to prevent dermatitis, especially if the breast milk is high in omega-3 fatty acids.

Did You Know …

Cholesterol and Heart Disease

Believe it or not, breast milk actually has more cholesterol than infant formula, but it is this exposure to cholesterol in the newborn that helps him handle cholesterol later in life. Just how is not clear, but programming is probably at play. Learning to deal with cholesterol as an infant may protect against developing heart disease later on in life.

Did You Know …

Bedwetting

Researchers have studied the incidence of bedwetting (two times per week) in children who were 5 to 13 years of age and found that those who were breastfed were less likely to experience bedwetting than their formula-fed peers. The reason for this protective effect is unknown, but may be due to the essential fatty acid composition of breast milk, which allows for improved cognitive and neurological development in children.

Did You Know …

Vaccine Enhancement

Breastfed infants, when compared to formula-fed infants, have a better response to vaccines. Components of breast milk (certain antibodies) may prime the infant's immune system to be able to deal with the harmful proteins or pathogens in vaccines.

Did You Know …

Duration

Studies in families both with and without a history of allergy show that the longer the duration of breastfeeding (with even as little as 3 months of breastfeeding), the less likely an infant is to develop atopy, or hypersensitivity to a substance, presenting usually as a skin rash, hay fever, asthma, food allergy, respiratory allergy or wheezing. Exclusive breastfeeding for at least 4 months provides protection from infancy through to at least the preschool years. Not introducing solid foods until 6 months of age while exclusively breastfeeding may also have a protective effect in preventing allergies.

One study found that increasing amounts of omega-3 fatty acids in breast milk was more protective against atopy (hypersensitivity to a substance) than breast milk that had a higher omega-6 to omega-3 fatty acid ratio. Supplementing the mother's diet with more foods rich in omega-3 fatty acids may be protective against developing eczema. Not all studies show that breastfeeding, or that diet during breastfeeding, prevents atopic dermatitis from occurring. Environmental effects also play a significant role.

Allergies

Does breastfeeding protect a newborn from developing allergies? Can a mother pass on allergies to her baby through her breast milk? These questions continue to occupy medical research scientists and clinicians, with no full consensus yet emerging.

Allergy Protection

Some studies show that the incidence of common hypersensitivities is about 50% lower in breastfed children. Even very small amounts of breast milk, such as the colostrum in the first few days, provide protection. Significantly, breastfeeding is the only way to decrease the incidence of atopy in children.

However, simply avoiding highly allergenic foods, such as milk, eggs, shellfish and peanuts, until a child is at least 2 to 3 years of age does not necessarily prevent allergy from occurring, according to current studies. This does not mean that avoiding allergenic foods is not helpful for some children; it just means that the studies have not shown that food avoidance is helpful for all children.

Allergy Transmission

Certain proteins in breast milk may cause an infant to become sensitive to that protein. When the immune system of the infant reacts to that protein (through immunoglobulin E, or IgE), then exposure to that protein through food causes a skin reaction (eczema), respiratory reaction (wheezing) or gastrointestinal reaction (diarrhea). Some studies have found that certain proteins taken in through the mother's diet and passed through the breast milk may sensitize a child to become allergic to these proteins, but other studies do not confirm any benefit to eliminating certain allergenic foods from the mother's diet while breastfeeding. Children who have some form of skin rash, such as atopic dermatitis, are at higher risk of developing a food allergy.

✳ Allergy Basics

What is an allergy? Allergies are usually defined as being IgE-mediated, with reactions, such as hives and swelling of eyes, occurring immediately; or non-IgE-mediated with delayed reactions usually affecting the gastrointestinal tract and causing diarrhea. Ig stands for immunoglobulins — these specific proteins are part of the immune system. IgE-mediated allergies occur when a patient has specific IgE toward a specific protein or particle. It is unknown why this happens in some people and not others.

Food Allergies: Responses to food allergy may be mild, such as diarrhea, or may be quite severe, causing life-threatening anaphylactic reactions that may block breathing. Food allergies occur in about 4% to 7% of children less than 5 years of age, but after this age, the incidence of food allergy decreases. Allergies to milk, wheat and eggs usually resolve in 90% of children by the time they are 5 to 7 years of age. Allergies to peanuts, tree nuts and seafood, however, can be lifelong, but do resolve in 10% to 20% of people by the time they reach adulthood. About 1% to 2% of adults have food allergies.

Many families believe their child to have an allergy when in fact they do not. Proper testing is required to diagnose a food allergy. Skin tests can be helpful in diagnosing an allergy to milk, eggs, peanuts, tree nuts, fish and shellfish when a clinical history exists.

Common Allergens: The most common food allergies in children are to cow's milk, soy products, wheat, shellfish, peanuts, tree nuts and eggs. Rates of allergy to cow's milk protein found in formula are significantly higher than allergy to the proteins found in breast milk.

Risk Factors: The highest risk factor for developing an allergy is if another family member has an allergy.

Environmental factors such as exposure to secondhand smoke and outdoor pollutants (car exhaust) are risk factors.

 Will avoiding certain foods while breastfeeding protect my baby from developing a food allergy?

There is no straightforward answer to this question, even among experts. The American Academy of Pediatrics suggests that breastfeeding women should try to avoid peanuts and nuts if there is a strong history of allergy in the family, and consider avoiding eggs, cow's milk and fish. However, the European Society for Paediatric Gastroenterology, Hepatology and Nutrition does not recommend that breastfeeding women follow any type of avoidance diet. Our advice? It would be best to discuss the issue with your family doctor or pediatrician and decide together which foods, if any, should be avoided, based on evidence at the time.

CHAPTER 2

Healthy Breastfeeding Nutrition and Lifestyle

WOMEN HAVE UNIQUE *nutritional needs while breastfeeding and may be lacking certain nutrients. For example, surveys indicate that 75% of women are not receiving an adequate intake of calcium, while more than 30% have an inadequate intake of folate and vitamin E from food sources. Almost 60% of women do not eat enough fruits and vegetables. In the United States, foods with poor nutritional quality make up about 30% of the daily total energy intake.*

Both the American Dietetic Association and the Dietitians of Canada recognize that women have specific nutritional needs. Women's nutritional issues are of special concern because women typically make the main decisions about home food purchases and tend to set the dietary habits of the family. If they themselves are not receiving adequate nutrition or adequate information about good nutrition, then their children may also not be making healthy food choices. Women clearly need to become better educated about nutritional requirements for good health, especially if they are breastfeeding and choosing foods to nourish themselves and their babies.

Nutrition Basics

Some nutrient requirements are higher during lactation than they were during pregnancy. A well-balanced diet is particularly important after the birth of your baby to support the needs of breastfeeding — and to help get your body back to its prepregnant size. Good nutrition will also help you to combat fatigue and promote general well-being.

Eating well during the breastfeeding period can be difficult, however, given the many other demands on your time. In this book, we have provided more than 100 recipes to help you or others in your family prepare nutritious meals. Many of these can be made ahead and frozen during pregnancy to provide healthy and ready-to-go meals in minutes for the first few months after your baby is born, when meal preparation time is limited.

Food Guides

One of the best ways to ensure a healthy diet during lactation is to follow the United States Department of Agriculture (USDA) Food Guide Pyramid guidelines or Canada's Food Guide for Healthy Eating. Each guide separates food into different food groups with similar nutrients. A healthy diet should consist of appropriate serving sizes of foods from the following four food groups: milk and milk products, bread and cereals, meat and alternates, and fruits and vegetables. If you are meeting your recommended daily intake of the different food groups, then you are likely balanced nutritionally and receiving the appropriate nutrient needs. During lactation, these needs change, but not dramatically. See the Resources section in this book for more information on these food guides.

Energy Needs

Food energy is commonly measured in calories. The energy requirements for breastfeeding are higher than they are for women in general. While a pregnancy may have required an additional 300 to 500 calories per day in the second and third trimesters, respectively, energy requirements for breastfeeding are about 500 calories per day in the first 6 months, reducing to about 400 calories extra per day in the following 7 to 9 months, depending on the amount of breast milk produced.

The additional 500 calories per day in the first 6 months takes into account that the mother has energy reserves stored in the body during pregnancy. The mother's energy needs usually fall after 6 months as her milk production rate falls. At this time, a baby usually begins to take in solids and reduces the intake of mother's milk.

✳ Estimated Energy Requirement during Breastfeeding (depending on activity level)

Months 1 to 6:	2,500–2,800 calories
Months 7 to 9:	2,400–2,700 calories
Months 10 to 12:	2,300–2,700 (depending on amount of breast milk produced)

USDA's Food Guide Pyramid

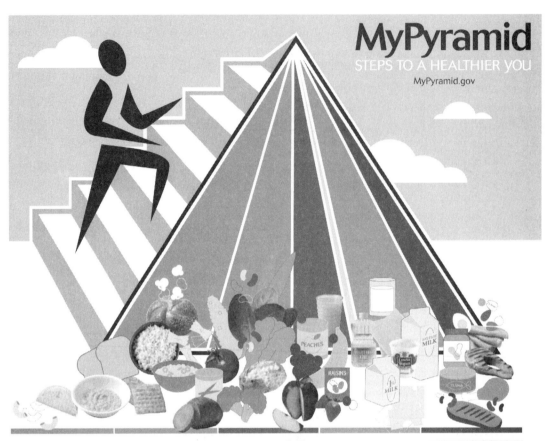

MyPyramid
STEPS TO A HEALTHIER YOU
MyPyramid.gov

GRAINS 6 ounces	VEGETABLES 2 1/2 cups	FRUITS 2 cups	MILK 3 cups	MEAT & BEANS 5 1/2 ounces
Make half your grains whole	**Vary your veggies** Aim for these amounts each week:	**Focus on fruits**	**Get your calcium-rich foods**	**Go lean with protein**
Aim for at least **3 ounces** of whole grains a day	**Dark green veggies** = 3 cups **Orange veggies** = 2 cups **Dry beans & peas** = 3 cups **Starchy veggies** = 3 cups **Other veggies** = 6 1/2 cups	Eat a variety of fruit Go easy on fruit juices	Go low-fat or fat-free when you choose milk, yogurt, or cheese	Choose low-fat or lean meats and poultry Vary your protein routine—choose more fish, beans, peas, nuts, and seeds

Find your balance between food and physical activity

Be physically active for at least **30 minutes** most days of the week.

Know your limits on fats, sugars, and sodium

Your allowance for oils is **6 teaspoons a day.**

Limit extras–solid fats and sugars–to **265 calories a day.**

Your results are based on a 2000 calorie pattern.

Name: _____

This calorie level is only an estimate of your needs. Monitor your body weight to see if you need to adjust your calorie intake.

Source: United States Department of Agriculture, MyPyramid.gov, 2005.

Canada's Food Guide for Healthy Eating

Recommended Number of *Food Guide Servings* per Day

	Children			Teens		Adults			
Age in Years	2-3	4-8	9-13	14-18		19-50		51+	
Sex	Girls and Boys			Females	Males	Females	Males	Females	Males
Vegetables and Fruit	4	5	6	7	8	7-8	8-10	7	7
Grain Products	3	4	6	6	7	6-7	8	6	7
Milk and Alternatives	2	2	3-4	3-4	3-4	2	2	3	3
Meat and Alternatives	1	1	1-2	2	3	2	3	2	3

The chart above shows how many Food Guide Servings you need from each of the four food groups every day.

Having the amount and type of food recommended and following the tips in *Canada's Food Guide* will help:

- Meet your needs for vitamins, minerals and other nutrients.
- Reduce your risk of obesity, type 2 diabetes, heart disease, certain types of cancer and osteoporosis.
- Contribute to your overall health and vitality.

Source: Food and Nutrition; Canada's Food Guide, Health Canada, 2007. Reproduced with the permission of the Minister of Public Works and Government Services Canada, 2007.

Phytochemicals, or phytonutrients, are considered to be a non-nutritive plant substance with some bioactivity. Flavonoids and carotenoids are phytonutrients, which are considered to have a beneficial effect on human health. Phytochemicals found in a whole fruit (including the peel) may provide the nutrients required to obtain their maximum benefit.

Flavonoids are compounds found in red, pink and purple plant pigments. Sources of flavonoids include berries, herbs and vegetables. Lycopene is a phytonutrient found, for example, in tomatoes (and in ketchup) in a concentrated form.

Carotenoids are natural fat-soluble orange/red pigments in plants and fruits and vegetables such as oranges, carrots, red peppers and tomatoes.

Total Calories

How many total calories a day does this translate to? If a woman is at her ideal weight before pregnancy, she would generally need about 2,500 to 2,800 calories a day. Level of activity will affect these requirements. The active woman may need more, about 2,900 calories a day, while the more sedentary mother would need somewhat less intake, about 2,300 calories per day.

Of course, these energy needs will depend on the amount of milk production. For example, if a mother decides to express her milk and feed her infant, energy needs may remain higher until she stops expressing.

The energy intake should be composed of nutrient-dense foods, including a variety of carbohydrates, fat and protein, eaten relatively evenly during the day in three meals and three snacks. Diets that eliminate certain foods or lack groups of foods may put an individual at risk of a nutrient deficiency.

Carbohydrates

Carbohydrates are required by the body for energy and for maintaining normal bowel movements. They should make up about 45% to 65% of total energy intake. Breads, grains and cereals, legumes, fruits and vegetables, and milk provide carbohydrates, as well as other important nutrients. While many highly processed foods also contain carbohydrates, they lack the nutrients — they simply provide energy and, often, an excess of calories.

Carbohydrates provide the energy we need for activity and for the normal functioning of organs. Red blood cells and cells in the brain also use carbohydrates as an energy source. If your diet does not contain enough carbohydrates, then the body's cells adapt by using protein or fat for its energy source.

Simple Carbohydrates or Sugars

Simple carbohydrates are made up of a short chain of molecules. Single sugars are also known as monosaccharides and include glucose, fructose and galactose. Disaccharides (two single sugars are connected) include sucrose (made up of glucose and fructose), lactose (made up of glucose and galactose) and maltose (made up of two molecules of glucose). Sucrose is found in fruits and vegetables, as well as in table sugar. Lactose is found in milk and dairy products. Maltose is found in cereals, such as wheat and barley.

Can I lose weight on a low-carbohydrate diet?
Are low-carbohydrate diets safe?

Generally speaking, any diet will work if enough calories are reduced and activity is increased enough to allow a lower overall ratio of energy intake to energy use. Because carbohydrates contribute more than 50% of energy intake, it makes sense that limiting these foods will reduce intake, but not if they are replaced by fats, for example. So a low-carbohydrate diet will work — if total energy intake is reduced.

However, the long-term benefits or risks of this diet are not known. Limiting intake of carbohydrate-containing foods, such as healthy grains, fruits and vegetables, could actually have a negative impact on health. These fiber-containing foods have been shown to decrease risk of heart disease, high blood pressure and constipation.

What has been shown to be effective in reducing weight is a balanced diet comprising all food groups with reduced calorie intake and increased physical activity.

Complex Carbohydrates or Sugars

The chain length of the sugar determines its classification. Long-chain carbohydrates are called polysaccharides and include the starches and modified starches, such as those found in plant foods or vegetables. Starch is found in rice, beans and potatoes, while modified starch (formed from starch) is used as a thickening agent in foods. Dietary fiber is a non-starch polysaccharide.

Fiber

Carbohydrates not digested in the digestive tract are called fiber. Fiber is found in all plants — fruits and vegetables, grains and legumes. Soluble fiber can easily be dissolved in water, while insoluble fiber does not dissolve in water. Oats and legumes, for example, are considered to contain soluble fiber, while carrots and whole wheat breads have insoluble fiber. These two different types of fiber work in different ways in the body, but both are important for maintaining normal bowel movements and preventing constipation and hemorrhoids, as well as for helping reduce risk of certain diseases.

Higher-fiber diets prevent or reduce incidence of colon cancer, heart disease, diabetes, high blood cholesterol levels and one of the most common causes of abdominal complaints in children, constipation.

Did You Know ...

Calories Per Gram

Carbohydrates contain 4 calories per gram, which is about the same as protein, while fat has about double this amount, at 9 calories per gram. This is why it may make more sense to restrict fat, rather than carbohydrate, in order to decrease energy intake if you are trying to lose weight. Keep in mind, however, that restricting too much fat is not recommended because a good variety of healthy fat is essential to a balanced diet.

✳ Lactose Intolerance

Lactose and Lactase: A person with a lactose intolerance has an inability to break down the lactose disaccharide due to a lack of the enzyme lactase. Lactase is found in the mucus lining of the small intestine. Lactase breaks down lactose from its disaccharide form to the monosaccharide or simple sugar forms of galactose and glucose. If this enzyme is missing or in limited amounts, then the undigested lactose is left in the intestine, where bacteria begin to digest it. As the bacteria digest the lactose, gas is produced, which often leads to abdominal discomfort, along with loose, watery stools or diarrhea. Sometimes this lactose intolerance is only temporary, following an illness that included diarrhea as a symptom.

Breast Milk: Although lactose is the main sugar found in breast milk, infants can tolerate it. However, some infants may develop a short-term lactose intolerance after a diarrheal illness, but lactose does not usually have to be removed from their diet. Breastfeeding should be continued.

Alternatives: Although people intolerant to lactose may not be able to drink cow's milk, they may still be able to eat fermented dairy products, such as cheese or yogurt. Milk that has been treated with the lactase enzyme and tablets containing lactase are also available for those who want to include foods that contain lactose in their diet.

Did You Know …

Legumes

Legumes are vegetables that include beans, peas and lentils. They also include soy, kidney, navy, fava, pinto and garbanzo beans (chickpeas). They are high in protein, folate, iron and potassium, with very low amounts of fat and no cholesterol. Legumes are an excellent source of fiber that can be easily incorporated into the diet.

Dietary Reference Intake for Fiber

For a breastfeeding mother, an adequate intake of fiber is 29 grams a day. What does this number mean in food intake? Twenty-nine grams of fiber, for example, equals 1 orange, $\frac{1}{2}$ mango, 1 cup (250 mL) bean salad, $\frac{1}{4}$ cup (50 mL) hummus, 1 cup (250 mL) blueberries, and $\frac{1}{2}$ cup (125 mL) green peas. Not that hard to take in every day!

Simple changes in the diet can boost fiber intake — for example, replacing white bread with whole-grain breads, choosing whole wheat pasta instead of white (or combining the two), adding legumes to salads and pasta dishes, snacking on fresh fruits and vegetables instead of drinking their juices and avoiding highly processed snack foods.

Good Sources of Fiber

By choosing the following foods more often, it is easy to take in the recommended 29 grams of fiber required daily by breastfeeding women.

Food	Serving Size	Total Fiber Content (grams)
FRUIT		
Apricots, dried	1 cup (250 mL), halves	9.5
Pear	1 medium	5.5
Blueberries	1 cup (250 mL)	3.6
Apple, with the skin	1 medium	3.3
Orange	1 medium	3.1
Strawberries	1 cup (250 mL)	2.9
Raisins	½ cup (125 mL)	2.7
Figs, dried	2 medium	1.6
GRAINS AND CEREALS		
Whole wheat spaghetti	1 cup (250 mL)	6.3
Bran flakes	¾ cup (175 mL)	5.3
Oatmeal	1 cup (250 mL), cooked	3.7
Rye bread	1 slice	1.9
Whole wheat bread	1 slice	1.9
LEGUMES AND NUTS		
Lentils, cooked	1 cup (250 mL)	15.6
Black beans	1 cup (250 mL)	15.0
Baked beans, canned	1 cup (250 mL)	13.9
Almonds	½ cup (125 mL)	6.3
Pistachios	½ cup (125 mL)	6.3
Peanuts	½ cup (125 mL)	5.8
Chickpeas	½ cup (125 mL)	5.3
VEGETABLES		
Corn	1 cup (250 mL)	4.6
Peas	½ cup (125 mL)	4.4
Tomato paste	¼ cup (50 mL)	3.0
Carrot	1 medium	1.7
Broccoli	½ cup (125 mL)	1.2
Green beans	½ cup (125 mL)	1.9

Glycemic Index for Carbohydrates

The glycemic index refers to how quickly a food containing a carbohydrate will raise blood sugar. Generally, those foods that raise blood sugar very quickly have a high glycemic index, while those that raise blood sugar more slowly have a low glycemic index. Eating a lot of foods with a relatively higher glycemic index may place you at risk of developing diabetes and perhaps heart disease, whereas lower-glycemic-index carbohydrates generally help people with diabetes keep their blood sugars under control, especially those with type 2 diabetes, where insulin is not generally required. In women who have gestational diabetes, appropriate food choices can help improve blood sugar levels, although insulin is sometimes required.

Processed or refined foods tend to have a higher glycemic index. For example, if wheat fiber or bran and the nutrient-rich inner germ are removed from the kernel during the processing of white flour, only the simpler sugars remain. Choosing less-refined foods and eating them in combination with higher-fiber grains or cereals is recommended, as is eating high glycemic foods in combination with protein. Protein foods can help decrease the absorption of simple sugars. Eat minimally processed grains, consume a healthy variety of fruits and vegetables, and choose brown rice (or a combination of brown and white) and whole wheat pastas (or a combination of plain and whole wheat).

Type 1 and Type 2 Diabetes

In two forms of diabetes — type 1, which is insulin-dependent, and type 2, which is non-insulin-dependent — the body is not able to regulate the level of sugar in the blood. In type 1, the insulin-producing cells of the pancreas are destroyed. Insulin is needed to bring sugar into body cells for energy; if this does not happen, the blood sugar, or glucose, stays in the blood. The body tries to rid itself of this excess sugar by increasing urination, which results in increased thirst.

Type 2 diabetes occurs most often in those who are very overweight (children included) and those with a family history of diabetes. In type 2, either the cells that produce insulin do not work properly or the insulin itself does not work properly. In either case, high blood sugar levels are the result.

In either type, uncontrolled high blood sugar levels can damage other tissues. Insulin injections are required for type 1, while a modified diet and weight loss can often help control type 2. Foods with a low glycemic index (that is, they raise blood sugar slowly) have been found to improve the symptoms

✳ Can I breastfeed if I have diabetes?

Yes. Regardless of your type of diabetes — type 1 (early onset) insulin-dependent or type 2 (late onset) non-insulin-dependent diabetes — you can breastfeed successfully. It does not matter if your diabetic condition predated your pregnancy or developed during your pregnancy (gestational diabetes). Because breastfeeding may decrease your insulin requirements, you will still need to monitor your blood sugar levels routinely.

Glycemic Index of Common Foods

Low Glycemic Index Foods (55 or less)
Skim milk, plain yogurt, sweet potato, oat bran bread, oatmeal, lentils, kidney beans, chickpeas

Medium Glycemic Index Foods (56–69)
Banana, raisins, split pea soup, brown rice, couscous, whole wheat bread, rye bread, popcorn

High Glycemic Index Foods (70+)
Dried dates, baked white potatoes, instant rice, plain bagel, soda crackers, French fries, ice cream, table sugar

of diabetes. For women who have gestational diabetes, appropriate food choices help improve blood sugar levels, although insulin is sometimes required.

Fat

Despite their bad reputation, fats are a vital component of a healthy diet. Among other functions, they transport fat-soluble vitamins — vitamins A, D, E and K — in the body. Fats are used for energy, as components of cell membranes, and for production of important hormones. Fat is an important part of the growth and development process in children. Because the type of fat mothers eat during breastfeeding is the type of fat used to compose the fat in her breast milk, mothers need to eat "good" fats and avoid "bad" fats.

There are various kinds of fat, all composed of smaller fatty acids. For example, triglycerides and phospholipids are combinations of fatty acids involved in fat storage and cell structure. A balanced diet will supply a variety of the different kids of fats, including saturated, monounsaturated and polyunsaturated fats.

Did You Know ...

Cancer-Fighting Fats

Choosing foods that contain monounsaturated and polyunsaturated fat will possibly reduce your risk of some types of cancer. Studies now reveal that the type of fat, not the total amount in the diet, is associated with different types of cancers. Some studies suggest that an increased intake of monounsaturated fats in the diet will help decrease the risk of breast cancer.

The recommended intake of fat is between 20% and 35% of total calories because high-fat food displaces other foods, such as grains, vegetables and fruits, which typically do not contain much fat, but are valuable sources of nutrients. A diet high in fat may also lead to excess energy intake, leading to obesity and its associated health risks, such as heart disease and diabetes. However, research now suggests that the type of fat making up the diet is even more important than the amount of fat eaten.

Saturated and Unsaturated Fat

The terms "saturated" and "unsaturated" fat refer to the number of double bonds in the chemical structure of the fat, with saturated fat containing no double bonds and unsaturated fat containing varying numbers of double bonds. Unsaturated fats can be monounsaturated or polyunsaturated. Dietitians recommend eating more unsaturated than saturated fats. Limiting saturated fats and increasing polyunsaturated fats in the diet can help improve overall health.

Dietary Sources of Good Monounsaturated and Polyunsaturated Fats

Monounsaturated Fats	Polyunsaturated Fats
• Olive oil	• Fish oils
• Canola oil	• Sunflower oil
• Avocado	• Walnuts, Brazil nuts, seeds
• Peanuts, hazelnuts, cashews, almonds	• Polyunsaturated margarines

Saturated Fats and Cholesterol

Saturated fats are found in high-fat milk and dairy products, as well as in meats and other animal products. A high intake of saturated fats can raise blood cholesterol levels, whereas monounsaturated and polyunsaturated fats lower blood cholesterol levels. High cholesterol levels in the blood can lead to heart disease.

However, some cholesterol plays an important role in cell membrane health and hormone circulation, including vitamin D (which is called a vitamin, but acts like a hormone). Cholesterol is naturally produced and regulated in the liver as well; in fact, the body manufactures more cholesterol than is derived from dietary sources. However, too much cholesterol in the diet can disturb its regulation.

Choosing foods that contain a variety of fats, eating a high-fiber diet and exercising regularly will help keep cholesterol in the blood at normal levels. Some people are genetically predisposed to having high blood levels of cholesterol, so they may also have to take medication to keep their blood cholesterol level in the normal range, thereby helping prevent heart disease.

Are eggs a healthy diet choice? Aren't they too high in cholesterol?

Eggs are a healthy part of the diet. Although the egg yolk does contain cholesterol, eggs are also an excellent source of protein, vitamin D and folate. One egg a day can be included in a healthy diet, unless otherwise advised by a health-care professional, for those people who cannot regulate their high cholesterol level.

Trans Fatty Acids

The location of the chemical double bond determines if a fat is a "cis" or "trans" fat. Fat with the cis conformation occurs more often in nature, while trans fats are more often manufactured or altered. While natural trans fats can be found in some dairy foods and meat products, manufactured or hydrogenated trans fats should always be avoided, not only during breastfeeding, because of their link to common disease conditions.

Naturally occurring trans fats are found in milk, cheese and beef, but only in small amounts. Hydrogenated trans fats are manufactured for use in some margarines and oils to make some foods, such as cookies, pastries and crackers, flakier and crispier as well as to increase their shelf life.

What is a safe intake of trans fats? At this time, researchers just don't know for sure, so limiting their intake as much as possible is recommended. Check the labels of processed snack foods, crackers, cookies and pastries for information on the trans fat content. If a product contains partially "hydrogenated fat" or "vegetable shortening," then the product will have trans fats.

Did You Know …

Trans Fat Risks

Trans fat can raise blood cholesterol levels in the same way saturated fats can by elevating LDL levels and lowering HDL levels. Trans fats also increase the inflammation process, contributing to chronic conditions such as heart disease and diabetes. Recently, the processed food industry has recognized these risks, and the use of trans fatty acids in food production is being eliminated.

Recommended Intake of Fat during Breastfeeding

The recommended amount of fat intake for women, including those who are breastfeeding, is between 20% and 35% of the total dietary calories. Young children and adolescents need slightly higher intakes of fat, between 25% and 40%, because they are still in a period of growth.

Essential Fatty Acids

Omega-3 and omega-6 fatty acids are considered essential because the body cannot make them on its own. They must be obtained from the fat we eat. These essential fatty acids (EFAs) are important components of cell structure and metabolic functions. The central nervous system contains a high amount. Development of vision in an infant depends on an adequate supply of essential fatty acids.

Omega-3

Omega-3 fatty acids help regulate inflammation, among other functions. This group of fatty acids includes linolenic acid, which is converted to docosahexaenoic acid (DHA) and eicosapentaenoic acid (EPA). DHA and EPA are important for heart health and for brain, nerve and eye development. Fatty fish, such as salmon, herring, sardines and trout, are the primary natural sources of DHA and EPA. DHA is found in breast milk and in some infant formulas. For breastfeeding mothers, DHA and EPA can be obtained in the diet and in preformed dietary supplements.

Omega-6

Omega-6 fatty acids tend to increase inflammation, but help keep blood cholesterol levels down. Linoleic acid, an omega-6 fatty acid, is converted to arachidonic acid (AA). Together, AA and DHA play a key role in normal brain development in a child.

 Are omega-3 fatty acid and fish oil supplements recommended during pregnancy and breastfeeding?

Instead of supplements, most national health agencies recommend the intake of fish that are low in mercury and PCB contaminants, along with other food choices high in omega-3 fatty acids. Some current research has shown benefits to the mother and the baby from taking omega-3 fatty acid supplements, but until further research is completed, supplements containing omega-3 fatty acids should only be taken if approved by a physician.

Foods High in Omega-3 Fatty Acids

- Fish: trout, salmon, herring, sardines, halibut, red snapper
- Shrimp
- Flaxseeds or flaxseed oil
- Canola oil, soft margarine made with canola oil
- Walnuts
- Soybeans and tofu
- Eggs enriched with omega-3 fatty acids (hens are fed grains containing omega-3 fatty acids)
- Bread, milk or juice enriched with omega-3 fatty acids
- Meat from grass-fed, not grain-fed, animals

Foods High in Omega-6 Fatty Acids

- Vegetable oils: soy, sunflower, corn
- Nuts and seeds
- Polyunsaturated margarines

Dietary Reference Intake of EFAs during Breastfeeding

The recommended amount of omega-6 fatty acids during pregnancy and breastfeeding is 13 grams per day, or 5% to 10% of total calories. The recommended amount of omega-3 fatty acids is at least 1.3 grams per day, or 0.6% to 1.2% of total calories.

What does this mean in food intake? To get double the recommended 1.3 grams (2.6 grams) of omega-3 fatty acids in one day, you could eat the following foods:

4 oz (125 g) of salmon (2.0 g) + 1 tbsp (15 mL) soy bean oil (0.9 g)

OR

½ cup (125 mL) firm tofu (0.7 g) + 2 tsp (10 mL) flaxseeds (1.6 g) + 2 eggs containing omega-3 fatty acids (0.8 g)

Protein

Protein is found in almost every part of the body — in hair, nails, muscle, bone and most tissue. Protein makes up important enzymes and serves as a carrier for vitamins and hemoglobin.

Protein is made up of many amino acids. Dietary intake of proteins is essential because the body cannot make some of the amino acids on its own. If the body lacks dietary protein, then serious negative consequences can occur. The body is constantly taking in and using protein, and losing some in hair, skin and excrement. Fortunately for those living in developed countries, lack of dietary protein is rare.

Protein Sources

Our food supply is varied enough to supply all the protein our bodies need. Protein is supplied by foods of animal origin, as well as by combinations of vegetables, grains and legumes. Animal protein should be trimmed of excess fat, with leaner cuts of meat chosen over higher-fat cuts. A high protein intake, above that recommended, is unnecessary and not beneficial.

Animal sources of protein are considered complete because they contain all of the amino acids needed. Proteins from grains, vegetables and legumes may be incomplete, but combining different plant sources will provide the right combination of amino acids.

 Are soy-based foods like tofu good sources of protein when I'm breastfeeding?

Some people who want to replace some of their animal protein sources with vegetable sources are choosing soy protein, often in the form of tofu. By doing so, you can improve your intake of fiber and many minerals and vitamins. However, too much soy protein may be associated with some negative health risks, though more extensive studies are needed to confirm this. Some dietitians suggest that two to four servings a week of soy protein food is safe. So soy protein can be a beneficial addition to a balanced diet that includes different sources of protein.

Dietary Reference Intake for Protein during Breastfeeding

Women who are not pregnant or breastfeeding need about 46 grams per day of protein.

During breastfeeding, a woman's protein needs are greater than normal, 71 grams per day, which is the same requirement as during pregnancy.

Folate

During pregnancy and breastfeeding, women have special needs for specific micronutrients, including folate (folic acid). Folate is a water-soluble B vitamin involved in numerous chemical reactions in the body that require the transfer of single carbon units or methyl groups. These reactions are essential in the formation of DNA (deoxyribonucleic acid), RNA (ribonucleic acid) and amino acids. At times in the life cycle, when the body is in a growing state, such as pregnancy and lactation, DNA, RNA and amino acid synthesis is greatly enhanced. Specifically during lactation, folate is not only an important component of breast milk, but also is required for milk synthesis in the mammary gland.

Folate Needs in Pregnancy

For some time now, women capable of becoming pregnant have been advised to consume a folic acid–containing supplement (400 mcg per day) until the end of the first trimester of pregnancy to reduce the risk of their babies being born with folate-dependent neural tube defects, such as spina bifida and anencephaly. These birth defects occur when the neural tube, later making up the spinal cord and brain, does not close properly during the first month of pregnancy.

Folate Deficiency

Despite folic acid fortification of the food supply, it appears that at least one-third of breastfeeding women still do not consume enough folate from dietary sources to meet their needs during lactation. Fortunately, the amount of folate in breast milk is generally unaffected by the folate nutrition of the mother, except on the rare occasion when maternal folate deficiency is severe (if, for example, the mother has megaloblastic anemia). So breast milk is a reliable source of folate for the nursing infant.

Nonetheless, given the important role of folate in a mother's own health and the possible impact that depletion of her folate stores could have on a subsequent pregnancy, it is important that woman continue to consume adequate amounts of folate during lactation when folate requirements remain elevated.

Recommended Folate Supplementation during Breastfeeding

Lactating women who consumed a folic acid–containing prenatal supplement for the duration of pregnancy, eat a well-balanced diet rich in folate-containing foods and are not capable of becoming pregnant again do not likely need a folic acid supplement. In contrast, women planning a subsequent pregnancy or not taking adequate precautions to prevent one should consume a folic acid–containing supplement (400 mcg per day) to reduce their future risk of neural defect–affected pregnancy.

There are situations where a larger folic acid supplement may prove worthwhile during lactation. These should be discussed with your doctor. For example, a woman who has lactated for a long duration, who has not taken supplemental folic acid and who has difficulty in remembering to take it every day may be a good candidate for a higher level of folic acid supplementation. Likewise, a woman who has had a previous pregnancy affected by a neural tube defect may quite rightly be advised to consume higher amounts of supplemental folic acid if she is capable of becoming pregnant.

In the event that a high folic acid supplement is recommended (greater than 1 mg per day), it is advisable that the first 1 milligram be consumed with a vitamin B_{12}-containing prenatal supplement and any folate above 1 milligram be consumed as a folic acid–only supplement to ensure that fat-soluble vitamin intakes (particularly vitamin A) do not reach unsafe levels.

Recommended Dietary Sources of Folate (based on usual serving size)

Excellent Source (55 mcg or more)	Good Source (33 mcg or more)	Source (11 mcg or more)
White bread, buns and rolls	Cooked lima beans	Cooked carrots, beet greens, sweet potato, snow peas, summer or winter squash, rutabaga, cabbage, cooked green beans
Pasta labeled enriched	Corn, bean sprouts, cooked broccoli, green peas, Brussels sprouts, beets	
Cooked fava, kidney, pinto, romano, soy and white beans, chickpeas and lentils		
Cooked spinach, asparagus	Oranges	Cashews, walnuts
Romaine lettuce	Honeydew melon	Eggs
Orange juice, canned	Raspberries, blackberries	Strawberries, banana, grapefruit, cantaloupe
Pineapple juice	Avocado	
Sunflower seeds	Roasted peanuts	Pork kidney
	Wheat germ	Breakfast cereals
		Milk, all types

Source: Nutrition for a Healthy Pregnancy, Dietary Sources of Folate; Health Canada, 2002. Adapted and reproduced with the permission of the Minister of Public Works and Government Services Canada, 2007.

Should I be taking a vitamin supplement while I breastfeed?

Most women will not need a vitamin supplement while they are breastfeeding, as long their diet is balanced. Breast milk content is usually not affected by low nutrient intakes by the mother.

However, some women have low iron, especially if they had low iron levels during pregnancy, and iron supplements may be recommended. If a mother's vitamin D levels are low because she lives in a northern climate or is not exposed to the sun for cultural reasons, then the baby's vitamin D intake may be low. Vitamin D supplements are usually recommended for fully breastfed infants unless they live in a warmer climate with regular sun exposure. Studies are underway looking at supplementing breastfeeding mothers with higher doses of vitamin D than usual as a possible substitute for giving infants vitamin D drops.

Did You Know ...
Folate Safety

Folate supplementation during breastfeeding is generally safe for the mother and the child, but is not without possible risks. For example, very high intakes of folic acid could mask a vitamin B_{12} deficiency by correcting its characteristic symptom, megaloblastic anemia. Undetected vitamin B_{12} deficiency may result in neurologic damage, which could be irreversible. The safety of very high levels of folic acid requires further study.

If there is not enough of this vitamin in the body, the nervous system can be affected and appetite and growth may be reduced in the mother and the baby. A deficiency of B$_{12}$ in women can result in megaloblastic anemia.

If a mother is a strict vegetarian, avoiding all animal products, then there may be an inadequate supply of vitamin B$_{12}$ to the breastfed infant. A vitamin B$_{12}$ supplement is recommended for strict vegetarian women who are breastfeeding. However, non-vegetarian women may be deficient in this vitamin — for example, if a woman is taking a gastric acid inhibitor, B$_{12}$ absorption may be affected.

Vitamin B$_{12}$

Vitamin B$_{12}$, also known as cobalamin, is another water-soluble vitamin that the body cannot produce. It is poorly absorbed by the intestinal tract, requiring an intrinsic factor (a protein) in the stomach for absorption. The intrinsic factor binds with the vitamin, and this compound is then absorbed in the small intestines.

Vitamin B$_{12}$ plays an important role in the development of red blood cells, acting in body tissues, including the liver, kidneys, brain, heart, blood and bone marrow. It is important for normal metabolism, especially in the cells of the nervous tissue and intestinal tract. Vitamin B$_{12}$ works with folic acid to produce important proteins.

Dietary Reference Intake for Vitamin B$_{12}$ during Breastfeeding

Breastfeeding women need about 2.8 micrograms of vitamin B$_{12}$ daily, while adult females need about 2.4 micrograms and pregnant women about 2.6 micrograms. Most prenatal supplements contain a source of vitamin B$_{12}$.

Good Food Sources of Vitamin B$_{12}$

- Animal products, especially the organ meats, such as liver
- Eggs
- Cheese
- Fish

Vitamin D

Vitamin D is known best for its role in bone health, improving the absorption of calcium from the diet. Vitamin D increases absorption of calcium by about 15%, from 10% to 15% absorption without vitamin D to 30% with vitamin D. This vitamin also functions like a hormone, affecting many systems in the body. Vitamin D is synthesized in the body when the skin is exposed to ultraviolet sunlight, and the vitamin is obtained from the diet.

Vitamin D Deficiency

A recent Canadian study found that almost 50% of women did not meet the recommend intake of vitamin D, 200 international units (IU) per day. (Some health-care professionals consider 200 IU per day far too low; field research is ongoing to determine the appropriate amount of vitamin D intake.) Vitamin D deficiency in a mother can affect her fetus, leading to an increased risk of developing diabetes later on in life. Studies have detected vitamin D receptors on the pancreatic cells, where insulin is produced. Vitamin D deficiency is also associated with osteoporosis and bone fractures, certain cancers (breast, colon, prostate and ovarian) and diseases of the immune system, such as multiple sclerosis.

If a pregnant woman's diet is deficient in vitamin D or she is limited in her exposure to the sun, her bone health and that of her fetus is at risk. Researchers from the United Kingdom reported that vitamin D deficiency during pregnancy can affect the bone health of the offspring almost 10 years later. Children of mothers with low levels of vitamin D had lower bone mass than those of mothers with normal vitamin D levels. Vitamin D transfers calcium from the umbilical cord to the fetus. Bones of infants whose mothers did not get enough vitamin D during pregnancy may be weaker and may have an increased risk of bone fracture. If infants do not get adequate vitamin D from breastfeeding or sufficient exposure to sunlight, they may show slower growth, with lower bone mass, and, in the long term, may even be at a greater risk for developing diabetes.

High-Risk Populations

High-risk groups for vitamin D deficiency include women with darker skin, because darker skin decreases the ability of the skin to produce vitamin D with sun exposure. Women and children living in northern latitudes, above the 55th parallel, are also at increased risk of being vitamin D deficient. This population

Did You Know ...

Vitamin D Status

At birth, the infant's vitamin D status is related to the mother's vitamin D status, so if a mother is deficient in vitamin D, this will affect the vitamin D levels of her baby. Although the blood levels of vitamin D in an infant are not always matched with the levels in breast milk, one study showed that if the mother is taking a high dose of vitamin D (2,000 IU per day), then her milk will have higher levels and the infant's blood levels may be higher as well. Mothers who are deficient in vitamin D during pregnancy may put their babies at risk for future development of allergies, type 1 diabetes and immune system disorders.

Recommended Dietary Sources of Vitamin D

- Fatty fish (salmon, trout, herring, sardines)
- Vitamin D–fortified cow's milk
- Fortified soy and rice beverages

If I'm breastfeeding, how much vitamin D does my baby need?

Although it would seem natural to assume that breast milk contains all the essential nutrients for a baby, research is indicating that vitamin D supplementation during breastfeeding should be recommended. In addition, for mothers and babies living in a northern climate or for those with dark skin, vitamin D production in the skin is limited, which can also influence the vitamin D content of the breast milk.

Vitamin D supplements are recommended for infants. The Canadian Paediatric Society recommends 400 international units (IU) per day (800 IU for infants in Far North communities), while the American Academy of Pediatrics recommends 200 IU per day until the infant has a regular dietary source of vitamin D, such as fortified formula and infant cereal, cow's milk, fish or other vitamin D–rich food.

may also have an increased risk of developing hypertension, heart disease, some forms of cancer and some immune disorders, such as multiple sclerosis, as well as osteoporosis.

Calcium

Calcium is best known as a component of bones and teeth, but also plays a role in the cardiovascular, nervous and musculoskeletal systems. Bone serves as storage for calcium, releasing it as needed by the body for normal function of these systems.

About 99% of calcium is stored in bones and teeth, while the remaining 1% is found throughout the body in muscle, blood and cells. Phosphorous, vitamin D, and protein also play important roles in bone health.

Did You Know …

Calcium Supplementation

During breastfeeding, mothers are advised to ensure adequate vitamin D intake to support calcium absorption by including in their diet vitamin D–fortified milk, which also contains protein, an important component of bone health. Some women may prefer to drink soy milk instead of cow's milk, but soy milk has less calcium than cow's milk and may not contain vitamin D. However, calcium supplementation is usually not required unless dietary intake is suboptimal.

Dietary Reference Intake for Calcium during Breastfeeding

The daily requirement of calcium for women is not increased during pregnancy or lactation (if more than 19 years of age). The requirement is 1,000 milligrams per day. The maximum safe upper limit of intake is 2,500 milligrams per day. Studies have shown that women who increase their intake of calcium while breastfeeding do not benefit in any way compared to women who do not supplement their intake.

✳ Calcium Deficiency

In the U.S. Third National Health and Nutrition Examination Survey, results indicated that 75% of women between 20 and 50 years of age were not receiving an adequate intake of calcium.

Osteoporosis, the most common bone disease, results from an inadequate intake of calcium. When calcium intake is inadequate, the body takes it from the bones to maintain normal blood levels so that calcium can then be used where necessary in the body. Over time, the bones become frail and weak, leading to fractures. New research suggests that an adequate intake of calcium can also help to prevent colon cancer and decrease risk of hypertension.

Studies show that women who breastfeed have lower bone density or a decrease in bone mass when compared to predelivery levels, and this can last for the duration of breastfeeding. Most studies reveal that when breastfeeding is stopped, bone mineral status returns to normal. Women who have prolonged breastfeeding periods in quick succession (pregnancies close together) may be at higher risk of developing osteoporosis later in life.

Dietary Sources of Calcium (based on usual serving size)

Excellent Source (275 mg or more)	Good Source (165 mg or more)	Source (55 mg or more)
Milk, all types	Mozzarella, Cheddar,	Creamed cottage
Swiss cheese	Edam, brick, Parmesan,	cheese, ricotta cheese
Tofu set with calcium	Gouda, feta cheese	Cooked or canned legumes
sulphate	Processed cheese spread,	(e.g., beans)
Plain yogurt	cheese slices	Cooked bok choy, kale,
Sesame seeds, whole	Yogurt	turnip greens, mustard
Fortified plant-based	Small sardines, canned	greens, broccoli
beverages	Salmon, canned with bones	Oranges
		Cooked scallops/oysters
		Almonds
		Dried sunflower seeds

Notes: Spinach, Swiss chard, beet greens, sweet potatoes and rhubarb are not good sources of calcium because these foods also contain oxalate or phytate, which inhibit calcium absorption. The calcium from vegetable sources is not as easy to absorb as that found in dairy foods. Certain elements found in vegetables (oxalates and phytates) can reduce the absorption of calcium. Intake of a variety of calcium-containing foods is recommended.

New products are coming on the market with added milk solids. Read labels to find out what amounts of calcium are added.

Source: Nutrition for a Healthy Pregnancy, Dietary Sources of Calcium; Health Canada, 2002. Adapted and reproduced with the permission of the Minister of Public Works and Government Services Canada, 2007.

A recent study revealed
that by delaying the
clamping of the
umbilical cord for a
minimum of 2 minutes
(it is usually clamped
within 5 to 10 seconds
of birth) in full-term
newborns, the risk
of anemia developing
in the infant can be
reduced. Iron stores
are boosted for up to
6 months through the
continued provision of
blood to the baby by
the umbilical cord.

Signs of iron deficiency
in infants and children
include slow weight
gain, pale skin, poor
appetite and irritability.
If iron deficiency is not
corrected in infancy,
then these children
can have learning
disabilities later on
in life.

Iron

Iron obtained from the diet is stored in the body, where the protein hemoglobin transports it. Together, the iron and hemoglobin carry oxygen to different cells of the body so that metabolic processes can occur.

If there is not enough iron, then hemoglobin levels may be decreased. In turn, this will decrease the ability of the body to carry oxygen to the needed destination. As a result, anemia can occur, leaving you feeling very tired and lethargic.

The type of iron found in different foods is not absorbed in the same way. Heme iron, found in foods from animal sources, is absorbed much better than non-heme iron, found in plant sources. Non-heme iron absorption can be increased by consuming food containing heme iron or with food containing vitamin C, such as oranges, mangoes and strawberries, which helps with the absorption of plant food sources of iron.

Iron Deficiency

Iron deficiency is the most common nutrient deficiency in both developing and developed countries. About 12% of women of reproductive age in the United States have iron deficiency. Because low iron stores have been associated with postpartum depression and milder forms of depression (which may be partly due to the increased tiredness that accompanies low levels of iron), breastfeeding women who feel more tired than usual and who feel they may be experiencing symptoms of depression should have their blood checked for low iron. Foods rich in iron, as well as iron supplements, may be recommended.

Dietary Reference Intake for Iron during Breastfeeding

The recommended amount of iron intake during pregnancy is 27 milligrams per day, but this decreases to 9 milligrams per day during breastfeeding, which is even lower than prepregnancy requirements for iron because menstruation does not occur during the first few months of breastfeeding. However, this level may be too low because a significant number of women may have low iron stores after pregnancy.

Recommended Dietary Sources of Heme Iron (based on usual serving size)

Excellent Source (3.5 mg or more)	Good Source (2.1 mg or more)	Source (0.7 mg or more)
n/a	Beef, ground or steak, cooked Blood pudding	Chicken, ham, lamb, pork, veal Halibut, haddock, perch, salmon, canned or fresh Shrimp, canned sardines, tuna Eggs

Recommended Dietary Sources of Non-Heme Iron (based on usual serving size)

Excellent Source (3.5 mg or more)	Good Source (2.1 mg or more)	Source (0.7 mg or more)
Cooked beans, such as white beans, soybeans, lentils, chickpeas Clams, oysters Pumpkin, squash, sesame seeds Breakfast cereals (enriched with iron) Tofu	Canned lima, red kidney beans, chickpeas and split peas Cooked enriched egg noodles Dried apricots	Peanuts, pecans, walnuts, pistachios, roasted almonds, roasted cashews, sunflower seeds Cooked pasta Bread Pumpernickel bagel, bran muffin Cooked oatmeal Wheat germ Canned beets, drained Canned pumpkin Dried seedless raisins, peaches, prunes

Source: Nutrition for a Healthy Pregnancy, Dietary Sources of Iron; Health Canada, 2002. Adapted and reproduced with the permission of the Minister of Public Works and Government Services Canada, 2007.

If I'm anemic, how will this affect my baby?

Most studies suggest that the iron content of breast milk is not affected by the mother's dietary iron intake, but if a mother has iron deficiency or insufficient iron stores, then an infant may also have an inability to store adequate iron. In this case, the child may require extra iron intake before the usually recommended age of 6 months.

Zinc

Zinc is required for healthy growth, metabolism and immune function. It is found in almost every cell in the body. Many enzyme processes require zinc for normal function. Zinc is also required for the senses of smell and taste.

Zinc absorption is higher in a diet containing animal products than in a diet based on plant products because one of the components of plant foods, phytates (found in whole-grain breads, legumes and cereals) can decrease absorption of zinc.

Zinc Deficiency

Zinc deficiency is very rarely seen in developed countries, but is identified in developing countries due to poor dietary intake of this mineral or its decreased absorption. Slightly more zinc is required during breastfeeding than during pregnancy and in women in general.

Dietary Reference Intake for Zinc during Breastfeeding

During breastfeeding, 12 milligrams daily are required, while 11 milligrams per day are required during pregnancy. In non-pregnant, non-lactating women, 8 milligrams per day are required. Women who are breastfeeding will supply their infant with enough zinc through breast milk, but by 7 to 12 months, as zinc needs increase, an infant will require an external source of zinc, usually found in solid foods, in addition to that found in the breast milk.

Recommended Dietary Sources of Zinc

- Meats and meat products
- Fish
- Dairy products
- Breakfast cereals
- Baked beans
- Cashews and pecans

Vegetarian Diets

Between 2% and 4% of the North America adult population currently follows a vegetarian diet. The health benefits of a vegetarian diet are many, including lower intakes of saturated fat and cholesterol with a higher intake of fiber, carbohydrates, antioxidants and phytochemicals. Vegetarians are also more likely to eat the recommended intake of fruits and vegetables, as advised by Canada's Food Guide and the USDA Food Guide Pyramid.

Some of the chronic diseases that are less likely to occur in those following a vegetarian diet include obesity, heart disease, diabetes and certain cancers (prostate and colorectal cancers). The type of fat in a vegetarian diet, the higher amount of fiber and the amount of antioxidants are all factors of a vegetarian diet that may protect against these chronic diseases. However, vegetarians have some special dietary requirements in general and especially in breastfeeding.

Special Nutrient Needs

Nutrients that require special attention in a vegetarian diet include protein, iron, zinc, calcium, zinc, vitamin B_{12}, and the essential fatty acid DHA.

Protein

Protein needs can easily be met with a vegetarian diet. Complementary proteins do not have to be eaten together at each meal, but vegetarians should make sure they consume all of the essential amino acids over the course of a day.

Calcium

Phytates and oxalates found in vegetables inhibit the absorption of calcium. While lacto-ovo vegetarians have an adequate intake of calcium, this mineral may not be adequately supplied in a vegan diet. Supplemented foods should be considered for those on a vegan diet. Vitamin D and protein also help with calcium absorption.

Vitamin B_{12}

Vitamin B_{12} is derived from animal sources, so this may be a concern in the vegetarian diet. Some B_{12}-fortified foods include soy milk, breakfast cereals, and nutritional yeasts or supplements. Lacto-ovo vegetarians can get enough B_{12} through dairy foods and eggs, as long as these foods are consumed regularly.

Did You Know ...

Vegetarian Diet Varieties

A vegetarian diet can vary from being very limited, such as a vegan diet, where only plant foods are consumed, to being more liberal, allowing some animal food sources, such as dairy and eggs for lacto-ovo vegetarians. Some self-described vegetarians also include fish occasionally as a source of protein.

Did You Know ...

Vitamin C Synergy

Foods containing vitamin C will increase the availability of iron from plant sources. When following a vegetarian diet, this is especially important for pregnant women, where iron deficiency is common, and an important consideration for children.

What are the risks of vitamin B_{12} deficiency in babies of vegetarian mothers who are breastfeeding?

A vegetarian diet that does not contain any animal products and no supplementation with vitamin B_{12} can result in B_{12} deficiency. For the mother, this can mean nerve damage that can cause tingling and numbness in the hands and feet and mental changes, such as confusion, irritability, and depression. For the breastfed infant of a vegan mother whose diet is deficient in vitamin B_{12}, deficiency can cause irritability, failure to thrive, refusal to eat, vomiting, and lethargy. Adults can store up to 3 to 5 years supply of vitamin B_{12}, but an infant does not have this storage capacity and so is more vulnerable to a diet deficient in vitamin B_{12}. Because vegetarian diets are often high in folate, it is possible that this will mask the signs of a vitamin B_{12} deficiency.

Did You Know ...

Iron and Zinc

Iron and zinc requirements are higher for those on a vegetarian diet because their bioavailability may be lower due to inhibitors of these minerals, such as phytates, which are found in cereals like bran.

DHA Essential Fatty Acid

DHA levels in breast milk of vegetarian mothers is lower than in the milk of non-vegetarian mothers. Because of the known importance of DHA for cognitive development and for eyesight in infants, it is recommended that vegan or vegetarian mothers include foods high in linolenic acid and other omega-3 fatty acids, which are converted to DHA. These foods include ground flaxseeds, flaxseed oil, canola oil and soy oil. Another choice may be a DHA supplement from a micro-algae source, if recommended by a physician. Consider limiting the intake of linoleic acid or the omega-6 fatty acids, since these can inhibit the formation of DHA. Food sources of linoleic acid include corn oil, safflower oil and sunflower oil.

Healthy Body Weight

The issue of weight after pregnancy is a sensitive one for many women. For almost 10 months during pregnancy, a woman watches her weight first go up slowly, then more rapidly at the end of term. Gaining 25 to 35 pounds or more in a relatively short time takes some adjustment. Most women want to get back to their healthy prepregnancy weight and the body image they desire. Some expect to be back to their normal weight within weeks of delivery.

This may be unrealistic, but a healthy body weight, or body mass index (BMI), can be achieved during breastfeeding. With time and sensible eating, in combination with a healthy level of activity, a woman's weight will return to normal, though it may take from 6 months to a year. Women who exercise and lose weight gradually after delivery are likely to benefit both physically and psychologically, perhaps helping to prevent postpartum depression.

Rushing weight loss may compromise breast milk production, especially if a severely reduced-calorie diet is followed in the hope of losing weight more quickly.

 Can I restrict certain foods in my diet and lose weight while I am breastfeeding?

You can safely lose weight while breastfeeding as long as you follow the USDA Food Guide Pyramid guidelines or Canada's Food Guide and include some form of exercise in your daily routine. Weight loss should be gradual. Do not restrict intake, however, to less than 1,500 calories per day on a low-fat diet, which can affect milk supply by decreasing the daily volume produced.

Research has shown that women who are overweight can safely follow a balanced restricted diet and enjoy exercising to lose weight while they breastfeed, without compromising the health of their baby. During a 10-week period, women in one study lost about 1 pound (0.5 kg) per week during their dietary restriction and exercise program, while their infants grew normally.

Body Mass Index

Your body mass index (BMI) helps to define a healthy target weight range. For women and men, BMI is calculated by measuring height and weight and then factoring them. For children, healthy BMI is different for different ages, and percentile charts are used instead. An accurate use of the BMI also needs to take into account the level of physical activity, growth and muscle mass.

Did You Know …

BMI Ranges

Normal BMI:
18.5 to 24.9

Overweight BMI:
25 to 29

Obese BMI: > 30

Underweight BMI: < 19

Weight Gain in Pregnancy

Did You Know ...

Body Image

According to the 1996/97 National Population Health Survey, about 20% of women in Canada in their childbearing years are overweight and therefore begin their pregnancy already at a less than ideal weight. Ironically, more than half of women in their childbearing years think that they should lose weight when in fact they are at a healthy weight. Many women constantly struggle to fit the right body image.

Following are recommendations for weight gain during pregnancy suggested by the Institute of Medicine's Food and Nutrition Board (1990) and the March of Dimes.

Normal Weight: If you are normal weight or at a healthy weight before pregnancy, with BMI at 20 to 25: Gain 25 to 35 pounds (11 to 16 kg) during pregnancy.

Underweight: If you are underweight before pregnancy, with a BMI < 19: Gain 28 to 40 pounds (13 to 18 kg) during pregnancy, though the gain may be more depending on actual prepregnancy weight.

Overweight: If you are overweight before pregnancy, with a BMI > 27: Gain 15 to 25 pounds (7 to 11 kg) during pregnancy.

In the first trimester, only a small amount of weight gain may be expected, about 2.2 to 8 pounds (1.3 to 3.5 kg). This increases to about 1 pound (0.45 kg) per week in the second and third trimesters. Weight gain should be slow and steady. A rapid weight gain, especially in the second and third trimesters, may indicate pregnancy-induced hypertension.

Weight Loss in Breastfeeding

The aim during breastfeeding is to return to your normal healthy BMI by 6 months to 1 year after pregnancy. The total weight gained during pregnancy does not automatically disappear after the birth of the baby. This weight gain is important for pregnancy and for breastfeeding. During pregnancy, extra weight gain allows for normal growth of the baby, and after pregnancy, extra weight "left" for the body helps a woman prepare for breastfeeding.

Studies reveal that most women retain about 7 to 15 pounds (3 to 7 kg) of the weight that they gained during pregnancy at 6 weeks after delivery. Fat stores that are laid down during pregnancy are not used during the first 2 to 3 months of breastfeeding. These stores are used once breastfeeding has continued for more than 3 to 6 months, when the maximum use of body fat stores takes place. This is another reason to continue to breastfeed for longer than 6 months.

Women who were above their recommended BMI before pregnancy or who gain more weight than is recommended during pregnancy are more likely to retain excess weight 1 year after delivery. Women who had a prepregnancy BMI above 25 or who gain more than the recommended amount during pregnancy may have a more difficult time losing weight unless they restrict their energy intake. New moms can follow a low-energy diet (but not less than approximately 1,500 calories per day) while breastfeeding in order to lose weight, without the need for a vitamin supplement, provided they select the proper foods.

Weight Loss Strategies

Protein Intake

For those interested in weight loss, protein can have added health benefits, in addition to providing an important supply of amino acids. Eating protein will increase satiety, or feeling of fullness, which means that you can reduce intake more easily.

✳ Top 12 Foods to Include in Your Diet

In no particular order, here are some foods important for health. This list applies to adults and children.

- Tomatoes
- Berries: blueberries, raspberries, strawberries
- Legumes
- Eggs
- Nuts and seeds
- Broccoli
- Whole-grain breads and cereals
- Fish
- Oranges
- Milk and cheese
- Olives and olive oil
- Carrots

Will exercising affect my breast milk?

Exercise is encouraged and will certainly help you get back to a healthy weight after pregnancy. It will also give you more energy and may help prevent fatigue. Lactic acid, which can build up in the blood during moderate exercise, does not seem to increase significantly in breast milk. Exercise does not decrease milk supply or change its composition or flavor. In a recent study of 24 women, moderate or even high-intensity exercise during breastfeeding did not decrease the infant's desire or acceptance of milk when taken 1 or more hours after exercise. Women who engage in a high level of physical activity while breastfeeding would be advised to increase energy intake accordingly.

Although certain types of carbohydrates provide more satiety than others, they are not as "satisfying" as proteins, and the same is true for fats. So the next time you have a meal of fish and brown rice, you will understand why it makes you feel less hungry afterward, compared to just having a bowl of ice cream or potato chips. Protein provides more satiety than carbohydrate, which provides more satiety than fat.

Increasing EFAs

In a study of the effects of a fatty acid supplement on weight loss, overweight subjects took the supplements, made up of two forms of conjugated linoleic acid, for 6 months. The researchers found that the supplement helped individuals lose weight. Other studies have suggested that including milk products as part of a diet helps people lose weight. Interestingly, conjugated linoleic acid is found in dairy

Will avoiding certain foods help settle my baby down? He seems to cry a lot, and friends have told me that certain foods I am eating may be the cause.

Generally speaking, no. Anywhere between 3% and 26% of newborns develop colic or irritability in the first 3 months of life. In general, foods eaten by the mother do not seem to have an effect on whether babies cry a lot or prevent them from becoming colicky. There are so many reasons that a baby is crying. Rest assured that, by providing your own milk, you are giving your baby the very best nutrition possible.

products (as well as in meat). Researchers suggest that conjugated linoleic acid keeps fat cells from increasing in number and reduces new production of fat cells. They still recommend an overall reduction in energy intake, as well as regular activity, in any weight reduction program.

Food Safety

A number of foods should be avoided or limited during breastfeeding, similar to the foods that should be avoided or limited during pregnancy. You should also follow certain food preparation guidelines while pregnant or breastfeeding or in any stage of life.

In the United States, approximately 76 million cases of food-borne diseases are reported annually, while about 11 to 13 million cases of food poisoning occur in Canada each year. Symptoms may be mild, such as gastroenteritis, or can be life-threatening, including neurologic, liver and kidney problems. Most causes of food-related illnesses occur because of improper storage or handling of food. Safe food practices mean that certain foods are avoided, that certain foods are eaten in moderation and that food preparation methods are clean and safe.

Foods to Avoid or Limit

Coffee and Tea

Coffee is safe to drink while breastfeeding, provided you do so in moderation. Caffeine does pass through breast milk, but only in small amounts. More than five 5-ounce cups (750 mL) of coffee per day may cause babies to be more fussy or restless. The caffeine may cause some disturbances in their sleep as well.

Herbal Products and Teas

Herbal products and teas should be consumed with caution. The labeling law on herbal products is not yet fully in place in Canada and not in place in the United States. This means that the actual content of the herbs is not known with certainty, and there is no quality control. Although many herbal products are probably safe, the consumer has no way of knowing for certain. Just because something is considered to be "natural" does not mean it should be considered "safe." It is best to check with your physician before taking any herbs while you are breastfeeding.

Did You Know ...

Natural Health Product Regulations

In Canada, natural health products, including herbs, vitamin and mineral supplements, traditional Chinese, Ayurvedic and other traditional medicines, and homeopathic medicine are in the process of being regulated by Health Canada. Each product will be given either a natural product number (NPN) or a drug identification number–homeopathic medicine (DIN-HM). This will let the consumer know that the product has undergone a review of its contents, labeling and instructions for use. Risks of using the products will also be provided. In the United States, natural health products are not yet regulated. They are considered to be dietary supplements, and their efficacy and safety do not have to be proven.

❋ Safe Daily Caffeine Intake

According to Health Canada's *Nutrition for a Healthy Pregnancy: National Guidelines for the Childbearing Years*, caffeine intake should be limited to 300 milligrams per day, while the Motherisk program at the Hospital for Sick Children recommends limiting caffeine to 150 milligrams per day. This is the equivalent of 1 to 2 cups of coffee, depending on the type, or 3 to 5 cups of tea. For example, 1 cup of brewed coffee has 135 mg of caffeine, while a cup of instant coffee has 76 to 106 mg. A cup of leaf or bag tea has 50 mg, while a cup of green tea has 30 mg. A 12-oz (355 mL) cola drink has 36 to 46 mg, and a cup of chocolate milk has 8 mg. Take-out containers at coffee bars have variable measurements, so be sure to check the amount of coffee in the usual size that you order.

Did You Know ...

Safe and Unsafe Sweeteners

Aspartame, which contains the amino acids phenylalanine and aspartic acid, is considered safe at 40 mg per kg body weight, which is equivalent to a 132-pound (60 kg) person drinking sixteen 10-ounce (355 mL) cans of diet soft drink daily. Other artificial sweeteners are also available, including sucralose and acesulfame potassium (ace K). However, saccharin and cyclamates are not permitted for use in Canada. They are not recommended during pregnancy and breastfeeding. They are sold as tabletop sweeteners, so be sure to read labels on sweeteners available at restaurants.

Herbal preparations contain active ingredients, so they can act as medicine in some cases. Some herbs have biological activity during pregnancy and breastfeeding, meaning they could adversely affect the mother and her baby. For a list of herbs and their safety, a recommended resource is the Motherisk program at the Hospital for Sick Children, which has published the book *Everyday Risks in Pregnancy and Breastfeeding*. See the Resources section for Motherisk contact information.

❋ Safe Herbal Teas

Several herbal teas have been recognized to be safe while breastfeeding, but at a maximum of 2 to 3 cups a day. As always, check with your physician if you have any concerns about your choice of herbal tea. It is probably wise to dilute herbal teas, especially if consumed daily. Among some of the better choices:

- Citrus peel
- Orange peel
- Ginger tea
- Lemon balm
- Rose hip

Artificial Sweeteners

The use of artificial sweeteners is not contraindicated during pregnancy or breastfeeding. However, foods containing these substances should be taken in moderation because excess amounts can replace other more important, more nutrient-dense foods rich in vitamins and minerals. Women who eat low-calorie and low-nutrient foods that contain artificial sweeteners in an effort to lose weight should critically evaluate their diet to ensure that they are receiving an adequate intake of calories and that they are meeting the recommended servings from the four food groups.

Mercury-Contaminated Fish

Fish provides an excellent source of protein, vitamins (vitamin A, D, and B), minerals (zinc and iron) and omega-3 fatty acids, both DHA and EPA. Some fish, however, are not recommended or should be eaten in moderation during pregnancy and lactation, due to the potential of environmental contamination from mercury. Other environmental pollutants can appear in fish, such as dioxins and polychlorinated biphenyls (PCBs), but the levels are generally low. The health benefits of fish, when eaten in moderation, outweigh the low health risk of the levels of these chemicals.

Mercury is a naturally occurring element in the environment. It is also a by-product created by some industries that released it into the air or the water as a pollutant. When this element enters waterways, it forms methylmercury, which, in high amounts, is harmful to our health. The fish we may eat absorb this methylmercury as they feed in polluted waters. Larger fish that swim and feed at the bottom of lakes and oceans typically accumulate more mercury than lighter

❋ *Is it safe to eat sushi while I am breastfeeding?*

The main component of sushi is sweet rice, seasoned with rice wine vinegar. Many different foods are used to make sushi, including raw fish, cooked fish and vegetables. Eating raw fish does carry a small risk of introducing microorganisms (for example, listeria) that can cause gastrointestinal upset. Though rarely reported, there are case reports of harmful microorganisms potentially being transmitted through breast milk.

If you are comfortable with the establishment that you frequent for your sushi, and know they practice safe food handling, then sushi should be safe to eat, from this perspective. Some of the fish used may also contain higher amounts of mercury, so check with your local or national food safety agency (such as Health Canada Advisories, Warnings and Recalls), the Canadian Food Inspection Agency (Food Facts) and the Environmental Protection Agency for guidelines on which fish have the lowest levels of mercury.

fish. Contact national health and environment agencies for advisories on safe fish consumption, and check with local agencies on the status of wild or game fish.

FDA and EPA Advisories

The U.S. Food and Drug Administration (FDA) and Environmental Protection Agency (EPA) recommend that larger fish, such as shark, king mackerel, tilefish, golden bass and swordfish, should be avoided or limited in the diet of pregnant women, breastfeeding women and younger children. Low mercury–containing fish, such as canned light tuna, salmon, pollack, sole, shrimp, haddock and catfish, can be consumed more regularly, about two times a week, to receive the beneficial omega-3 fatty acids.

Health Canada Advisory

Health Canada suggests that women who are pregnant or breastfeeding and younger children can consume a maximum of one meal per month of top predator fish that may contain higher levels of mercury, including shark, swordfish and fresh or frozen tuna (excluding canned tuna, which contains much lower levels of mercury than these predatory fish). Health Canada recently recommended limiting canned albacore tuna (which has higher levels of mercury than canned light tuna, but still well below standard cautionary mercury levels) in women who are pregnant or breastfeeding to four servings per week. One serving = 2.5 oz (75 g) or ½ cup (125 mL). Children who are between 1 and 4 years can eat up to one serving per week, and children between 5 and 11 years of age can eat up to two servings of albacore tuna per week. There are no restrictions to the consumption of canned light tuna.

 If I eat spicy food, will my baby taste it in my breast milk?

Yes, spices and some foods will affect the flavor of your milk, but this is to your baby's and your advantage. Your baby has already experienced "flavors" through your amniotic fluid, which was affected by the different foods you consumed during the pregnancy. By experiencing different flavors through your milk, your baby will be ready to make the transition to different-flavored solid foods. Perhaps you may even be able to decrease the chances of having a picky eater by providing variety and interesting flavors through your milk.

Can bacteria be transmitted through my breast milk to my baby?

Although a rare occurrence, it is possible for microorganisms ingested by the mother to be passed on to her baby through breast milk. There was one reported incidence of _Salmonella enterica_ being transmitted by the mother to her premature twins through breast milk. Food safety measures should always be followed in order to help avoid food contamination.

✳ Food Preparation Safety Guidelines

During food preparation, including preparing your own baby food, food safety guidelines must be followed. The home is the first place to practice safe food handling. Practical considerations when handling food include the following:

- Wash your hands thoroughly, as well as any surface area to be used for food preparation.
- If you are unsure how long food has been stored, throw it out. Organisms that grow on foods do not usually smell, and may not even taste bad.
- Avoid eating raw meat and animal products (including raw hot dogs, raw fish, raw poultry, raw eggs and unpasteurized dairy products).
- Keep raw foods and cooked foods separate to avoid contamination of the cooked food by the raw one. Keep this in mind while preparing recipes with multiple ingredients. Use separate cutting boards for raw foods and clean thoroughly before using again for another food. Keep utensils used to prepare foods separate. For example, knives used to cut poultry should be washed before being used to cut vegetables or fruit.
- Wash all fruit and vegetables well under cold running water, even those with a thick peel that you won't eat, such as melons and oranges. Pay special attention to vegetables that are leafy or flowered, such as lettuce, broccoli and spinach.
- Remove bruised or damaged areas of fruit or vegetables because organisms can grow in these areas.
- Reheat leftover meats until they are at least 165°F or 73°C (until they are steaming).
- Defrost frozen foods in the refrigerator overnight, not at room temperature on the counter.
- Hot foods should be kept at warmer than 140°F (60°C) and cold foods should be kept at lower than 39°F (4°C).
- Clean the surface of canned foods before opening, and clean the can opener after each use.

Remember to check your local or federal food regulatory agency for any health alerts on contaminated foods. In Canada, check the Canadian Food Inspection Agency site, and in America, check the United States Food and Drug Administration. See the Resources section in this book for contact information. You can also sign on for e-mail alerts.

Storage Tips for Fruits and Vegetables

Food storage is an important part of food safety. Here are recommended storage practices for fruits and vegetables.

Fruit or Vegetable	Storage Method: Time	Tips
Apples	Room temperature: 1 to 2 days Refrigerator crisper: up to 1 month	Ripen apples at room temperature. Once they are ripe, store them, unwashed, in plastic bags in the crisper.
Bananas	Room temperature: 2 to 3 days	Ripen bananas at room temperature.
Berries (blackberries, raspberries, strawberries)	Refrigerator crisper: 2 to 3 days	Before storing berries, remove any spoiled or crushed fruits. Store the berries, unwashed, in plastic bags or plastic containers. Do not remove the green tops from strawberries before storing them.
Broccoli	Refrigerator crisper: 3 to 5 days	Store broccoli, unwashed, in plastic bags.
Beets, carrots, parsnips, radishes, turnips	Refrigerator crisper: 1 to 2 weeks	Remove green tops and store the vegetables, unwashed, in plastic bags. Trim the taproots from radishes before storing.
Corn	Refrigerator crisper: 1 to 2 days	For best flavor, use corn immediately. Corn in husks can be stored in plastic bags for 1 to 2 days.
Grapes	Refrigerator crisper: 3 to 5 days	Store grapes, unwashed, in plastic bags.
Herbs	Refrigerator crisper: 2 to 3 days	Herbs may be stored in plastic bags.
Lettuce and greens	Refrigerator crisper: 5 to 7 days for lettuce; 1 to 2 days for greens	Store them, unwashed, in plastic bags in the refrigerator crisper.
Melons (watermelon, honeydew, cantaloupe)	Refrigerator: 3 to 4 days for cut melon	For best flavor, store melons, unwashed, at room temperature until ripe. Store ripe, cut melon, covered, in the refrigerator.
Nectarines, peaches, pears	Refrigerator crisper: 5 days	Ripen the fruit at room temperature, then refrigerate them, unwashed, in plastic bags.

Fruit or Vegetable	Storage Method: Time	Tips
Onions (red, white, yellow, green)	Room temperature: 2 to 4 weeks for dry onions Refrigerator crisper: 3 to 5 days for green onions	Store dry onions loosely in a mesh bag in a cool, dry, well-ventilated place away from sunlight. Store green onions, unwashed, in the refrigerator.
Oranges	Room temperature: 2 weeks	Best stored at a cool room temperature.
Potatoes	Room temperature: 1 to 2 weeks	Store unwashed potatoes in a cool, dry, well-ventilated area away from light, which causes greening.
Tomatoes	Refrigerator crisper: 2 to 3 days for fully ripe tomatoes	Ripen tomatoes at room temperature away from sunlight. For best flavor, store them, unwashed, at room temperature and eat them immediately when ripe. Store fully ripened tomatoes, unwashed, in the refrigerator.

(Adapted by permission from Van Laanen, Peggy, and Scott, Amanda. *Safe Storage of Fresh Fruits and Vegetables.* Texas Cooperative Extension, The Texas A&M University System.)

Food Contamination

Foods can become contaminated from improper food handling procedures that may result in cross-contamination. Following food safety practices is of paramount importance. Although federal, state and provincial agencies inspect foods before they reach the consumer, we cannot always rely on them. In Canada alone, about 11 to 13 million cases of food poisoning occur each year.

Some bacteria, such as *Listeria monocytogenes*, are particularly dangerous to a fetus. This bacterium can be found in dairy products, leafy vegetables, fish and meat products. Toxoplasmosis is a parasite found in raw meat or other raw foods, including fruits and vegetables. Both listeriosis and toxoplasmosis can cause flu-like symptoms. Both are harmful to a fetus.

Other harmful food-borne illnesses can be caused by more familiar bacteria, such as salmonella, campylobacter, and *Escherichia coli* (E. coli). These microorganisms can be harmful.

Did You Know …

Detoxification and Cleansing

Many people are under the false impression that the body needs to be cleansed periodically to rid it of toxins and pollutants. There is no scientific evidence that any detoxification regime or cleansing diet works. Some may even be harmful. The body is well equipped to rid itself of toxins through its own detoxification systems — the liver, kidneys and colon.

Food Additives

Nitrates

On their own, nitrates are non-toxic, but about 5% of ingested nitrate is converted in the body to nitrites, which can have negative effects on health. Nitrates are found in water, soil, and food, mostly in vegetables. Nitrates are also a food additive used as a preservative in raw and processed meats, processed fish, and in cheese products. It is desirable to limit intake of nitrates. Nitrates are generally less common in most organic foods.

While these nitrite compounds are often linked to cancer and other diseases, it has also been suggested that they may be of benefit to health. Nitric oxide is formed in the stomach from the nitrates, which, in this form, have an antimicrobial effect on gut pathogens and may play a protective role in the body.

Pesticides

Research has not proven definitively that pesticides used in our food supply are harmful. Stay well informed by contacting your local food inspection or environmental agency should questions about food additive safety arise.

Organic Food Safety

Organic foods have become popular because it is believed they are more nutritious and safer, especially for growing infants and children. Some studies have shown organic food is higher in vitamin C, but B vitamins and vitamin A in organic foods are generally the same as found in conventional foods. The nutrient status of these foods depends on the soil conditions where the product is grown. Organic food remains generally more expensive than conventional food products.

Certainly, infants and children are vulnerable to environmental toxins, regardless of the source, because they are still in a period of rapid development. The degree to which organic food reduces the exposure of individuals to pollutants is not known.

What is known is that food safety depends on safe handling and proper cleaning practices, whether the food is certified organic or not. Organic or not, a healthy diet must include a good variety of foods, with plenty of fresh fruits and vegetables, healthy grains and adequate fiber, with a focus on iron-containing foods for new mothers and toddlers.

Regulations

Both non-organic and organic food production are regulated by federal agencies in North America. In the United States, the USDA National Organic Program certifies foods grown and processed with organic farming methods. The organic sticker makes it easier for consumers to identify organic foods.

In Canada, the Canadian Food Inspection Agency (CFIA) is the single certifying body for organic food. The CFIA issues licenses to manufacturers to use the official "organic" logo. Food must be made up of at least 95% organic materials in order to be assigned the Canada Organic logo.

✺ Is cow's milk safe to drink when I'm breastfeeding?

North American milk supplies are safe to drink, organic or not, because there are strict regulations regarding use of hormones and antibiotics during milk production, though there are regulatory differences between the United States and Canada. The use of synthetic hormones is prohibited under the Canadian Food and Drugs Act, and milk containing any antibiotics cannot be sold.

Safe Water

Water makes up more than two-thirds of body weight and is required for the body to function. Women who are breastfeeding should drink water. Women who are pregnant need extra water to support the increase in blood volume that occurs during pregnancy and to prevent dehydration. Adequate hydration may also help relieve the symptoms of constipation. Women who are breastfeeding need this water for the extra demands of lactation.

To ensure that you receive enough fluids while you are breastfeeding, you should drink when you are thirsty and carry water with you when traveling.

Fresh Water Supplies

Women who are pregnant should let tap water run freely in the morning before drinking it in order to prevent excess intake of lead or copper, which may have accumulated in the pipes overnight. This is true for older and newer houses. Higher amounts of lead or copper are carried from the hot water tap because heat can release these substances. Lead or copper can interfere with the health and well-being of the fetus. It would seem prudent for women who are breastfeeding and for children to also consider these precautions.

Did You Know ...

Municipal Water

In Canada and the United States, the municipal water is considered to be safe for breastfeeding women. However, the safety of local tap water is dependent on the disinfection process, which usually involves chlorination of the water. Disinfection is necessary to kill the microorganisms and viruses that cause serious illnesses or even death.

Dietary Reference Intake of Fluid during Breastfeeding

While the recommended intake for liquid from all food sources (that includes water from food, beverages and drinking water) is about 11 cups (2.75 L) per day for women, those who are pregnant require 12 cups (3 L) per day, and breastfeeding women require 15 cups (3.75 L) per day.

Information on the safety of individual municipal or tap water is available from the local water supplier (which can be found on your water bill or at your local tax office). General information about drinking water can be obtained from the Environmental Protection Agency and Health Canada. Well water should be tested at regular intervals by licensed agents of local government agencies. For anyone accessing water from lakes, streams or rivers, treatment using a specially designed water kit should be completed before consumption.

 ## Do I need to give fluoride supplements to my breastfed baby?

Infants who receive breast milk do not need fluoride supplements, at least for the first 6 months. The American Academy of Pediatrics suggests that babies older than 6 months may require fluoride supplements if the source of water usually used does not contain fluoride. According to the Canadian Paediatric Society, fluoride supplements are only recommended for infants older than 6 months of age if the drinking water has less than 0.3 parts per million (ppm) of fluoride, and then 0.25 mg per day of fluoride is recommended as a daily supplement. It is best to check with your family doctor or pediatrician for advice. If you are using a water filtration system in your home, check with the company to see if fluoride is also removed in the filtration process. It would be prudent to have your water checked for the fluoride content.

Bottled water may not contain any fluoride, unless indicated on the bottle. If this is the case, and bottled water is the sole source of water intake, fluoride may be lacking in the diet. This is especially important for young children. Inform your physician if this is the case, and supplementation may be required. Most prenatal vitamin supplements do not contain fluoride.

Bottled Water Supplies

Many people believe that bottled water is safer than tap water, but there are no scientific studies to date that indicate that bottled water is any better for a person's health than tap water. Bottled water is not necessarily sterile.

Bottled water is subject to government regulations, and the World Health Organization has established international standards for bottled drinking water. For example, bottled water that claims to be from a spring or mineral source must come from an underground source. Bottled water usually has a 2-year shelf life.

Should I drink more water when I am breastfeeding? Does my baby need water?

Most breastfeeding mothers find that they are thirsty more often, and if they "drink to thirst," they will increase their fluid consumption naturally. Because breast milk is 90% water, there is no need to give extra to your baby. If your baby were to fill up on water, she wouldn't receive the nutrients available in breast milk needed to grow and develop normally. Give her more breast milk if she seems thirsty.

Lifestyle-Related Risks

Besides possible food-related risks to mother and baby during breastfeeding, there are other lifestyle risks, including smoking, drinking alcohol and taking drugs — over-the-counter, prescription or illegal.

Smoking

Did You Know ...

If You Can't Quit

If a mother cannot quit smoking while she is breastfeeding, she should continue breastfeeding, but smoke away from her infant, smoke outdoors as much as possible and smoke after, not before, breastfeeding. This will give her body more time to eliminate nicotine and other substances before they can enter the milk.

Smoking is not recommended for women in general and can be especially harmful to a fetus or a breastfed baby. Mothers who smoke increase the risk of their infant developing asthma. Smoking also increases the risk of SIDS and low birth weight. Nicotine can reach the infant from both the milk and the air. Secondhand smoke can have long-term health effects on infants, possibly predisposing them to more respiratory infections by damaging the respiratory cells, causing an increased incidence of infection. Smoking may also decrease the mother's milk supply.

Alcohol

Alcohol does appear in breast milk. It can interfere with milk supply and harm the infant. High intakes of alcohol can affect the letdown of milk, resulting in a decreased supply of milk.

However, the occasional drink, consumed at least 2 hours before breastfeeding, is considered to be safe, according to Health Canada's guidelines for the childbearing years. For more information on alcohol and breastfeeding, see the Resources section in this book for the Hospital for Sick Children Motherisk program and its book *Everyday Risks in Pregnancy and Breastfeeding*.

Drugs

If you are sick and need prescription drugs, check with your doctor about the safety of breastfeeding. Only a small amount of prescription drugs pass through breast milk. Many will not harm your baby. There are a few exceptions, including

Can I drink alcohol if I'm breastfeeding?

Yes, provided you follow some practical guidelines. For each drink consumed, breastfeeding should be delayed by about 2 hours, but this may be sooner for women who weigh less and later for women who weigh more. One drink is the equivalent of 5 ounces (150 mL) of wine, 12 ounces (360 mL) of beer and 1.5 ounces (45 mL) of liquor. As with medications, breastfeed just before having a drink and wait at least 2 hours before breastfeeding again or expressing your milk. Babies who are hungry during this time can be bottle-fed mother's milk that has been previously expressed.

cyclosporine, methotrexate, bromocriptine, cyclophosphamide, doxorubicin, ergotamine and phencyclidine. Breastfeeding is also contraindicated if a woman is undergoing chemotherapy treatment. For further information on drugs and breastfeeding, see the Resources section in this book for the Hospital for Sick Children Motherisk program and its book *Everyday Risks in Pregnancy and Breastfeeding*. Street drugs, such as cocaine, heroin and marijuana, are all contraindicated during breastfeeding. Professional counseling is strongly recommended in such situations if you cannot stop using these substances.

Postpartum Depression

It is hard to believe at first that many women become depressed after delivering their baby, but 50% to 80% of mothers experience a mild mood disturbance, often called baby blues, while 20% of these women go on to develop a significant depressive episode within a year of their baby's birth. Symptoms can include anxiety, forgetfulness, fatigue, irritability and headaches, to name a few. These symptoms may affect the mother's ability to care for her baby, including breastfeeding.

These disturbances can begin within 2 weeks after the delivery and may last for a few hours, days or weeks. Women who are likely to develop depression may have been more stressed during their pregnancy, may have a relative with similar symptoms and may have been more fearful of the pregnancy and delivery. The most highly affected group is adolescents, in part because of their inexperience, immaturity and economic circumstances.

✳ Strategies for Preventing Postpartum Depression

- Ensuring adequate iron intake is important because iron losses during delivery may cause anemia. If the anemia is corrected, you may feel less tired and irritable, and better able to handle the demands of caring for a new child. See Iron, page 40.
- Ensuring adequate carbohydrate intake provides adequate insulin secretion, which may help prevent depression.
- By balancing the ratio of omega-3 to omega-6 fatty acids in your diet, you may decrease depression.
- Increasing intake of DHA, an omega-3 essential fatty acid, can reduce the chances of depression. The concentration of DHA in a woman's breast milk is associated with a decrease in prevalence or occurrence of postpartum depression.
- Staying active with regular exercise will help you return to your normal weight and improve your self-image.
- If severe depression is suspected, alert your family physician. Antidepressant medications may be required.

CHAPTER 3

Healthy Breastfeeding Basics

WOMEN'S BODIES ARE *well prepared to provide breast milk for their babies. The production of breast milk occurs as a natural continuation of pregnancy in most women after delivery. About 85% of women will produce as much milk as their baby requires, while that percentage increases to at least 97% with proper assistance and advice on the techniques of breastfeeding.*

While most women have no problems with initiating and continuing breastfeeding, some rare conditions may cause a delay in the initiation of a milk supply. When some of these conditions are properly treated, milk production generally increases. While it takes about 4 to 6 weeks to establish breastfeeding fully, the first week after delivery can be the most challenging. Some women may feel anxiety about breastfeeding and a lack of control. Encouragement from your partner, immediate family and health-care providers will be most welcome as you become more comfortable breastfeeding your baby.

Can I use birth control pills when I am breastfeeding?

It is generally considered safe to take low-estrogen birth control pills once your breastfeeding is well established at about 4 to 6 weeks after delivery, although some mothers report that they feel their milk supply is diminished once they start the pill. Progestin-only birth control pills have less effect on milk supply. Ask your health-care provider to recommend the best birth control method while you are breastfeeding.

Breastfeeding Physiology

Some women may describe having poor success with breastfeeding because they don't fully understand how breast milk is made and how they should feed their babies. They often lack good information and strong support from their family and health-care workers. Breastfeeding myths abound; for example, when a mother experiences problems initiating breastfeeding, some will advise them to substitute breast milk with formula to get started. This seems like an easy solution, but it may create more problems than it solves for subsequent efforts to breastfeed the baby. Dispelling these myths with knowledge of how breastfeeding works and giving clear guidelines on how to breastfeed should help most women succeed in this rewarding maternal role.

Does the size or shape of my breasts affect my ability to breastfeed?

The size or shape of breasts generally does not matter when it comes to breastfeeding. The frequency of feeding and effective removal of milk from the breast determines milk supply. Women with smaller breasts can successfully breastfeed, but may need to feed more frequently because they are not able to store as much milk as women with larger breasts, not because they can't produce a sufficient amount. Even women who have had breast reduction or breast augmentation (enlargement) may be able to breastfeed successfully, depending on the surgical procedure, but they may need guidance from a lactation specialist, preferably before delivery.

Anatomy of the Breast

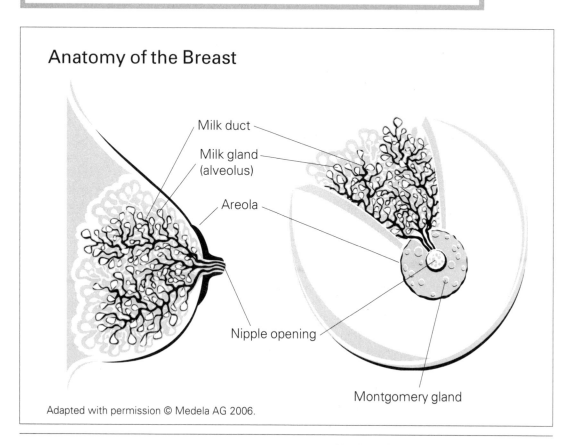

Milk duct

Milk gland (alveolus)

Areola

Nipple opening

Montgomery gland

Adapted with permission © Medela AG 2006.

Hormone Interactions

Breastfeeding (also known as lactation) is influenced by the secretion of specific hormones, chiefly progesterone and estrogen, prolactin and oxytocin. Both the neurological and the endocrine system are involved.

Progesterone and estrogen are released initially by the ovaries, and then by the placenta during pregnancy. They are responsible for the development of the ducts and milk-producing glands in the breast, which results in an increase in breast size (usually one bra size or more.) The levels of these hormones decline sharply after delivery of the infant, when the placenta is removed. Once progesterone and estrogen levels decline, the hormone prolactin, which is responsible for the production of breast milk, is able to reach its target cells in the breast tissue.

Prolactin is at increased levels in the blood during pregnancy, but breast milk is not released until after delivery because estrogens and progesterone produced by the placenta prevent prolactin from reaching its target cells in the breast.

Prolactin

Prolactin is produced in the pituitary gland in the base of the brain. It stimulates cells in the breast to produce milk proteins, milk sugar (lactose) and fats. The constant production of prolactin depends on continued breastfeeding or breast milk expression through pumping. Prolactin is produced during pregnancy, but this does not result in breast milk being produced until after delivery.

✳ Breast Milk Production Flow Chart

Increased prolactin after delivery
➡
Breast milk produced
➡
Baby feeding
➡
Increased prolactin
➡
More breast milk produced

Oxytocin

Oxytocin is another hormone involved in breastfeeding that is also produced by the pituitary gland. Oxytocin plays a role in the release of the milk from the breast, which is commonly known as letdown. Oxytocin is released during stimulation of the areola and nipple by the baby suckling or through expressing your own milk.

Oxytocin works in the breast, causing contraction of the cells that surround the alveoli (milk-producing cells in the breast), releasing the milk into the milk ducts. Some women can feel a tingling sensation in their breasts or nipples when oxytocin "triggers" the release of milk for breastfeeding.

Oxytocin also causes the uterus to contract, allowing the uterus to return to its more normal prepregnancy size. Women in the first few days postpartum may feel these contractions or cramping during breastfeeding, and sometimes they can be quite uncomfortable. Doctors generally prescribe pain medication to deal with these common post-delivery contractions, called afterpains.

 Will stress and anxiety prevent the letdown of my milk?

Breast milk production itself is not normally affected by the state of the mother after delivery. However, the extreme stress of a prolonged labor or the emotional upheaval of an unplanned Cesarean section or preterm delivery may delay milk production. The release of prolactin can then be affected by emotional triggers. After most deliveries, milk production continues no matter how tired or emotional you are.

Emotions can also affect the letdown of milk by influencing the release of oxytocin. Extreme stress or a negative psychological state can decrease or inhibit the production of oxytocin, resulting in less stimulus to release the available milk. This can become a vicious cycle, with a new mother worrying about not being able to produce enough milk for a crying baby, and the decreased milk release caused by this anxiety. Understanding the psychology and physiology of breastfeeding will help a new mom realize that she is entirely capable of producing enough milk for her baby with the proper guidance during those first few weeks of uncertainty.

Breast Milk Composition

The breast glands produce water, amino acids (small parts of proteins), proteins, fats, vitamins, lactose (sugar), minerals and other substances that are taken from the mother's blood and body to produce milk.

There are three stages of milk production: colostrum (first milk), transitional milk and mature milk. The milk produced in each stage has a different composition and function. Infant formulas, on the other hand, are a uniform liquid that cannot provide the same specific benefits to the changing needs of babies.

Colostrum

The milk initially produced after delivery is called colostrum. It may be whitish to yellowish orange in color. Colostrum is produced by all women after about 16 weeks of gestation, even if they are not breastfeeding, because the production of colostrum is hormonally driven. Production of more mature milk is driven mainly by the demand for milk by the baby.

Produced in small quantities, colostrum is thick and sticky, rich in protein and minerals and lower in carbohydrate, fat and some vitamins than mature milk. Colostrum helps to promote the growth of the beneficial *Lactobacillus bifidus* organism in the gastrointestinal tract and promotes the passing of meconium, the thick, sticky stool that collects in the baby's intestines during pregnancy.

Only about 1 to 2 ounces (30 to 60 mL) of colostrum are produced each day in the first few days, which match the small capacity of the baby's stomach, depending on the baby's size and weight. Colostrum contains about 67 kcalories per 3 ounces (90 mL).

Transitional Milk

Transitional milk is produced from about 6 days after birth (ranging from 4 to 8 days after birth) for about 2 weeks. White in color, this milk arrives in greater volume than colostrum, rising from 2 ounces (60 mL) per day of colostrum to about 16 ounces (500 mL) per day of transitional breast milk by day 5. Milk volume then increases more slowly to 20 to 32 ounces (600 to 950 mL) per day of mature milk during the next 3 to 5 months.

Mature Milk

About 2 to 3 weeks after birth, breast milk is referred to as mature milk. Studies show that about 16 ounces (500 mL) per day of breast milk is produced by about 5 days after delivery, going up to about 27 ounces (800 mL) per day, with a wide range of 18 to 40 ounces (550 mL to 1.2 L) per day once breastfeeding is established.

About 90% of mature breast milk is water, which is essential for the hydration of the infant. This milk contains between 67 and 75 kcalories per 3 ounces (90 mL). While the amount of immunoglobulins and proteins in the milk declines at this time, there is an increase in lactose, fat and energy in mature milk. The protein content of mature breast milk is easily digested. About half of the volume of milk the newborn drinks will have already been emptied from his stomach by 50 minutes after the feeding.

Foremilk and Hindmilk

The first part of breast-milk-feeding or expression is called the foremilk, followed by the hindmilk as the breast is emptied. The foremilk contains a higher amount of water for thirst quenching and lactose (sugar), but a lesser amount of fat than the hindmilk. Both parts of the milk should be taken in by an infant for a balanced feeding.

Feeding Sequence

If babies receive the foremilk of both breasts without hindmilk, they may not be receiving enough of the richer, fatty hindmilk. Switching breasts during breastfeeding before the first one is emptied may cause a baby to have increased gas and looser,

How much milk should my body be making and how much milk should my baby be taking?

Once your milk supply is established after the first 2 to 3 weeks, your body will be producing milk in the range of 18 to 40 ounces (550 mL to 1.2 L) a day for one baby. Breastfeeding is regulated by the baby, so she takes what milk she wants, when she wants it, to meet her needs. It is not uncommon to find that some feedings during the day are small thirst quenchers of 1 to 2 ounces (30 to 60 mL), while other feedings are a full meal of 3 to 6 ounces (90 to 180 mL).

usually green and watery stools because of the higher sugar load. The lower-fat foremilk empties from the baby's stomach faster than the hindmilk, providing a higher lactose load to the baby's small bowel than it can handle, resulting in undigested lactose, producing gas and diarrhea. If this pattern continues to occur, the baby may not grow well and may seem to be hungry all the time.

Gently compressing or squeezing the breast during the feed will assist in the release of more hindmilk, ensuring a good mix of foremilk and hindmilk. This may help decrease the gas and eliminate looser or watery stools caused by the high lactose load of the foremilk.

Infant Weight Gain

In the first few days of feeding, when a baby receives the colostrum, he is not likely to gain weight because the energy demands are not yet being met for growth. This is not something to be concerned about; rather, it is a natural transitional process. Once the whiter, transitional milk comes in, providing more volume and containing a higher amount of fat, the baby's weight gain starts to occur.

Concern is raised when infants lose more than 10% of their body weight in the first 5 days of life or at any time thereafter. If mature milk has not yet come in (for some women it takes longer), then this weight loss is likely due to inadequate volume (thus inadequate energy intake), not because the baby is not feeding well. By day 7 of life, a baby should start to gain weight, with birth weight regained by 2 to 3 weeks.

Macronutrient Content

Breast milk is composed of the three macronutrients — carbohydrate (lactose), protein and fat. The contribution of calories by each of the macronutrients is approximately 42% carbohydrate, 6% protein and 52% fat.

Carbohydrate

Lactose is the main carbohydrate found in human milk. There is a much greater quantity of lactose in transitional and mature breast milk than there is in colostrum. Breast milk changes with time in order to adapt to the changing needs of the infant. While the initial milk, colostrum, is very high in immunoglobulins and complex carbohydrates called oligosaccharides, the later milk or mature milk has a higher amount of lactose and fat.

Lactose

Lactose provides a large amount of energy to the rapidly growing brain of the infant. Lactose also plays an important role in the absorption of calcium and iron by helping to increase their absorption in the intestine.

It is very rare for infants to have a lactase enzyme deficiency leading to lactose intolerance. Lactase is found in the mother's breast milk and in the baby's small intestine. Infants have the ability to digest lactose and break it down into the simple sugars (monosaccharides) galactose and glucose.

Oligosaccharides

Although oligosaccharides are carbohydrates that cannot be digested, they are considered to be prebiotics, helping with the growth of the beneficial bacteria in the small intestine. Oligosaccharides are highest in colostrum and then decrease in quantity in mature milk.

Did You Know ...

Breast Milk Protein

There are 7 to 10 grams of protein in each liter of breast milk. Whey and casein are the two main proteins found in breast milk.

✳ Protective Factors in Breast Milk

Some proteins in breast milk have immunological properties. These factors decrease the incidence of otitis media, bacterial infections, gastroenteritis and respiratory illness in breastfed infants and have a preventive effect on heart disease, celiac disease, some forms of cancer and diabetes. Infant formulas do not have these protective factors.

Lactoferrin: Lactoferrin attracts and carries iron, making it easier for infants to absorb iron from breast milk. Lactoferrin also prevents other organisms found in the intestines from using this iron for their growth. This protects the infant from gastrointestinal illnesses, perhaps accounting for the fact that breastfed infants get fewer diarrheal illnesses than formula-fed babies.

Secretory IgA, IgG, and IgM (Ig stands for immunoglobulin): These proteins found in breast milk help protect the baby from bacterial and viral infections. They may also protect the baby from developing allergies.

Lysozymes: These proteins protect the baby's intestines from potentially harmful microorganisms, such as E. coli and salmonella. These enzymes also help the good microorganisms, or flora, to grow in the intestines and have an anti-inflammatory effect.

Bifidus factor: Found in breast milk, this factor helps with the growth of lactobacillus that helps prevent other, more harmful bacteria from growing in the baby's intestines.

Other components of the protein are amino acids and nucleotides, both important for many metabolic functions, as well as growth factors and hormones that help with the development of the intestines, promoting maturation of the cells. The intestines contain a large part of our immune system. Proteins of the immune system protect the surface of the intestinal cells.

Did You Know ...

Fat Content

The fat content of transitional breast milk (the first 2 weeks of breast milk produced after colostrum) contains slightly less fat than mature milk, with 3.5 grams of fat per 3 ounces (90 mL) compared to 3.9 grams of fat for the same amount. Colostrum has even less, at 2.6 grams of fat per 3 ounces (90 mL). In preterm milk (from mothers who have delivered babies before 37 weeks gestation), the fat content is 30% higher than in mature milk.

Protein

The high-quality protein found in breast milk meets all of the infant's needs for growth. Some of the protein taken in is not absorbed by the infant, but serves to provide protection for the gastrointestinal tract. Overall protein quantity decreases in breast milk with time. The changes in protein content of breast milk match the developmental needs for the baby.

Whey and Casein

Initially, about 60% of the protein in breast milk is whey and 40% is casein. Whey is easier to digest, while casein requires more energy for digestion. As milk matures, the amount of casein increases, so the ratio for whey to casein becomes about 50:50. The whey and casein proteins found in breast milk are easier to digest than those found in cow's milk formula. Calcium and iron are also easier to absorb from breast milk than from formula.

Fat

Fat makes up about one-half of the energy of breast milk. The fat found in breast milk is easy for the baby to digest because it comprises specific fats and triglycerides (palmitic acid) ideal for the baby's digestive system. Breast milk also contains lipase, an enzyme that helps to digest the fat in the breast milk. Pancreatic enzymes of the infant also help to digest fat. The fat in breast milk carries the fat-soluble vitamins and a complex matrix of fatty acids, including essential fatty acids, such as docosahexaenoic acid (DHA) and arachidonic acid (AA), which the infant needs for brain growth and visual (retina) development.

The total fat in the mother's diet does not affect the amount of fat in breast milk, but the type of fat consumed in the mother's diet will affect the type of fat in breast milk. Studies have shown that an increased intake of DHA through the diet will increase the amount of this fatty acid in breast milk. If dietary intake of omega-3 fatty acids is low, then it may be prudent to consider including a source of this fatty acid in the diet while breastfeeding (and, ideally, before and during pregnancy).

Cholesterol in Breast Milk

Although unaffected by the mother's dietary intake, cholesterol levels are high in breast milk. Studies suggest that it is this early exposure to cholesterol in breast milk that may have a protective effect against coronary heart disease later on in life. By exposing infants to a higher level of cholesterol early in life through breast milk, their enzyme systems for handling cholesterol are developed, perhaps providing this protection against heart disease.

Micronutrient Content

Vitamins

Breast milk contains both fat-soluble vitamins (vitamins A, D, E and K) and water-soluble vitamins (B vitamins, vitamin C). Fat-soluble vitamins in breast milk are not affected by the mother's diet (but mothers still need vitamin D), but water-soluble vitamins are. It may be important for a mother to enrich her diet with foods containing these vitamins.

Vitamin D Supplements

There is very little vitamin D in human breast milk, possibly due to health warnings to decrease exposure to the sun and to the increased use of sunscreens by the mother. In rare cases, in those infants who are not exposed to sunlight, vitamin D deficiency has been reported. The Canadian Paediatric Society and the American Academy of Pediatrics both recommend vitamin D supplementation for all breastfed infants. The CPS recommends 400 IU of vitamin D daily, while the AAP recommends 200 IU daily.

Minerals and Electrolytes

Breast milk provides all of the minerals, including sodium, calcium, iron, zinc and magnesium, required by the infant for normal growth and development. The diet of the mother has little influence on the mineral content of breast milk because maternal body stores regulate the amount of minerals in human breast milk. Because 90% of breast milk is water, there is no reason to give infants water in addition to their feeding to maintain electrolytes. The sodium content of breast milk decreases with time.

Hormones

Human growth factors, insulin, prolactin, thyroxine, cholecystokinin and cortisol are hormones found in human breast milk. They help strengthen the intestines of the infant, promote digestion and enhance the immune system.

Enzymes

Lipase and amylase are components of breast milk that help with the digestion of fat and polysaccharides (long-chain carbohydrates), respectively.

Did You Know ...

Vitamin K

Vitamin K is found in small amounts in breast milk and is a component of blood clotting. Because a baby has minimal milk intake after birth, vitamin K supplements are usually given at birth, by needle, to prevent hemorrhage, or uncontrolled bleeding. Bacteria in the intestines are not yet present in the gut of the newborn; these bacteria become an important source of vitamin K as the infant grows.

Did You Know ...

Food Restriction and Elimination

Women who severely restrict their intake are still able to produce breast milk because the nutrients needed for milk production will be taken from the mother's own body stores. The breast milk composition will be the same as in women who do not restrict their diets, but the fat component of this breast milk may be altered.

Do my food choices affect my child's food preferences?

What a mother eats during her pregnancy and during breastfeeding can influence preference for certain flavors by the baby. This may explain the immediate acceptance of different cultural foods. The same is true during breastfeeding and weaning to solid foods. If the mother eats a diverse diet, the child may be more interested in a greater variety of foods later in life. This should motivate mothers-to-be and breastfeeding mothers to eat a variety of foods in their diet, including herbs and spices. Studies show that by 4 to 5 months of age, food preferences may already be set.

Growth Patterns

It is important for a health-care professional to track the pattern of growth for your child over time. The pattern of growth is often more important than the absolute weight of your child.

World Health Organization Standards

Recently, the World Health Organization (WHO) documented the growth and weight gain of breastfed infants. No matter what the cultural background, exclusively breastfed babies grew in the same pattern, although this growth can be quite different from growth patterns in formula-fed or combined formula-fed and breastfed babies that have been followed on previous growth charts.

Growth of breastfed babies is more rapid in the first 2 to 3 months and slows down in the following 12 months. Sometimes, this slower growth can result in false concern by family doctors. Parents of a breastfed infant may be instructed to introduce formula or increase solids in the diet in an attempt to increase their baby's rate of weight gain. However, by plotting infants using the new WHO growth charts, fewer breastfed children should appear to be falling off their growth curves after 6 months of age and to be growing normally without the need for formula supplements.

Will breastfeeding lead to obesity if my baby overeats?

On the contrary. With the increased prevalence of childhood obesity, which is caused by many factors (such as insufficient activity and excessive energy intake), one way to help decrease the chances of a child being obese is by breastfeeding. In recent studies by the World Health Organization (WHO), children between 9 and 14 years of age were less likely to be overweight if they were breastfed. It did not matter if mothers were overweight or if they had diabetes while they were breastfeeding.

One explanation for this effect is the role of leptin. A hormone that helps with control of weight gain, leptin from the mother is transferred to breast milk. Another explanation is the control the baby has over the amount of milk needed to satisfy hunger and thus avoid overeating.

WHO growth charts show that exclusive breastfeeding results in a greater weight in the first 6 months of life, but lower weight in the next 6 months of life. Infants included in the development of the new growth charts came from different parts of the world, and, interestingly, there was no difference in growth between races or countries of origin.

✳ How to Read WHO Growth Charts

The baby's actual height and weight at his corresponding age are plotted on the chart. The line along which height and weight are plotted indicates the percentile for that height and weight. Weight should be at about the same percentile as height.

The 50th percentile indicates the average height and weight of a breastfed baby at that age. If a child's height and weight are plotted on a higher percentile (for example, the 97th), it does not necessarily mean that there is a problem. Nor is there necessarily something wrong if a child's height and weight are plotted on a lower percentile (for example, the 3rd). This usually just means that they have larger or smaller parents. It is growth over time — the growth pattern — that is most important.

Feeding can be assessed by tracking growth and weight gain. If there are any significant deviations from the growth curve over time, your family doctor or pediatrician will discuss this with you. If you are worried about the size of your baby, growth charts can help determine whether you have cause for concern, provided that growth over time has been charted. The growth pattern is more important than single measurements.

To properly assess the growth rate of a breastfed infant, WHO growth charts should be used. Other charts include formula-fed infants, for whom the growth pattern is slightly different. Breastfed infants grow more quickly in the first few months and more slowly later in the first year. For more information on WHO growth charts, see the Resources section in this book.

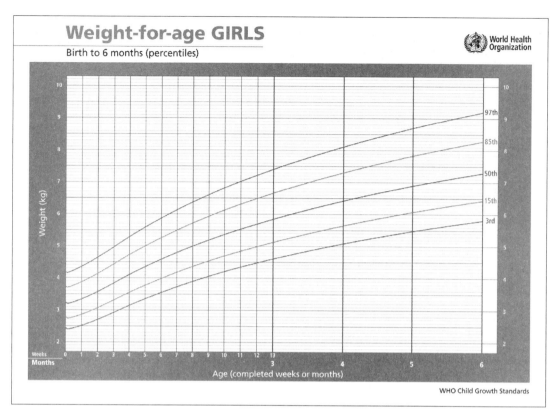

Weight-for-age GIRLS
Birth to 6 months (percentiles)

World Health Organization

WHO Child Growth Standards

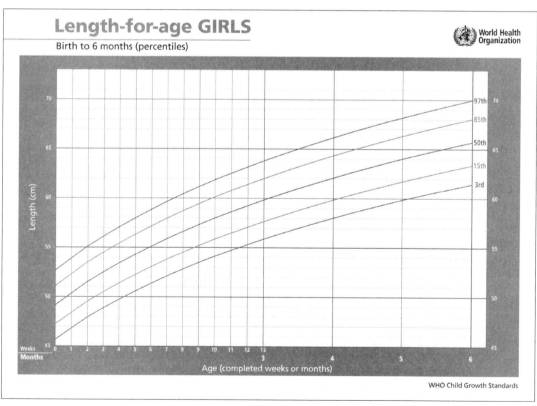

Length-for-age GIRLS
Birth to 6 months (percentiles)

World Health Organization

WHO Child Growth Standards

Weight-for-age BOYS
Birth to 6 months (percentiles)

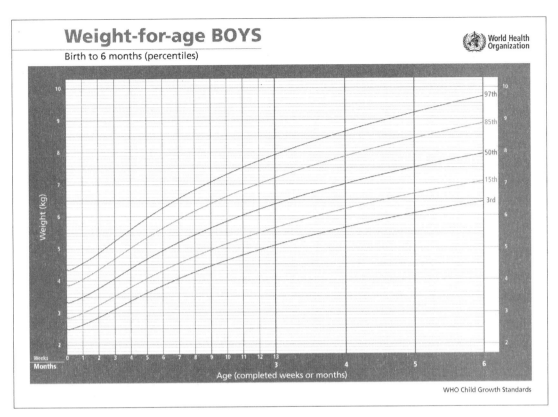

World Health Organization

WHO Child Growth Standards

Length-for-age BOYS
Birth to 6 months (percentiles)

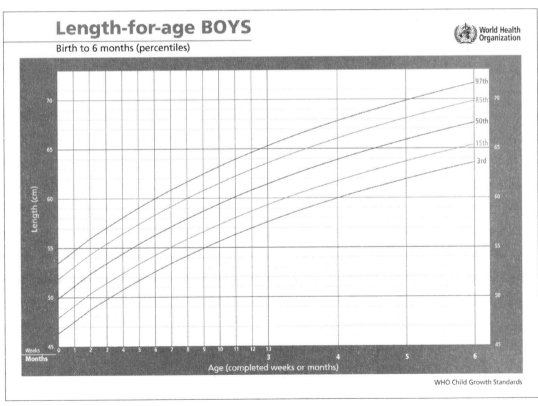

World Health Organization

WHO Child Growth Standards

CHAPTER 4

Strategies for Healthy Breastfeeding

THERE IS NO SUBSTANCE made that can provide your baby with the unique constituents of human milk. Exclusive breastfeeding for the currently recommended period of 1 year and beyond, with the introduction of solid foods at 6 months, is the optimum goal, but this may not always be possible. When treated as a special medicine rather than just daily nutrition, the immunities provided by even a small volume of mother's breast milk help ensure your baby's health. There is nothing more satisfying than knowing that you are doing something to contribute to the well-being of your child that only a mother can provide. And even if you only offer a "comfort" breastfeed at bedtime and expressed breast milk from a bottle during the day, you are sharing a bonding and trusting relationship with your baby that may last a lifetime. In this chapter, we present strategies for breastfeeding successfully.

Breastfeeding Support

Learning to breastfeed is like learning to ride a bicycle. You may fall off many times before you master the technique required. Breastfeeding is an interactive process for both you and your baby, though your learning curves may be different. Be patient with both yourself and your baby.

Breastfeeding is not always easy without support from your family and health-care workers. Reach out for support whenever you need help with this learning experience.

✳ The Measure of Success

For some women, success at breastfeeding means a pain-free, trouble-free experience that is relaxing and pleasant for both mother and baby for many months. For other mothers, the measure of success is breastfeeding comfortably for a specified period of time before returning to work. Some mothers are very happy and comfortable with expressing their milk and bottle-feeding it to their baby for either a short term or long term. For mothers who have struggled with illness, either their own or their baby's, or who have had difficulties establishing a milk supply, success may be measured by every teaspoon of breast milk consumed by the baby.

Family Support

Father's Role

Breastfeeding is nature's way of providing the best possible start for your baby and provides your partner with long-term health benefits as well. A father's attitude toward breastfeeding has a direct impact not only on the choice of how to feed his child, but also on his partner's success in breastfeeding. One study of the factors affecting a mother's decision to breastfeed found that a father's approval and knowledge of the benefits of this feeding option were associated with a high incidence of breastfeeding.

For the first few weeks of the baby's life, the father can best help by comforting and nourishing his partner while she comforts and nourishes their newborn baby. Fathers can do the grocery shopping, prepare nutritious meals, clean the house, do the laundry — and change diapers, bath their baby, and cuddle and rock their baby while mother has a nap or takes a shower. The more time a mother has to spend with a newborn baby, the quicker she can establish good breastfeeding habits. Her confidence in breastfeeding will increase as she learns to care for her newborn baby. The father's opportunity to spend long hours with his baby will come in time.

Grandparents' Role

Grandparents, too, can support their daughter or daughter-in-law in the decision to breastfeed and offer encouragement during the first few weeks of adjustment when mother and baby are learning how to breastfeed together. While many new parents want to be alone with their new baby for the first few days at home, the household tasks begin to pile up and the call goes out for help. Grandparents can take over some of the household chores while the mother can rest and focus on caring for her baby.

Grandparents also need to be doubly careful in making comments that link breastfeeding to their grandchild's behavior. When the baby cries, such comments as, "There must be something wrong with your milk," or "Are you sure you have enough milk?" are a sure way to make a mother doubt her natural ability to feed her baby. Gone are the rigid feeding schedules that came with formula-feeding. Babies know best when they want to feed and how much they want to take at each visit to their mother's breast, so frequent feedings may be normal for a new grandchild.

If I'm not feeling well, can I still breastfeed?

If you're not feeling well, your baby has likely been exposed to the same bacteria or virus. Your body will make antibodies to fight whatever you have been exposed to, and this protection will be passed on to your baby in your breast milk. If you are too ill to breastfeed, your milk can be pumped and fed to your baby by an alternative method until you are well enough to put your baby back to the breast.

Health-Care Resources

Every new mother will be faced with sifting through the well-meaning advice of everyone who is trying to assist her in breastfeeding her baby. Much of this advice may be conflicting, and at some point, the mother will seek professional advice.

Depending on the county, province, state or country, there may be different paths to finding health-care resources for new baby care. In most communities, the public health system will have professionals trained to assist you or will provide referrals to appropriate agencies or individuals. These public health programs, dedicated to the healthy development of infants and children, include the Women, Infant and Children (WIC) programs in America and the Healthy Babies, Healthy Children programs in Canada. See the Resources section at the end of the book for contact information.

If I had problems breastfeeding my first baby, will I have problems with my next baby?

A knowledgeable lactation professional can help you overcome the problem you had with your first baby, whether it was related to the mother or baby. No two babies are alike. Each will have a distinctly different personality and, very likely, different feeding behaviors.

Starting Out

The first week of breastfeeding is an important time for a mother and her baby as they learn how to breastfeed and establish a feeding routine. If you and your baby are doing fine, start breastfeeding as soon after birth as possible.

First Hours

The delivery room staff will likely place your baby on your chest immediately after your baby is born. Your baby now has the chance to find his own way to your nipple. The gradation of color of the areola and nipple catches your baby's eye and acts like a target.

✳ Feeding Cues

Common feeding cues indicate your baby is hungry. Offer your baby your breast whenever you observe these feeding cues. Don't wait until your baby cries, because he may get too upset to latch easily. Crying is a late-stage hunger cue.

1. **Rapid eye movement (REM):** If you watch your baby, you will notice the eye moving underneath the eyelid. This means the baby is in a light sleep and ready to wake for feeding.

2. **Movement:** Your baby will start to move, stretch and put hands to mouth.

3. **Sounds:** Your baby starts to make sounds.

4. **Sucking motions:** If you continue to watch, your baby will start sucking motions with her lips and tongue.

5. **Rooting:** Your baby will "root" if something comes near her mouth. When the lips or the area around the mouth are touched, the baby's mouth opens wide and the tongue drops, preparing for the nipple to be drawn in.

✳ How to Promote Milk Letdown

In some circumstances, it can help to promote letdown before you latch your baby. Once breastfeeding is well established, your baby's sucking is all that is needed for letdown to occur.

1. Take a hot shower or use warm compresses for 5 minutes before feeding to help with letdown.

2. Try wrapping your breasts in warm hand towels covered by a bigger towel to keep in the heat.

3. Gently touch your nipple or areola in a circular motion with the tip of your finger for 1 to 2 minutes.

4. Present your breast to your baby. Some babies may not be interested in feeding right after delivery, but continue to present your breast. When your baby is near your breast, milk production hormones are stimulated. This will promote milk letdown.

5. Continue to offer the breast whenever the baby shows feeding cues.

Allow for an uninterrupted time after birth to help achieve the first successful breastfeeding. Your baby may take an hour or more after birth to latch on to your breast and begin sucking or may need some gentle assistance.

You are now off to a good start in the "art" of breastfeeding — and in providing your baby with good nutrition and immunity against infections. This first feeding is made up of colostrum, which is very nutritious and high in infection-fighting factors. Colostrum immediately coats the intestine to aid in digestion and absorption.

Comfortable Positions

It is important that you and your baby are comfortable while breastfeeding. Take your pain medications as prescribed by your physician if you are experiencing pain from your episiotomy stitches or afterbirth cramping. If your bottom is tender, use pillows to sit on or lie on your side to breastfeed.

✳ Guide to Good Positioning

1. You should feel comfortable.

2. A straight-back chair with arm supports is usually best for breastfeeding. This prevents problems with back discomfort and allows your arms to support your baby more easily. Depending on your height, your feet might need to be supported on a stool. Your knees should be slightly higher than your hips for comfort.

3. Breastfeeding pillows help to support your baby, but you can use ordinary pillows as well. You should not feel that you are supporting the weight of your baby during the feeding.

4. Your baby's head should be tilted slightly back as if sniffing the air. This position makes it easier for your baby to swallow.

5. Your baby's head should not be turned toward her shoulder, but remain in alignment with her body. Turn your head toward your shoulder and try swallowing. It is difficult! Your baby should not lie on her back in the cradle or side-lying position with the head turned to the side. In the cradle and side-lying positions, your baby should be totally on her side with her chest, tummy and knees touching you. The baby's ear, shoulder and hips should be in a straight line.

6. You should line up your baby's nose and your nipple so they are opposite each other, with your breast in its normal position. This allows the lower jaw to come in contact with more of the areola when latching.

7. You should always bring your baby to the breast. It is very difficult to get sufficient areolar tissue in your baby's mouth if you try to put the nipple in the mouth.

✳ Breastfeeding Positions Guide

There are four main positions women find comfortable for breastfeeding, but there are many other ways you could hold your baby. Experiment to find out what works best for you. In whatever position you choose, you should feel relaxed and your baby should have easy access to your breast. As your baby gets older, you will have figured out what works best for you.

Cross Cradle

This is a good learning position, allowing you good control of your baby's head. Sit with your baby totally on his side and close to you, well supported on pillows, so his chest, abdomen and knees are facing and touching you. If you are feeding on your left breast, you will use your right arm to support your baby's body and your right hand to support your baby's head. How you support the head is important because babies generally fuss if you hold them around the top of their heads. Open your hand up wide and hold your baby's head low down at the base of the head, with your thumb on one side of the head and your fingers on the other side. Your left hand supports the left breast.

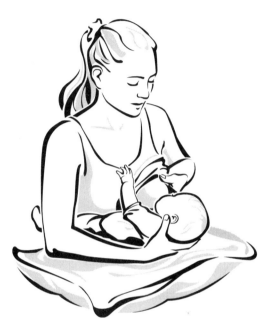

Football Position

This is also a good learning position, preferable for many mothers after a C-section. The upright football position keeps your baby more awake. Put a pillow vertically behind your back to move you forward in the chair. This allows more room for your baby's legs behind you. Hold your baby at your side, supported on pillows. If you're breastfeeding on your right breast, you would seat yourself as far to the left side of the chair as possible. Use your right arm to support your baby at your side, with your right hand supporting the baby's head at the base of the head. Your left hand will support the breast.

Side-Lying Position

This position is often used during the first feeds and at night and when you want to rest as your baby feeds beside you. It is best if you and your baby are able to latch well before trying the side-lying position, because it is a little harder to have both hands accessible in this position. To feed on the left breast, lie on your left side with your back well supported. You might find it easier in this position to have your head and shoulders well supported on a pillow so that you can see your baby. Lay the baby on the bed on his right side facing you, with his chest against your chest. A pillow or roll behind him will also keep him positioned on his side. Your right arm will support your baby's body and your right hand will support the baby's head, bringing your baby toward your breast. Some mothers are more comfortable with the baby supported in the crook of the arm.

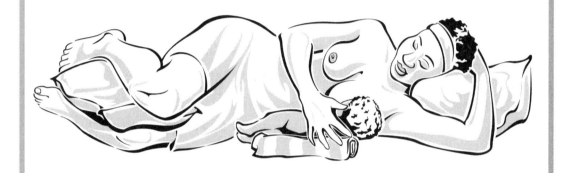

Cradle Position

This is a common position for older babies who can easily latch. You can use it initially if it works for you. It is a little harder to control the head in this position. You are sitting with your baby well supported on pillows on your lap. Turn your baby totally on her side and close to you so her chest, abdomen and knees face and touch you. If you are feeding on the left breast, your left arm supports her head, with her head being supported by the forearm but not over the bend in your arm. Her nose should be opposite the nipple to begin. You should not feel you need to move the breast sideways for your nipple to reach her mouth. Your right hand supports the breast.

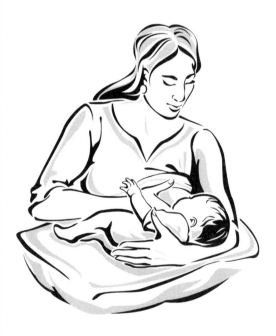

✳ How to Hold the Breast

To take adequate milk from the breast, the baby needs clear access to the nipple and the areola (darker area around the nipple).

1. When you support the breast with your hand, it is important you are not covering the areola with your fingers. Try holding the breast with your thumb on one side of the breast well back from the areola and the other four fingers on the opposite side. If you are small-chested, some of your fingers may rest more comfortably on the chest wall.

2. Support the breast well for a small baby or a baby with a weak suck throughout the feeding. If your breast is large, you may need to support it so there is not a lot of weight on the baby's chin. If your baby maintains the latch well throughout the feeding and your nipples are not sore, you can choose whether or not to support the breast during the feeding.

3. Here are two holds that work well:

C Hold
In the C hold, the thumb is on the top of the breast and the four fingers are underneath, creating the shape of a C. This hold can be used in any position to support the breast. A small towel roll placed under a large breast may help with support.

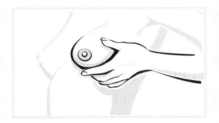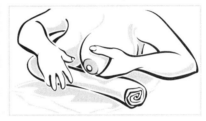

Modified from the original image © Childbirth Graphics®, www.ChildbirthGraphics.com.

U Hold
In the U hold, the thumb is at the outside of the breast and the fingers are on the other side between the breasts. This hold often makes the latch for cross cradle position easier.

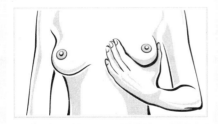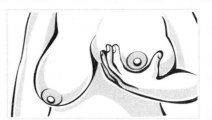

Adapted with permission by Diane Weissinger.

When the breast is held in a U hold, the breast is an oval shape vertically. When the breast is held in a C hold, the breast is a slightly oval shape horizontally. Your baby's wide-open mouth will be able to latch more easily when the breast is held in these oval positions.

✳ How to Establish a Good Latch

There are different ways to achieve a good latch. There is no right or wrong way — only what works best for you to achieve comfortable breastfeeding and ensure a good milk transfer.

1. If you have correctly positioned your baby, she may come to the breast and latch all by herself with minimal assistance. When babies self-latch, they are generally rooting well and draw the nipple and areola well back in their mouth.

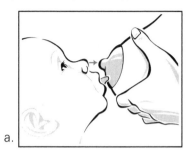
a.

2. If your baby doesn't self-latch, gently touch your nipple along her lip from one corner to the other once and move her slightly back as you wait for the mouth to open wide and the tongue to drop (rooting). Bring your baby's chin to touch the breast first and the nipple to the roof of the mouth in a quick but gentle motion. The more of the breast you get in the baby's mouth, the more successful the latch will be.

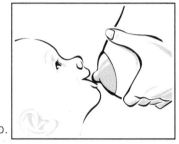
b.

3. You can also think about placing the baby's mouth onto your breast as if taking a bite out of a big sandwich. **a)** First, line your baby up with the nipple opposite the nose. **b)** Touch your baby's lip with your nipple. Immediately move your baby about an inch away from the breast so you can see her mouth. Your baby's nose is opposite the nipple, and the head is tilted back. **c)** Wait for the baby to open wide. **d)** Bring the chin and then lower lip to the areola as far from the nipple-areola junction as possible. **e)** Then aim the upper lip over the nipple, covering as much of the areola as you can on the other side of the nipple.

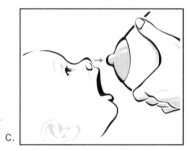
c.

4. Support your breast until you feel your baby latch and start to suck and swallow. If you remove your hand immediately, your baby may not have enough time to bring the nipple and areola well back in the mouth. The nipple's pushing up against the palate at the back of the mouth stimulates sucking. Most newborns need the breast held throughout the feeding.

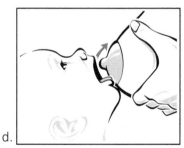
d.

5. Always remember to bring the baby to your breast. Trying to push the nipple into your baby's mouth does not achieve an effective latch.

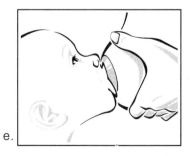
e.

Modified from the original image © Childbirth Graphics®, www.ChildbirthGraphics.com.

❋ How to Care for Your Breasts

Be sure to care for your breasts to ensure that the breastfeeding process is not only successful but also enjoyable.

1. Wash your hands before touching your breasts to prevent infection, especially if you have sore nipples.

2. Wash your nipples once a day with warm water only (no soap) and apply breast milk to the nipple and areola after breastfeeding. Air-dry the nipples for 10 minutes after each feeding. If privacy is an issue, try leaving your nursing bra open under your clothing.

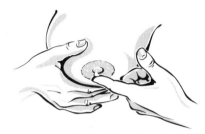

(Adapted by permission of Amy Spangler © 2006.)

3. Wear 100% cotton bras and reapply dry nursing pads frequently. Most women have some leaking, especially in the first weeks as the milk supply regulates. Your nursing pads should not have a plastic backing to prevent air circulation. Reusable, washable breast pads are a better choice. Folding your arms and pressing against your breasts if you feel your milk letting down can prevent leaking when you are out in public. Lighter colors and patterned clothing hide wet patches more easily if you have chosen not to wear breast pads.

4. Generally, avoid creams and ointments unless recommended by your health-care provider, because they may aggravate sensitive skin.

Latching

Getting a proper latch is the key to effective breastfeeding. Although there is some difference of opinion, an asymmetrical latch is most recommended. This means the baby's lower jaw covers more of the areola than the upper jaw. If there is any areolar tissue visible when your baby is latched, you want to see more above the upper lip than below the lower lip. Positioning your baby so the nipple is opposite the nose ensures that the baby takes in more of the areola by the lower jaw than if you start with the mouth opposite the nipple.

This maximizes the amount of areolar tissue the tongue comes in contact with to "milk" the breast, and allows the nipple to extend further back in the mouth, where it will feel more comfortable. If your baby's mouth is positioned correctly on the breast, the nipple tissue itself should be far back in his mouth and away from the intense pressure of the tongue and jaw at the opening of the mouth.

Did You Know ...

Feeding Schedule

Most newborns will want to feed 8 to 12 times in 24 hours. They will usually feed about 15 to 45 minutes each time. As they get older, the feedings will decrease to 6 to 8 feedings a day. The baby generally falls into a fairly predictable schedule as breastfeeding is established at around 6 weeks.

Correct latch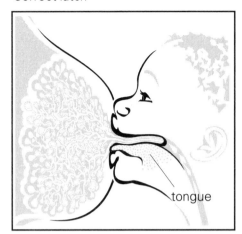

Incorrect latch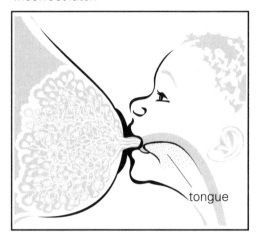

tongue

tongue

Modified from the original image © Childbirth Graphics®, www.ChildbirthGraphics.com.
Anatomy of the breast adapted with permission © Medela AG 2006.

Nipple Readiness

Did You Know …

Diaper Only

For sleepy babies, remove their clothing and feed them with only their diaper on. Newborn babies get very sleepy feeding at the breast, especially if they are too warm from wearing too many clothes or from being wrapped in a blanket. When your baby is next to your skin, your body warmth will keep her warm. Research and experience show that babies are very content held on their parent's chest, right next to their skin.

Even though pregnancy prepares the breast tissue for greater elasticity for the suckling infant, there is no doubt that the first few days of intense suckling at pressures rarely experienced by the breast tissue may cause some discomfort or pain for the new mother. This initial discomfort, as the nipple elongates to proper feeding position, should only last for the first few minutes of a feeding and then subside, provided that the baby's mouth is latched properly on the breast. Breastfeeding that continues to cause pain throughout the feeding should be assessed by a breastfeeding specialist to correct the latch and solve the discomfort. There is really no recommended way to prepare your nipples or "toughen them up" during your pregnancy.

Most cases of breastfeeding discomfort are caused by a latch problem. Be sure to have a lactation consultant or experienced maternity nurse check the latch before you are discharged home from the hospital. Even if a mother has difficulty latching her baby to her breast, does not enjoy breastfeeding or is unable to nurse her baby at the breast, there are very efficient breast pumps that allow the mother to express breast milk to feed her baby via alternative feeding methods, such as bottles, spoons or finger-feeding. This may be a good solution for some working mothers who rely on caregivers to feed their infants.

✳ Latching Troubleshooting

Most important for you is how comfortable it feels when your baby is sucking.

1. Is your baby tucked in close to you with his chin pressed close to the breast and the nose just touching or close to the breast?

2. Does your baby have a good amount of the areola in the mouth and more of the areola showing above the upper lip than the lower lip?

3. Are your baby's lips flared outward, not rolled in?

4. Are there hollow areas in your baby's cheeks, like sucking on a straw, indicating the nipple and areola are not filling the mouth?

5. Are you hearing any clicking or smacking noises while your baby sucks? If so, take the baby off and relatch.

 Should I offer one or both breasts to my baby at each feeding?

Remember that breast milk is not the same throughout the entire feeding. The first milk (foremilk) is higher in water and lactose (sugar) and satisfies the baby's thirst. As the baby continues to feed, the milk (hindmilk) becomes higher in fat content. Also remember that milk production increases when the breast is more completely emptied. It is best to leave your baby on the first breast until you hear very minimal swallowing, indicating that he has swallowed the higher-fat-content milk. The baby can be burped at this time, although unless he's been crying a lot before feeding, a breastfed baby doesn't swallow a lot of air, so he may not need to burp.

Now offer the second breast. Some babies will want to feed on the second breast for as long as the first, some for 5 to 10 minutes, but others will be satisfied with the first breast only. If so, at the next feeding start with the breast last offered, so that for every feed, one breast is being more completely emptied. Some women switch a ring from hand to hand to help them remember or place a pin in the bra strap of the side they should start on next. When mothers only need to feed from one breast, they may choose to pump the other breast to provide a supplement at another time or for when they return to work.

Sucking and Swallowing

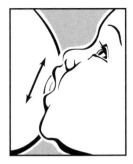

Now that your baby is properly latched, check to see if she is sucking and swallowing. Your baby could be sucking, but not getting milk. When your baby starts to suck, you will notice the sucking is fairly rapid, and then, after 1 to 2 minutes, you may feel sensations in your breast that signal your milk is letting down or starting to flow. As the milk starts to flow, the rate of sucking slows down.

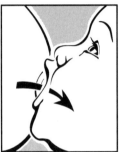

You will start to hear her making a "kaa-kaa" sound, which is the swallowing sound. If you have a large milk supply, you will probably hear your baby gulping milk. If you look carefully, you will notice a brief pause as the mouth opens the widest with sucking just before the mouth closes. This brief pause marks when the baby swallows. When the milk is flowing, you should hear swallows with every suck or every two to three sucks as the milk flow slows down before the next letdown.

First Week Urine and Stool Patterns

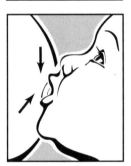

Keeping track of the number of soiled and wet diapers is especially important in the first week of breastfeeding. This is always a good guide to let you know your baby is receiving enough breast milk. For the first 6 days after delivery, your baby should have as many wet diapers per day as he is old — one on day 1, two on day 2, etc. The diapers should get heavier every day, especially after day 3 to 4, once your milk volume increases. If you are unsure about the weight of a "wet" diaper, measure out 2 to 4 tablespoons of water (30 to 60 mL) and pour this amount into the center of a diaper.

Pull the plastic backing of a disposable diaper to observe the urine. The urine should be odorless and clear in color, though it may be pinkish in the first few days. If the pink color persists beyond day 3, if the urine is very yellow in color or if your baby is not passing urine in amounts expected, check with your health-care provider. After the baby is 1 week old, continue to expect 6 to 8 heavy wet diapers every 24 hours.

You can expect to see a dark green or black sticky stool, called meconium, in the first day of feeding. The first day, there may only be one stool. Remember, the amount of colostrum taken in on the first day is very little. This colostrum milk, however, helps with the passing of the sticky meconium. By days 2 and 3, the stool should be turning greenish brown, but by day 4 and 5, it will become lighter in color (yellowish) and may be pasty, runny or seedy. If your baby is still having black meconium stools on day 5, contact your health-care provider.

Once a baby reaches 4 to 6 weeks, the bowel pattern may change. Your baby may continue to have several bowel movements a day or change to one a day, one every other day or even one a week. These patterns are all normal, provided the baby has 6 to 8 very wet diapers in 24 hours, eats well, gains weight and otherwise appears healthy and happy.

✳ First Week Urine and Stool Output Minimums for a Baby Exclusively Breastfeeding

Day	Urine Minimum (24 hours)	Stool Minimum (24 hours)
1	1 light wet diaper	1 blackish green
2	2 light wet diapers	1 blackish green
3	3 heavy wet diapers	2 greenish/brownish
4	4 heavy wet diapers	2 greenish/brownish getting more yellow
5	5 heavy wet diapers	2 yellow
6	6 heavy wet diapers	2 yellow

Note: A light wet diaper feels like 2 tablespoons (30 mL) of water and a heavy diaper feels like 4 to 5 tablespoons (60 to 75 mL) of water. Some babies may stool at every feeding.

✳ How to Do Breast Compressions

This technique helps get extra milk to your baby. Gently compressing or squeezing the breast during the feed will assist in the release of more hindmilk. Breast compressions can be used in situations when your baby is sleepy or can't suck strongly enough to get sufficient milk.

1. Support your breast well with your thumb on one side of the breast and your four fingers on the other side, back far enough on the breast so that you are not touching the areola.

2. Compress or squeeze your breast gently between your thumb and fingers as the baby is sucking, until the baby stops sucking and you release the pressure on the breast.

3. Apply pressure again once the baby sucks. You will notice your baby swallow more frequently.

4. Alternatively, try a more rhythmical compression, as if you were hand-expressing milk into your baby's mouth to keep milk flowing.

✳ How do I know if my baby is getting enough milk?

There are many ways to tell how well your baby is breastfeeding. Do an objective assessment of your breastfeeding by asking these questions:

1. Is your baby waking regularly or otherwise giving you hunger cues to breastfeed? This signifies a baby who has energy enough to waken.

2. Do you hear your baby swallow well throughout the feeding and finish looking satisfied? A baby who continues to root and wants to suck and is fussy and crying is indicating hunger.

3. Is your baby having adequate bowel movements and wet diapers? If your baby is receiving adequate breast milk, expect six to eight heavy diapers every 24 hours. Expect a minimum of two bowel movements every 24 hours up to 4 to 6 weeks.

4. Is your baby gaining weight normally? Babies may lose 5% to 7% of their weight in the first few days. While a 10% loss of body weight is considered normal, this may indicate a delayed milk response or feeding difficulty and should be assessed by a health-care provider or breastfeeding specialist. Weight loss is expected as the baby loses excess fluid and meconium. Babies receive only small amounts of colostrum in the first few days, which allows the immature kidneys to prepare for processing more urine as the breast milk volume increases. Babies should be back to their birth weight 2 to 3 weeks after delivery.

   In the first 1 to 2 months, the average weight gain expected is 1 to $1\frac{1}{2}$ ounces (30 to 45 g) per day for a breastfed baby. This works out to about 7 to 11 ounces (200 to 320 g) per week. Weight gain is more moderate after 3 to 4 months, up to a year.

   See the "Growth Patterns" section in chapter 3 for further details.

Jaundice

Jaundice, a condition that makes your baby's skin yellow, can affect breast milk intake. Normal jaundice may start 48 to 72 hours after birth with many babies, and peaks 3 to 5 days after birth.

Encouraging feeding is important if your baby has jaundice. If your baby gets sufficient breast milk, this helps the baby have stools, which helps eliminate the bilirubin causing the yellow skin color characteristic of jaundice. However, if the jaundice is severe, hospital treatment may be required. Be sure to consult your health-care provider if you notice that your baby is showing any signs of becoming jaundiced.

Settling into a Routine

Babies respond well to structure and routine. Just as your body should be feeling "back to normal" about 6 weeks after delivery, so too should your breastfeeding be settling into a problem-free, enjoyable and quiet time with your baby. By now, you and your baby have learned what feeding positions are most comfortable for you. No longer should your baby need much assistance to latch correctly. At this point, your breast size may begin to decrease to your prepregnancy size, which may coincide with a greater demand for breast milk from your baby as he experiences a growth spurt. A good routine will help you cope with this situation.

Breast Size and Growth Spurts

Be assured that the decrease in breast size that naturally occurs from about 4 to 6 weeks is rarely an indication that your milk is going away. This is just a decrease in hormonal swelling of the breast tissue from birth. Your breast tissue is now prepared to release milk on demand when your baby requires it.

Unfortunately, this decrease in breast size often coincides with a growth spurt around week 6. Babies have periods when they grow more quickly. These growth spurts tend to occur around 2 to 3 weeks after delivery and then at 6 weeks and 2 to 3 months. When your baby needs more milk to meet his increased growth, he will want to feed more frequently. This is your baby's way of telling your body that it needs to make more milk. Increased feeding behavior usually lasts 2 to 3 days, until your body has increased production to satisfy the baby, and then reverts to your usual feeding routine.

Feed your baby on demand. If you allow the clock and not the baby's new temporary schedule to dictate your feeding times, he will be fussy and your milk supply will not increase to meet your baby's new demands.

Baby Talk

For many mothers, the most frustrating part of caring for their new baby is learning what their baby is trying to say. Like us, newborns try to communicate through their gestures and their voice, but their language can be hard to learn. Be patient, watch and listen carefully, and you will soon be able to understand your baby.

Do I need to supplement my breast milk with water in a bottle?

No. Babies should not be given water to drink in place of breastfeeding. Breast milk is 90% water. Plain water has no nutritional value and makes the baby feel full, so she may not take in the amount of breast milk needed for optimal growth and development.

Sucking Motions

Right from birth, your baby will let you know that he wants to suck by putting his hand or fist to his mouth or by making sucking motions with his mouth and lips. In the first few weeks of life, any effort to suck should be rewarded with breast milk. Put your baby to your breast if he shows any motions to suck. These are early feeding cues.

Sounds

If the baby's first hunger cues are not answered, his vocal communication begins. Very quickly, your baby will turn a whimper into a screaming cry that says, "You didn't answer my first request, and now I'm really angry with you." Establishing a good latch with a screaming baby who has lost his focus can be difficult, resulting in an infant who becomes even more distressed because he can't get his food.

Feeding Styles

Babies often have distinct feeding styles that tend to match their personalities. We affectionately refer to some of them as barracudas or gourmets. As the terms suggest, the barracuda-type baby latches on to the breast, suckles voraciously and may completely empty a breast in 5 to 7 minutes, ready and raring to get going on the second breast without a rest break or burp.

The gourmet-type feeder may latch on eagerly, but feeds slowly, savoring the food and contact with his mother, taking routine pauses to rest between sucking bursts. This baby may take 30 to 40 minutes to feed the same amount of milk. Both the barracuda and the gourmet baby are perfectly normal feeders, only with different personalities and styles.

Like adults, sometimes a baby is only thirsty and wants a little drink. At other times, the baby is ready to have a larger meal, consuming a much larger volume of milk, and will likely settle in for a long sleep. No different than adults, babies need time for the bulk portion of their feeding to settle in their tiny stomachs. For a stomach the size of a golf ball, that 2- to 4-ounce (60 to 120 mL) feeding has stretched it enormously in that tiny body. And just like adults, babies may take a break after dinner before having dessert. If your baby wakes up crying 20 to 30 minutes after being put down, place him back on your breast. These babies will almost always fall asleep within 2 to 5 minutes of suckling or come off the breast with a "drunken stupor," contented look.

Sleeping Styles

Don't be concerned if your baby doesn't fall asleep after every feeding. Within a few short weeks of birth, many babies will have times during both the day and the night when they are content to lie quietly after a feeding and gaze around their new environment. Other babies may fall asleep at the end of their feeding, get their diapers changed, nicely settle into bed, and then 20 minutes later awaken crying, asking to be fed more or comforted before going back to sleep.

Did You Know …

Longer Sleep Stretch

In the first month of life, most babies will have one longer sleep stretch of about 4 to 5 hours each day. As long as the baby is generally feeding well, passing adequate urine and stool, and gaining weight, there is no reason to be concerned.

❋ ### What if my baby will only feed from one breast?

Some baby's develop a preference for one breast because they are positioned more comfortably on that side or they like the way the milk flows. Some mothers will purposely feed from one breast and pump the other breast to freeze breast milk for later use.

Troubleshooting Problems

The following sections help you with some of the issues women experience when breastfeeding. The earlier you intervene, the more likely the concern will be resolved successfully.

Crying

For new parents, soothing a crying baby can be frustrating. You know your baby is fed and changed, but he does not settle and begins to cry or wakes up crying after settling. What's wrong? Every well-meaning friend and relative has an answer: "You don't have enough milk." "Your baby is still hungry." "Give the baby a soother." "Here, I'll take the baby and rock him until he settles." Everyone means to be helpful, but these comments can undermine the mother's self-confidence and make her think that she doesn't know what she's doing with her baby. Most of the time, there is a very easy explanation for this common baby behavior.

✳ Causes of Crying

1. Your baby ate too much food and is feeling uncomfortable.

2. There is too much activity going on and your baby is overstimulated.

3. Your baby has just passed a large stool or is trying to have a stool.

4. Your baby has a very wet diaper that may cause a burning sensation on her tender skin.

5. Your baby needs to have a burp.

6. Your baby is having difficulty latching or getting milk from the breast at the rate she wants.

7. Your baby is crying due to colic.

 If my baby is well fed, clean and dry but continues to fuss and cry, what should I do?

Perhaps your baby ate too much food and is feeling uncomfortable. When you lay the baby down, his full stomach may push upwards and cause some reflux or spitting up of excess food. Keeping your baby in an upright position for a while after feeds may solve the problem, or settle him in a car seat or baby chair where he will sit more upright. Some babies like to lie face down, cradled across your forearm, or be gently rocked back and forth. For other babies, a gentle rhythmic patting on the bottom distracts them from whatever is distressing them and settles them.

Some babies cry in response to overstimulation — too much activity around them, too much light and noise. Try to change the environment surrounding your baby and see if that helps him to settle. Other babies love the noise and chaos, learning to eat and sleep very nicely, never bothered by the dog barking or by vacuuming under their crib. Many health-care professionals feel that learning to sleep in a noisy environment when you are an infant makes you a much better sleeper when you are older.

Colic

Some babies have periods of inconsolable crying around the same time each day, which is often referred to as colic. Colic tends to develop as early as 2 to 3 weeks of age and often lasts through 4 to 6 months. There are several theories about the possible causes of colic, including latching or feeding frustration, food sensitivities or intolerances, gas pains or gastric discomfort caused by gastroesophageal reflux.

✳ How to Manage Colic

The key to managing colic is to address the possible cause. Solving this problem may involve considerable trial and error. The problem may spontaneously resolve as quickly as it started.

1. A clue to why the baby is crying might be to recognize when your baby cries. Has the baby just had a large stool, or is he trying to have one? Is your baby crying during or just after a feed because he needs to burp or is too full? Was your baby taken off the breast and is protesting that he wasn't finished? Has the baby had repeated difficult latching on the breast and is crying in frustration?

2. If you have addressed these possible causes and your baby continues to cry and can't be comforted, a sensitivity or reaction to something in your diet could be the problem. Are you drinking excessive amounts of caffeine beverages (coffee or soft drinks)? Did you eat anything other than your usual diet in the past few days? Trace amounts of all foods you ingest pass through into your breast milk. If you suspect a food sensitivity, discuss this with your doctor, a lactation consultant or a dietitian. They may suggest that you try to eliminate that food from your diet for a week or so, and see if you notice a difference in your baby. There is no evidence that suggests that eliminating foods such as onions, cauliflower or garlic is necessary.

3. If your baby continues to cry for long periods, refuses to eat, has decreased urine or stool, appears very sleepy and develops a fever or rash, you should seek medical attention. Babies can become dehydrated very quickly, so don't let more than 24 hours go by if these symptoms occur in the first few months of life.

Refusing to Latch

Colic is not the only cause of discomfort for your baby while trying to breastfeed. Your baby may refuse to latch or be unable to latch correctly to your breast. Usually, when babies won't latch, it is because they can't get milk easily from the breast and they become frustrated. Babies, unless they are ill, want to suck and satisfy their hunger. If your baby can't latch properly, he may cry when you bring him to your breast.

Every baby should anticipate that being at his mother's breast will be a pleasant experience that leads to a satisfying feed. Some mothers feel a sense of rejection or guilt if their baby becomes obviously distressed as they are being positioned for a feed. Fortunately, this problem can be managed before it reaches this critical impasse and you and your baby are both upset and frustrated. While you work on solving this problem, your baby's intake, weight gain and milk volume need to be closely monitored.

✳ How to Help a Baby to Latch

1. If your baby cries going to the breast, stop! Don't make the frustration worse. Put your baby into what we call neutral or kangaroo position. Your baby is held upright between your breasts with her skin against your skin. Offer your finger for your baby to suck on. Let your baby settle before she shows feeding cues and try again. Some women have had success latching after holding their baby skin to skin while together in warm bathwater. Be sure you have another adult who can take the baby from the bath.

2. Offer your breast when the baby shows the first signs of hunger.

3. Make sure the areola is very soft. Hand-express milk as necessary. For some babies, the areola has to be very soft to entice them to latch.

4. Give your baby time to get used to the breast — time to lick at the nipple, to smell and taste the milk. Express drops of milk and watch what your baby does. Don't try to latch the baby before she is ready.

5. Try not to give a bottle with a nipple or a pacifier to your baby when she is learning to breastfeed, to avoid confusing her. To breastfeed, her tongue needs to cup the nipple and areola, moving in a wave-like motion backward to get the milk from the breast. However, this type of sucking is not necessary to get milk from a bottle nipple. Babies also do not have to root or open very wide when a bottle nipple is placed in their mouth. They may then find it difficult to root as they go back to the breast. Bottle-fed babies tend to bring their tongue to the roof of their mouth to stop the fast flow of milk, which may not help as they try to go back to breastfeeding. If your nipple and areola do not stretch out easily, it is even more important not to confuse your baby with bottle nipples.

6. Consider feeding your baby by an alternative method while she learns to breastfeed. Pump your breasts regularly at feeding times until your baby latches, and feed this milk to your baby using a spoon, cup or

bottle (if nothing else works). When your baby is fed and you are both feeling more relaxed, lie down with your baby skin to skin near the breast where she can see, feel, and smell it. Once the baby feels more comforted and less threatened by the breast, you can gently offer her the breast again. After one or two good comfortable feeds that satisfy her hunger, you should be back on track.

7. Offer your baby your finger to suck on to quiet her, and then try again to latch.

8. Pump your breast for a few minutes before latching your baby to help draw out and shape the nipple for an easier latch. Make sure the areola is soft. Sometimes the baby is having difficulty latching because the nipple is flat or turns inward. Remember, the baby latches to the areola, not the nipple.

9. If needed, wear breast shells between feedings to help bring out the nipple. Nipple shields, soft silicone nipple coverings, are sometimes recommended by lactation consultants to help shape the breast for a feeding when a baby can't latch. The baby's intake and weight gain and the mother's milk volume need to be closely monitored when using a nipple shield.

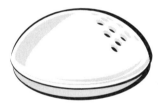 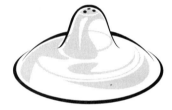

Breast shell   Nipple shield

10. Avoid bottles and pacifiers in this situation until your baby latches well. You may need to use an alternative method of feeding and pump your breast with a hospital-grade pump if the baby continues to have trouble latching.

11. If your baby has a very tight frenulum, the little tissue that attaches the tongue to the bottom of the mouth, it may not allow the tongue to move properly over the gum line to remove the milk from the breast. If this may be the case, consult your health-care provider.

12. Try latching your baby when she is still sleepy. Don't change the diaper first, which may wake her.

13. If your baby is not latching before you go home from the hospital, ensure you have an appointment at a breastfeeding clinic or with a lactation consultant to assess why your baby won't latch. For many babies, they just need a little more time, as do some mothers for their milk to come in.

Sore Nipples

Nothing takes away from the enjoyment of breastfeeding more than sore nipples. While experts differ concerning the prevalence of sore nipples among breastfeeding women, many women do experience some degree of nipple tenderness in the first week as they begin to breastfeed. It is normal in the first week for you to feel nipple tenderness and a pulling sensation as the baby sucks. This resolves normally around the third to sixth day after delivery.

However, if this initial tenderness persists or you ever feel you can't breastfeed due to soreness, seek help immediately. This is not normal. It is important to find out why the nipples are sore. The earlier the intervention, the more easily the problem can be solved.

✳ How to Prevent Sore Nipples

The best treatment for sore nipples is prevention. Here's how.

1. Position your baby comfortably for feeding and be sure the latch is correct. Good positioning and successful latching are the keys to preventing soreness. When the latch and sucking are normal, the nipple shape is round, not pinched or blanched (white) after the feeding.

2. Wash your nipples once a day with warm water. Apply breast milk to the nipple and areola after each breastfeeding. Air-dry the nipples for 10 minutes after each feeding. If privacy is an issue, try leaving your nursing bra open under your clothing.

3. Wear 100% cotton bras and reapply dry cotton nursing pads frequently. Your nursing pads should not have a plastic backing that prevents air circulation. Many disposable pads do, so washable ones are a better solution.

4. Avoid creams and ointments because they may aggravate sensitive skin and need to be wiped off for feeding, causing further damage.

5. Make sure the areola is soft before latching your baby.

6. Take your baby off the breast by inserting your finger between the baby's lips and gums. Remove the nipple before removing your finger from the baby's mouth.

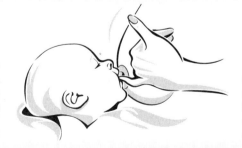

Occasionally, there may be some bleeding with a cracked nipple. This will not harm your baby. Your nipples may need a healing time before you resume breastfeeding. You can pump your breasts and provide your milk by alternative methods until they heal.

Causes of Persistently Sore Nipples

Some women have very sensitive nipples, and even with the best care, they are not able to tolerate the sensation they feel with breastfeeding. Check with your doctor or a dermatologist to see if there is an underlying medical condition. If it is too painful to nurse your baby, the next best choice would be to consider pumping your breast milk to provide all the same health benefits to you and your baby.

Incorrect Positioning and Latching

Incorrect positioning and latching are the primary causes of sore nipples. If your nipple is sore with the initial latch and improves once the baby is sucking and swallowing, then you probably have a good latch. However, if the nipple is sore throughout the feeding, you see a blister, cracks or a bruise on your nipple, or the nipple looks pinched, blanched or misshapen when the baby comes off the breast, poor positioning and latching may be the cause. Be sure to get help immediately from a health-care provider to correct the position and latch.

Poor Sucking

Even though the baby is well positioned and latched, the way a baby sucks at the breast can also cause sore nipples. If you pull gently back on the lower lip, you should be able to see the tongue coming over the lower gum line. This tongue placement is essential to cushion the nipple from the pressure of the lower jaw and to cup the nipple and areola properly. The nipple and areola are compressed between the roof of the mouth and the tongue. The wave-like motion of the muscles of the tongue compresses the nipple and areola, moving the milk from the breast into the mouth.

Some babies need help to get the tongue in the proper position and to suck properly. A lactation consultant can help you see if your baby has this problem. Suck training and finger feeding are used as interim measures until your baby sucks properly at the breast.

Plugged Nipple Pore

This is a plugged pore opening right at the surface of the nipple. It shows as a white dot on the nipple and can be very painful.

Did You Know …

Tongue Tie

The frenulum is a band of tissue that attaches the tongue to the bottom of the mouth. A tight frenulum, commonly called tongue tie, may prevent the tongue from coming over the lower gum line to cushion the nipple from the lower gum during a feeding. This can be painful for the mother and frustrating for the baby.

If the frenulum is preventing the baby from getting milk and the mother is experiencing soreness, a simple procedure can be done to clip the frenulum, enabling the tongue to then cup the nipple and areola. While this procedure is somewhat controversial, the Canadian Paediatric Society suggests considering clipping of the frenulum if breastfeeding is compromised.

Try warm compresses right before feeding and frequent breastfeeding or hand-expressing. If there is no improvement in a few days, your doctor can gently insert a sterile needle into the blocked area, often giving immediate relief. If the nipple pore releases, it often looks like a string of spaghetti coming out of the pore.

Yeast Infection

Mothers and their babies can pass yeast infections back and forth. Yeast infections can cause thrush or white patches in the baby's mouth and a reddish rash on baby's bottom. Your baby may be more irritable than usual. Yeast infections can also cause you great discomfort. You may suddenly develop very sore nipples with burning or itching pain during and after breastfeeding. You may also have a vaginal yeast infection.

Both mother and baby need to be treated with antifungal medications prescribed by your doctor. To prevent reinfection, bras should be washed daily, nursing pads should be kept dry, and soothers and toys that come in contact with the baby's mouth should be boiled daily. Most mothers should find relief within 24 hours with antifungal medication. If it is too painful to breastfeed, you can pump for a few feedings or days until feeding is painless again.

Vasospasm

A vasospasm of the nipple can cause burning and soreness. It can be caused by a constriction of the arteries due to a difference in the temperatures between baby's warm mouth and the air after feeding. Women notice the nipple is white after the feeding and then turns red and sometimes blue before returning to its normal color. Vasospasm can also be experienced with poor latch or with a baby who clenches the jaws, compressing and decreasing the blood flow to the nipple. This can happen more frequently if mothers have Raynaud's phenomenon, where their fingers and toes can turn white due to constricted arteries, then pink again when circulation improves.

Applying warm compresses to the breasts before and after breastfeeding and making sure the position and latch are correct can be effective treatments. There are medications your doctor can prescribe to alleviate this condition if symptoms persist.

Pulling on the Nipple

Sometimes a crack can develop in the area where the nipple joins the areola because the baby pulls when coming off the breast. Be sure to insert a finger in the baby's mouth through

✳ How to Treat Persistently Sore Nipples

1. Promote letdown by applying heat to your breasts with a warm hand towel or gently touch the areola in a circular fashion for 1 to 2 minutes. This saves the 1 to 2 minutes of sucking the baby does each feeding to get the milk to flow.

2. Consider creating a moisture barrier over the sore or cracked nipple to promote healing. You may want to consider this especially if you have dry skin. Lansinoh and PureLan are ultra-pure, hypoallergenic, non-toxic forms of modified lanolin that do not have to be removed before feeding and should be reapplied after feeding to maintain the moisture barrier.

3. Try different feeding positions that place pressure from the baby's mouth differently on the nipple.

4. Breastfeed on the less sore breast first, when the baby is hungrier and sucks more vigorously, and then switch to the sore side.

5. Try to feed more frequently and not as long at each feeding. Your baby won't be as hungry and feed as vigorously.

6. Support your breast throughout the feeding, and hold your baby close so there is no unnecessary pulling on the nipple.

7. Try to get to a breastfeeding clinic or call for breastfeeding help the same day if you feel you can't correct the latch or you have corrected the latch and you are still experiencing pain.

8. If you feel that one breast is just too painful for a feeding, shift to the other breast and hand-express or pump the sore breast. You can feed the baby on one breast and offer the expressed milk by an alternative feeding method, if he is still hungry.

9. If both nipples are too sore or very cracked or bruised, express both breasts every 2 to 3 hours and allow them to heal until you feel comfortable enough to try again, usually within 24 hours.

10. Try wearing hard plastic breast shells between feedings to protect the nipples from immediate contact with clothing. This prevents the outer healing layer of the nipple from being removed if your bra or nursing pad sticks to the nipple. If this should happen, soak the pad or bra first with water and carefully remove it from the breast. Breast shells are worn over the nipples and held in place by your bra. Nursing pads can be worn over the shells if leaking is excessive. Bra straps will need to be adjusted. Wearing a bra one size larger will prevent the breast shells from leaving a red mark on the breast. Some women like to wear breast shells to collect small amounts of leaking milk instead of using breast pads. This leaking milk should be discarded. Shells should be washed well with hot soapy water, rinsed well and dried before being reapplied. Breast shells are not recommended when you are sleeping for long periods because they can place excessive pressure on your breasts. Breast shells are usually available in maternity hospital drugstores.

the baby's lips and gums and then ease the nipple out before removing your finger from the baby's mouth.

Sometimes babies will pull back on the nipple when they want more milk to flow. Support your baby at the breast or remove him if the feeding is completed.

An older baby will sometimes try to take the nipple with him when he is distracted and turns his head to see something. Teach your baby not to do this. Gently take the baby off the breast and say no. The same procedure can be used if an older baby tries to bite you. Their teeth are not involved with the sucking process and rarely cause mothers any feeding distress.

Breast Pumps

Breast pumps that are used improperly or that apply too much pressure can damage your nipples. Please see the section on breast pumps for more information.

Breast Fullness and Engorgement

About $1\frac{1}{2}$ to 4 days after your baby is born, your breasts feel different. They are warm, tender and heavy. This fullness indicates your breasts are now producing more milk volume. If your milk is not expressed, either by feeding or pumping, your breasts may become engorged. The breasts can also become engorged at other times if the baby is not being breastfed regularly or is not feeding effectively.

Engorged breasts feel hard and painful. Because there is milk-producing tissue under the arms in many women, this area may also develop hard lumps that can become tender. The areola can become very hard and the nipples may flatten, making it difficult for your baby to latch. Instead of emptying, the breast becomes even more engorged. As engorgement is relieved by regular feeding, hand-expressing or pumping, your breasts will then feel softer and smaller. This does not mean your breast milk is gone, but that the amount your baby is taking from each breast equals the amount of milk your breasts are producing.

Plugged Ducts

Plugs of milk can block a milk duct. If the duct stays blocked, the area behind the plugged duct also becomes hard. You may notice a small hard lump that may feel tender and painful or cause no discomfort. The breast may be red, but you will have no fever and generally feel well.

✳ How to Prevent and Relieve Engorged Breasts

The following suggestions will help prevent and relieve engorged breasts. Begin as soon as possible and you will soon feel better.

1. Breastfeed frequently right from birth, usually every 1 to 3 hours, whenever your baby shows feeding cues. Try not to miss, delay or restrict feedings. Resist the temptation to sleep all night without breastfeeding, even though you are tired. Instead, sleep when your baby sleeps.

2. Help milk flow with a hot shower or warm compresses for 5 minutes before feeding. Wrap your breasts in warm hand towels covered by a bigger towel to keep in the heat. If heat doesn't help the milk to flow, switch to cold compresses before feeding. You can massage your breasts gently as well.

3. Gently touch your nipple or areola in a circular motion with the tip of your finger for 1 to 2 minutes to help your milk letdown.

4. Soften your areola first before feeding. This is the key to relieve engorgement. Once the areola is soft, your baby can again latch effectively. To soften the areola, place your thumb at the edge of the areola and your forefinger on the opposite side of the breast. Push with your thumb and forefinger back toward the chest wall, and then, without coming forward, compress the breast tissue between your thumb and forefinger. Continue to work your way around the areola until the areola is softened in all directions. If you find this too uncomfortable, try softening your areola with a breast pump, although hand-expressing generally works better.

5. Latch your baby to the softened areola. Check for an effective latch. Let your baby suck and swallow on this breast until you hear no more swallowing. You can gently use breast compressions or massaging in a circular motion to help soften the breast as baby feeds.

6. If your baby is breastfeeding well and your baby does not want the other breast, you can hand-express or pump this breast until you feel comfortable and then start on this breast at the next feeding.

7. After feeding or pumping, apply cold to your breasts. You can wrap your breasts with hand towels soaked in cold water or apply frozen bags of ice or vegetables wrapped in a cloth to your breasts in between feeds for comfort. This helps relieve some of the tissue swelling that comes with engorgement. You can also apply cold raw green cabbage leaves to your breasts (not the nipple) and remove them when they are wilted, usually about 10 to 15 minutes. Discontinue using the cabbage leaves when the engorgement subsides, because continual use may decrease milk supply. The exact ingredient in cabbage leaves that helps with engorgement is unknown, and although not scientifically proven, it is a home remedy that many women find comforting.

8. Continue to drink to satisfy thirst. Restricting fluids does not decrease engorgement.

9. If you are very uncomfortable, take pain medication as prescribed by your doctor.

10. If your baby is unable to feed effectively, pump both breasts every 2 to 3 hours with a hospital-grade electric pump until your baby is breastfeeding well again. These pumps have intermittent pumping pressures that will not damage the breast tissue. They mimic the sucking pressures of a normal newborn infant.

The exact cause of plugged ducts is unknown, but they are thought to be the result of pressure on the breast, ineffective emptying of the breast or a large milk supply that does not drain sufficiently. With appropriate treatment, plugged ducts usually feel better in 24 to 48 hours. If the hard area persists for more than a few days or if you develop signs of mastitis, see your health-care provider.

✳ How to Prevent and Treat Plugged Ducts

1. Avoid underwire bras and bras that are too tight. Pay attention to the amount of pressure you are applying on your breast with your finger or thumb when feeding. Front baby carriers can also apply too much pressure.

2. Apply warm compresses directly to the affected area for 5 minutes before and between feedings. A warm shower or bath feels wonderful. You can combine heat with gentle massage toward the nipple. Relaxing helps your letdown.

3. Check for effective emptying of the breast. Ask yourself:

   - *Is my baby latched correctly?*
   - *Am I letting my baby feed on the first breast until there is no more swallowing before I offer the second breast?*
   - *Am I using different positions at different feeds to empty different parts of the breast?*
   - *Am I breastfeeding according to baby's hunger cues throughout the day and night?*
   - *Have I delayed a feeding longer than usual?*

4. Try different feeding positions to better drain your breast. At some feedings, place your baby's chin next to the plugged area to drain that area more effectively. This may be difficult, depending on the area.

5. Massage your breast gently during the feeding and when applying heat. Starting at the outside edge of your breast, gently move over the hard area toward your nipple.

6. Offer the first breast until there is no more swallowing before offering the second breast. To ensure adequate emptying, start the next feeding with the breast offered last. Pump or hand-express your breasts if your baby is not latching and swallowing well.

7. As a last resort, try placing your baby on some pillows on the floor. Kneel on your hands and knees over your baby so the breast falls unimpeded into the baby's mouth. This has helped many women unblock a persistent plugged duct. If the milk flows too quickly, allow some to flow out first. This gravity technique also works well using heat and massage.

Mastitis

Mastitis begins with inflammation in a part of the breast tissue, which may progress to an infection. Typically you notice a hot, painful, red area on a part of your breast. There may be red streaks on the breast. You start to feel unwell and experience chills, a fever and a flu-like feeling. Mastitis usually affects only one breast but can be found in both breasts.

Women who develop mastitis report previous fatigue, increased stress, plugged ducts, unrelieved engorgement, sore, cracked nipples and breasts not draining regularly or effectively. Your breast milk may taste saltier due to a temporary increase in sodium and chloride. This does not cause harm, but your baby may refuse this breast because of the altered taste. As the mastitis clears, the breast milk resumes its former taste.

Mastitis can be effectively treated with antibiotics. Seek medical treatment promptly if you experience symptoms. Symptoms begin to resolve in 24 to 48 hours of treatment. There is no risk to mother or baby with continuing to breastfeed on the affected breast.

✳ How to Treat Mastitis

1. Keep emptying both breasts regularly. Offer the unaffected breast first to get your milk flowing. If it is too painful to breastfeed or your baby is not effectively emptying the affected breast, pump instead and give this milk to your baby. Resume feeding on the affected breast as soon as you are able.

2. Get lots of rest. The best idea is bed rest until you are recovered. Feed your baby while in bed.

3. Apply warm, moist compresses before feedings and in between feedings. Soaking in a warm tub or under a warm shower can get milk flowing from the affected breast. Cold applications also provide relief for some women between feedings.

4. Apply gentle massage during feeding or while applying heat or cold.

5. Increase your fluids and eat a varied, nutritious diet to boost your immune system.

6. Complete the course of all the medication prescribed by your doctor to ensure the mastitis is cleared. You can continue to breastfeed while taking almost all antibiotics. If you and your doctor are unsure if the antibiotic is safe, check with the Motherisk program at the Hospital for Sick Children (Toronto) or a local breastfeeding clinic. Acetaminophen or ibuprofen prescribed by doctors for pain can ease the discomfort and are safe for your milk and your baby. Remember, with treatment, you will soon start to feel relief. On the rare chance that this does not happen, seek further medical help.

❋ *Can I still breastfeed if I have mastitis?*

Yes, it is strongly recommended that you continue to breastfeed to empty the breast. If you are uncomfortable breastfeeding, your milk can be pumped and safely fed to your baby by an alternative method. The antibiotics prescribed by your doctor for this condition present no risk to your baby.

Overactive Letdown and Large Milk Supply

Some mothers find their milk flows very fast, sometimes with a forceful spray. The baby may not be able to swallow quickly enough and may cough or choke. In response to this, some babies start to push away from the breast when feeding or refuse to go back onto the breast.

When you have a large milk supply, your baby can get too much milk with high lactose content. Breast milk is higher in lactose and water at the beginning and fat at the end of the feeding. Some of the excess lactose can remain undigested in the bowel, making your baby uncomfortable. Your baby may cry and pull up his knees in discomfort. He may also have explosive green stools.

The situation is made worse when a fussy baby is moved from one breast to the other, where more high-lactose milk is consumed. As the baby gets less fat content, he gets hungry more quickly and continually wants to go the breast. The latch may be poor since the baby can so easily get milk. Over

❋ How to Manage Overactive Letdown and a Large Milk Supply

1. Let the initial milk spray or drip out before latching your baby. Your baby will then want to stay at your breast. Try to get a good latch.

2. Feed only one breast and sometimes even two feedings on the same breast before returning to the other breast. Put your baby back to the same breast if your baby wants to feed within an hour from the last feed.

3. If the breast not being fed on becomes uncomfortable, hand-express some milk until you are more comfortable.

4. Lie down or lean back so your baby is above the breast when in a sitting position so gravity is not increasing the flow.

the long term, many mothers will lose their milk supplies when the baby forgets how to latch and suck properly to more fully empty the breast.

Insufficient Milk Supply

Most mothers have lots of milk for their babies, and almost all mothers can provide some breast milk for their babies. We would not have survived as a species if this were otherwise. However, there are some mothers who do not have enough milk. This is a situation where a thorough assessment by a lactation consultant is very helpful. The sooner the problem is identified, the faster the problem can be corrected.

Insufficient Milk Supply Symptoms

The lactation consultant will try to determine if the milk supply is adequate, and then determine if the baby, for whatever reason, is not removing the milk available in the breast.

- If the milk supply is, in fact, inadequate, the baby will feed for long and frequent intervals and never seem satisfied.
- Some babies getting insufficient milk intake will not have enough energy to awaken for feeds and instead sleep long stretches of 5 to 6 hours and then feed listlessly.
- Diapers will not be heavy and fewer than the expected six to eight in 24 hours. Bowel movements will be decreased and scanty.
- The baby will not gain weight appropriately.
- If all of these signs are ignored, babies can become dehydrated, with a dry mouth and a sunken "soft spot" on the top of her head. There is need of immediate medical attention for the baby.

Did You Know ...

Milk Supplementation

If, for some reason, the milk supply can't be increased, the mother should supplement her breast milk with pasteurized donor milk, if available, or with infant formula recommended by her health-care provider. For more information on donor milk banks, see the Resources section in this book.

✳ How to Help Your Baby Swallow More Milk

1. Use breast compressions to ensure your baby gets all the milk available.

2. Try for more frequent feedings, at least 8 to 12 in 24 hours, to increase milk supply.

3. Offer both breasts at each feeding if you have not already been doing this.

4. Remember not to change breasts until there is minimal swallowing on the first breast and your breast feels soft.

5. Pump after each feeding. You can use an alternative method to give your baby expressed breast milk or formula after breastfeeding.

✴ How to Increase Milk Supply

1. Drink to satisfy your thirst and have a varied, nutritious diet.

2. Review your medications. Some medications, such as birth control pills, can decrease milk supply. Progestin-only contraceptives have less effect on milk supply. If your supply is low, you can speak to your doctor about an alternative method of birth control. Make sure your doctor is aware you are breastfeeding when discussing any medications.

3. If you have undergone breast enlargement or reduction surgery, consider supplementing your breast milk with pumped milk if possible. These surgical procedures can affect total milk supply. While some women may be able to breastfeed exclusively, others may need to supplement with some formula as recommended by their health-care provider. Close follow-up of the baby is very important, especially in the first weeks as breastfeeding is established.

4. Consider medications designed to increase breast milk if more frequent feedings and pumping do not increase your milk supply. Ask your doctor if these medications are appropriate for you. Herbal remedies, such as fenugreek and blessed thistle, have been recommended for many years to increase breast milk volume; however, these substances are not regulated, so it is not possible to know with certainty their active ingredients or accurate dosage. Many cultures have their own dietary remedies or myths to enhance maternal milk supply.

 Are there any foods that will help improve my breast milk supply or ensure that I have enough breast milk?

There are no specific foods that will help increase breast milk supply. The best method to keep milk supply sufficient is by breastfeeding or expressing milk frequently — the more often the breasts are emptied, the more signals you give to your breasts to make more milk. Milk supply is usually established by day 7 after delivery. However, it usually takes about 4 to 6 weeks to establish breastfeeding fully.

Measuring Milk Supply

If the mother's milk supply appears to be adequate, the amount of milk taken by the baby at a feeding can be measured quite accurately with electronic scales. Based on the equation that one gram of weight gain is closely equal to one milliliter of fluid intake, the difference between the before and after breastfeeding weight of an infant will give a measure of the milk he consumed at the breast. The mother can then pump after the feeding to see how much the baby did not take at the breast. This gives an idea of the baby's intake and the mother's total milk volume at a single feeding. Because a baby's intake will vary from feeding to feeding, this would need to be repeated several times.

Treatment of inadequate milk supply involves improving the mother's supply or the baby's intake. If the mother pumps a large volume of milk not taken by her baby at the breast, then she needs to supplement the breastfeeding with her pumped milk until her baby starts taking sufficient amounts from the breast. If supply issues are identified early, many mothers will still have a good supply.

✷ Special Breastfeeding Challenges

For some women, breastfeeding presents a special challenge because of physiological or health problems. In most cases, these problems can be overcome with assistance from health-care professionals.

Hormone Imbalance: Women with an endocrine disorder that affects the pituitary gland and the secretion or production of hormones that regulate breast milk production and release may have breastfeeding difficulties. If you were unable to become pregnant naturally or required hormone therapy to become pregnant, there is the possibility that the hormones regulating lactation may be affected as well. A physician or lactation professional should monitor your progress in establishing an adequate volume of milk during the first week.

Inadequate Glandular Tissue: One of the primary factors in true lactation failure is inadequate glandular (milk-secreting) tissue, although it is a rare occurence. This condition is suspected when there is a history of little or no breast development during puberty and no breast changes noted during the pregnancy. Tenderness is usually felt in the breasts in the first month or two of pregnancy, and the breast size usually increases one bra size. When there is insufficient glandular tissue, it is possible for one breast to appear much smaller and be less developed than the other, or both breasts may be equally affected. The mother's ability to produce adequate milk volume for her baby will be limited. Nevertheless, the mother can use a lactation aid with a feeding supplement if she still wishes to breastfeed her baby.

Breast Surgery: Lactation insufficiency has been reported in women who have had breast surgery that involves incisions around the areola. In most cases of breast enlargement, where the breast is lifted from a bottom incision at the chest wall to place an insert, there should be minimal effect on the ability to provide sufficient breast milk for the baby. If the mother has had a breast reduction, it is quite possible that she will not be able to produce sufficient milk to meet the baby's growth needs by exclusive breastfeeding. In this case, a breastfeeding specialist can show you ways to provide a feeding supplement at the breast.

Alternative Feeding Methods

If you are having difficulty breastfeeding your baby, you can hand-express or pump your breast and then feed your milk to your baby using alternative feeding methods, such as bottle-feeding, finger-feeding or cup-feeding. In this section, we provide you with information about these alternatives, but you will likely need the assistance of a lactation specialist for instruction, appropriate equipment and follow-up.

✳ Can I feed my baby by both bottle and breast?

This is never an easy answer and difficult to research. Some babies have no difficulty switching from breast to an occasional bottle, some babies will not breastfeed again after a few bottles and some babies will never accept a bottle nipple. They only want their mother's breast. The most common advice is to introduce an occasional bottle, if necessary, only after breastfeeding is well established and problem-free, usually by 4 to 6 weeks.

Bottle-Feeding

Feeding expressed breast milk by bottle may be necessary in some situations, but this may create problematic nipple confusion or nipple preference for some babies, though not all.

By virtue of its design, a bottle must allow air back into it to allow milk to flow from the nipple opening. We have all turned a bottle upside down and watched the milk drop instantly from the nipple. When pressure is applied to the nipple, a significant stream of milk will shoot out of the hole in the nipple.

Nature's model of feeding has an infant go to mother's breast and let the breast know that it's time to release milk by completing a series of rapid suckling movements (non-nutritive sucks) before the mother's breast releases milk and the sucking settles into a nutritive suck and swallow pattern. If the baby does this normal rapid sucking pattern on a bottle nipple, the baby would instantly receive large volumes of milk that would likely cause coughing and choking due to the baby's inability to swallow the large volume of milk. Not wanting to choke on this fast flow of fluid, the baby quickly learns to change his feeding behavior and creates fluid-blocking mechanisms by forcing his tongue to the roof of his mouth to stop the rapid flow of milk from the bottle nipple until he is ready to swallow it safely.

It may take only a few or several bottle-feedings, but once this new fast-flow feeding behavior is learned, there can be problems getting some babies back to nature's way of supplying milk.

Bottle Designs

Bottles generally come in two designs: those that use a collapsible, disposable bag, and wide-base nipple system and standard glass or plastic bottles with universal threads to fit a variety of bottle nipples. The collapsible-bag-design bottle is promoted as a system that limits the amount of air the baby can ingest with the feeding, therefore requiring less burping. The use of disposable bags requires no bottle sterilization.

Nipple Designs

Babies generally seem to adjust well to a long, firm silicone nipple that graduates in size from the tip to the base. One recent study reports concerns about the nipples with a small tip that increases quickly to a very wide base. If the baby's lips do not get fully open around this wide base, the baby will learn to short-suck on the narrow tip of the nipple only. If this technique is transferred to latching at the breast, the mother could experience nipple pain very quickly.

If the mother has a good milk supply that flows quickly and the baby feeds well, he will likely manage with a nipple hole size that is recommended for his age on the nipple package. If the baby is a slow feeder and does not gulp milk rapidly, a nipple hole recommended for newborns will likely be better, to slow down the milk flow.

Because there are increasing concerns about developing latex sensitivity with repeated exposure during a lifetime, we recommend silicone rather than latex bottle nipples.

Finger-Feeding

With bottle-feeding creating a flow dilemma for some breastfeeding babies, finger-feeding may provide a solution. Your lactation consultant will provide you with instruction, equipment and adequate follow-up.

Finger-feeding means nothing more than using an available finger as a nipple. A finger maintains its shape and doesn't collapse like a bottle nipple, therefore allowing babies

Did You Know ...
Orthodontic Nipple

There is considerable controversy among lactation experts concerning the orthodontic-type nipple. The shape of this nipple seems to promote a biting-down motion as soon as it slips over the baby's gum line and touches the roof of the mouth. This creates a very short nipple that doesn't elongate over the tongue surface as the breast does, therefore promoting a different sucking mechanism.

Did You Know ...
Adoptive Mothers

Lactation devices were originally developed by adoptive mothers who, although able to stimulate some milk supply from the breasts, wanted a vehicle to allow them to provide the necessary nutritional supplement while nurturing their new babies at the breast to enhance bonding.

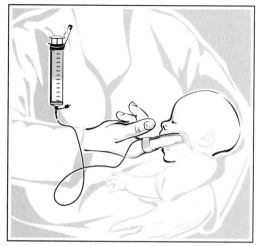

Finger-feeding

to use the wave-like motion of their tongue on the finger as they would on the breast nipple. A tube is taped to the finger, with one end placed in a container of expressed breast milk. The baby suckles on the finger and tube while feeding.

This technique of feeding closely resembles breastfeeding because the milk will only flow when the baby sucks as he would on the breast — that is, the baby does several rapid suckles to get the milk flowing through the tube, and once the milk reaches the baby's mouth, he settles into a suck and swallow pattern as he would on the breast. When the baby stops sucking, the milk stops flowing.

Cup-Feeding

You may find that in the nursery for newborns your baby has been given a feeding supplement using a cup. This method of feeding was designed not to interfere with the inside workings of a baby's mouth, but rather to encourage an infant to actively use her tongue to lap up milk from a cup placed against her lower lip, much like a cat licking milk from a bowl.

This exercise can be very useful if the breastfeeding specialist determines that the baby needs to learn to extend the tongue beyond the lower gum line, as she would in breastfeeding.

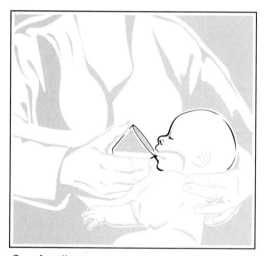

Cup-feeding

Lactation Devices

It may be necessary for you to supplement your baby with pasteurized donor milk or infant formula if your milk supply is low or if you have been given instructions by a health-care professional to prepare a feeding supplement for your baby. If your baby latches well to the breast, supplementation can be achieved by using a lactation device

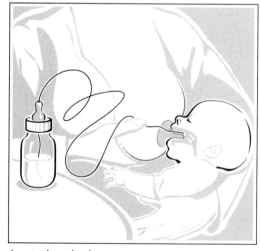

Lactation device

at the breast. A lactation consultant can provide you with instructions, equipment and follow-up required to monitor the use of this device.

A lactation device, or aid, is a flexible plastic, rubber or silicone feeding tube positioned or taped on your breast so that the end of the tube rests on your nipple and becomes an external milk duct. Just as with finger-feeding, the small end of the tube is the outlet into the baby's mouth, while the wider end of the tube is placed in a container of breast milk or baby formula. The milk container can be placed on a table beside you or pinned with a rubber band and safety pin to your sleeve, as long as the milk remains at the baby's head level.

This simple idea works quite well when introduced to infants during the first month or two of life, after which they get too smart and realize that something strange is happening at mom's breast and will likely refuse to latch with the tube on the nipple. The young baby that adjusts well to the lactation aid latches well to mom's breast and, as he suckles, draws alternative milk up the tubing and drinks that milk at the same time as he gets breast milk from the breast.

Nipple Shields

In the hospital environment, your baby may have already been introduced to bottle-feeding if you haven't been able to stay with her around the clock for breastfeeding. If there are problems latching, a lactation professional may suggest the use of a nipple shield. This soft, hat-shaped silicone device covers your nipple and provides the same texture to the baby as she has experienced with a bottle nipple or pacifier.

When used correctly, a nipple shield has been shown to increase milk intake in premature babies. Often the nipple shield will help transition the baby from bottle-feeding back to the breast. But a word of caution. If used incorrectly, a nipple shield can decrease a mother's milk supply if the baby does not get enough breast tissue (covered by the nipple shield) into her mouth to stimulate the breast to empty efficiently. The breast may need to be gently compressed to keep the milk flowing down to the nipple. Once the baby latches without difficulty to the nipple shield for repeated feedings, the mother can remove

Did You Know ...

Finger-Feeding Benefits

Finger-feeding allows any caregiver to feed the baby in a way that provides the least interference with the mother's attempts to latch her baby. Finger-feeding is also very helpful as a transition back to the breast if the baby has developed a bottle-feeding suck, where the tongue tends to go to the top of the mouth quickly. Finger-feeding promotes the baby to keep the tongue relaxed and cupped nicely under the finger to allow the backward wave-like motion to suck properly and obtain milk as in breastfeeding.

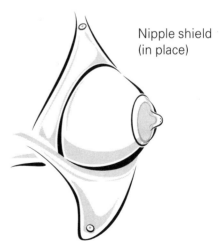

Nipple shield (in place)

Adapted with permission © 2006 by Amy Spangler.

the nipple shield and try to latch directly to the breast. The use of any device to assist you with breastfeeding should be assessed by a lactation professional so that its proper use and care can be discussed.

✳ *Should I use a pacifier if I am breastfeeding?*

Pacifiers, also known as soothers or dummies, have been used to calm babies by allowing them to use their own natural self-soothing mechanism — sucking. However, they should never be used instead of feeding, so they should be delayed until breastfeeding is well established.

When pacifiers are used frequently while you're establishing breastfeeding, nipple confusion or preference between your nipple and the artificial soother nipple may be detrimental to the comfort and ease of breastfeeding. The use of soothers promotes a tight mouth and biting behavior by the baby so that the soother doesn't fall out of the mouth. When this behavior is transferred to the breastfeeding model, you might find yourself complaining of the baby biting or sore nipples from a tight-mouth latch.

Pacifiers have been implicated in causing early weaning, increased frequency of ear infections and dental problems, according to the Canadian Paediatric Society. Appropriate care and cleaning of pacifiers by washing in warm soapy water and rinsing well is important to limit contamination. There have been a few published studies that show an association between pacifier use and the reduced risk of sudden infant death syndrome (SIDS), but they are not conclusive.

Special Babies and Mothers

Having a healthy newborn infant is a total lifestyle change for new parents. When there are complications at birth, such as an unexpected Cesarean section, or the baby is premature, near term part, or part of a multiple birth, there are special challenges to overcome for the infant, the mother, and the entire family during breastfeeding.

Breastfeeding after a Cesarean Section

For the safety and well-being of you or your baby, your doctor may perform a Cesarean section (C-section) birth or you may have a preplanned C-section in a non-emergency situation based on your health history.

If you give birth by this surgical procedure, you will need to attend to your own healing, as well as the needs of your newborn. Be sure to ask your health-care providers and family to help you establish breastfeeding. Focus on feeding your baby and let your helpers do everything else, including feeding you. For the sake of the mother's recovery, relatives, friends and other visitors should give mother and baby about a week to get settled at home.

Positioning

Once you are at home and possibly alone with your baby, finding a comfortable position for breastfeeding may not be easy at first. Some mothers prefer to breastfeed while lying somewhat on their sides in bed with a pillow behind their back and another beside them to raise the baby to breast level. Other mothers are more comfortable in a sitting position with a pillow across their abdomen to support the baby. You can also use the upright football hold, where your baby is sitting on a pillow beside you being held along your same side arm and facing the breast. See the Breastfeeding Positions Guide on page 81.

Breastfeeding Multiples

If you have multiples, be confident that you can supply enough breast milk for their needs, though the whole process of feeding two or more hungry babies may need extra planning and a sense of humor.

Positioning

The easiest way to nurse twins at the same time is to use the football hold for both babies. Prop up some pillows to support each baby, which will leave your hands free. You can also try the regular cradle position for both babies, with their legs overlapping. Your babies may decide for themselves which breast they prefer, and you will quickly learn which baby prefers what position. Some moms say that they can identify which baby is which by the strength of their suck or the speed they eat.

If one baby is larger or stronger than the other, you can alternate breasts to maintain an adequate milk supply in both breasts. Whether or not you choose to nurse your twins together or separately is a choice you should make based on what works well in your daily routine. Mothers of twins will tell you that either way is fine. Try various techniques to find what works best for you.

Did You Know ...

Feeding Twins

In the case of twins, each baby will stimulate sufficient milk supply from one breast to supply all her growth needs. Although enough milk can be produced to feed more than two babies, most mothers with triplets plan on a revolving feeding pattern in which, at every third feeding, one baby is fed previously expressed breast milk or formula by bottle while the other two babies feed from the breast.

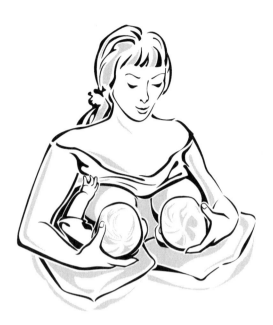

Football position for multiples

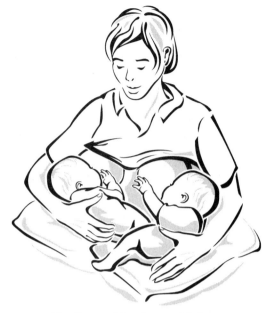

Cradle position for multiples

Breastfeeding Premature Infants

Did You Know ...

Doubly Healthy

If breastfeeding is healthy for full-term babies, it is doubly so for premature infants, though feeding at the breast may not be possible and alternative methods will need to be used at first.

Prematurity is defined as any infant born before 37 weeks' gestation. If born several weeks early, these babies are typically cared for in a newborn intensive care unit. This is a stressful experience for new parents, who are often confused by the technology of an intensive care nursery and worried about their baby's long-term health. If the mother herself is unwell due to the complications of the pregnancy or delivery, the father has a double burden of concern for two very important individuals, his partner and their new baby.

From about 16 weeks of gestation, your breasts have been preparing colostrum in preparation for your delivery day, so if you have delivered a premature baby, rest assured that you will be able to produce breast milk to protect and nourish your tiny baby. In fact, your breast milk has a distinct composition that helps your baby grow and develop as he would have if he were still in the uterus. Premature milk consistency lasts for about the first 6 weeks after your early delivery, and then your milk changes to more-mature-term milk. Your baby may require special premature feeding supplements, such as human milk fortifier, added to your breast milk to supply extra protein and minerals needed for growth.

✳ How to Nurse a Premature Baby

If your baby has been born very early in your pregnancy, between 25 and 30 weeks of gestation, and needs assistance to breathe, it could be several days or weeks before you are really able to hold him in your arms. Up to that point, the baby is keenly aware of sensory stimulation — your touch, your voice or the taste of your breast milk on his lips. The more time you spend with your premature baby, the more you get to know his likes and dislikes.

1. **Kangaroo care:** When the medical team has determined that your baby is stable enough to be moved out of his incubator for short periods, the first place he should be placed is on your chest, skin to skin, in an upright position, between your breasts. This position is appropriately called kangaroo care, with your baby nestled between your breasts just like a baby kangaroo nestled in his mother's protective pouch.

   During kangaroo care, the baby hears and feels your heartbeat just as he did in the uterus. Studies have shown that a mother's body temperature can rise up to 2°F to keep her baby warm. The rise and fall of your chest teaches breathing rhythm to your baby. Most babies will continue to be connected to their heart monitors, where you can watch the marvel of the baby's heart rate, breathing and oxygen levels achieve normal or stable levels, possibly for the first time.

   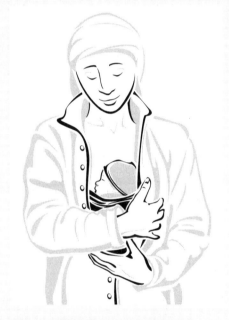

   Kangaroo care becomes the first step in familiarizing your baby to breastfeeding as your baby progresses to breathing on his own and you begin to position him closer to the breast and nipple, where he becomes aware of the smell and taste of your milk. Once your baby takes an active interest in licking your nipple and opening his mouth in an attempt to latch, you are on your way to learning breastfeeding. For the premature baby born at 30 to 36 weeks, the transition from tube-feeding to sucking at the breast will occur sooner, as your baby matures at a much faster rate and learns to coordinate the actions of sucking, swallowing milk, and breathing.

2. **Positioning:** You may want to use some pillows to elevate your premature baby. Provided your premature baby has his head well supported, you can hold your baby across your chest and facing your breast in a cross-cradle position or hold him in an upright football position directly facing your breast for first introductions to the breast.

Continued on next page…

✳ How to Nurse a Premature Baby
(continued)

3. **Latching:** Depending on the size of your nipple area, it might not be possible for your baby to latch for several weeks until he grows, but his awareness of your warmth and heartbeat and the taste of your milk at the nipple facilitate the process of latching to your breast. Premature babies will attempt to lick the milk from the end of the nipple and open their mouths just like full-term babies. Your baby may not have a strong nursing reflex yet, so you may need to pull down his chin and direct your nipple into the back of his mouth.

4. **Nipple Shield:** Try using a nipple shield. When used correctly, a nipple shield has been shown to increase milk intake in premature babies. Often the nipple shield will help transition the baby from bottle-feeding back to the breast.

✳ *Can I feed my preterm baby breast milk?*

Yes, by all means. Expressed mother's milk is beneficial for the health and survival of these babies. Preterm milk is quite different than full-term milk. It is richer in energy, protein, lipids, some vitamins, minerals and some immune factors — all needed for a premature infant to grow. Often, very premature babies need to be supplemented with minerals and vitamins to optimize their growth. By adding nutrients to the mother's milk, energy and electrolytes are adjusted to meet the extra needs. The immune system of the premature baby is especially at a disadvantage compared to healthy term babies. The protective immunities in breast milk make it very important for the preterm baby.

Coordination

Although sucking has been shown to develop between 18 and 24 weeks of gestation, a baby's ability to feed effectively depends upon the coordination of his suck, swallow and breathing reflexes. Most premature babies have developed this coordination by 33 to 34 weeks of gestation, although it may take several days to several weeks before babies can take the full amount of feeding they require for growth. If your baby is too immature to learn how to coordinate sucking, swallowing and breathing, your breast milk will be placed directly into his stomach through a small feeding tube placed in his nose or mouth.

It is normal for premature babies to be alert and active for a few feedings a day, but often they don't have the energy to participate actively in every feeding session. At these times, they will be fed through a feeding tube while they rest and gather energy for the next feeding.

Breastfeeding the Near-Term Infant

When babies are born healthy at 35 to 37 weeks' gestation, they provide a unique feeding challenge. These babies typically weigh within the range of babies who are discharged home, but because they are still premature, they require some extra attention when breastfeeding and should have close follow-up.

To support the growth and development of your baby's needs at this stage, she may require some encouragement to breastfeed as often as she needs. Born prematurely, your baby may not be ready to cope with the outside world, including the sensory stimulus of sights, sounds, smell and touch around her. When the stimulus becomes too much for babies to deal with, they tend to close their eyes and pretend to go to sleep. This sleepy behavior might carry right through feeding times. Often, just removing some clothes or unwrapping the baby from a blanket and exposing her to slightly cooler air will arouse her.

Expressing Breast Milk

If your baby can't feed at the breast or you are not available to breastfeed him, you can express your milk with your hand or with a pump for finger-feeding, bottle-feeding or cup-feeding. This may be necessary or desirable, depending on the circumstances. The baby may have been born too early or too ill to feed at birth. Despite the best efforts of all concerned, some babies can't latch or suck effectively at the breast. Due to financial concerns and other responsibilities, mothers may need to return to work very soon after their baby is born and can't be with their baby 24 hours a day, 7 days a week. If you find yourself in any one of these situations, you can still provide your baby with the nutritional and protective benefits of breast milk by expressing it.

Can I go back to work and still breastfeed?

Yes, you can. Depending on your work schedule and ability to pump your breast milk during your working hours, you may still be able to provide all the breast milk your baby needs. Some mothers are happy to breastfeed before work and bedtime only during the week, while giving the baby expressed breast milk via alternate methods during the day, and then revert to all-day breastfeeding on the weekends.

Expressing with a Pump

Frequent stimulation and adequate emptying of the breast with a hospital-grade pump are needed for good milk production if your baby is not feeding at the breast. When you pump your breasts, the milk-producing hormones prolactin and oxytocin are released, causing the milk to flow from your breasts. Oxytocin release can be decreased if you are feeling stressed, so make yourself as comfortable as possible for pumping. Take care of yourself as well as your baby. Try to stay rested, well nourished and calm. Find a private place to pump, if desired. Take any pain medication prescribed by your doctor.

Recommended Breast Pumps

There are many pumps available, but not all are appropriate for establishing and maintaining a milk supply when a baby is not feeding at the breast. We recommend a hospital-grade, double-electric pump, usually available in hospital drugstores or gift shops, but you may want to contact your birth hospital or lactation consultant for recommendations about the type of pump to rent or buy and where they are available. These pumps cycle at approximately the same rate as a normal healthy baby would suck at the breast. The pressures on the pump, mimicking the intraoral pressures of a healthy newborn, are enough to make the milk flow from the breast, but not enough to cause nipple soreness when used properly.

You will need two pump kits that fit over each breast and connect you to the breast pump. The flange, or part that fits over the nipple, should easily let the nipple move in and out without discomfort. Flanges come in different sizes.

Pump Costs

The initial cost of buying or renting a pump can seem high. The monthly cost of renting is still less than the cost of purchasing regular formula, bottles and nipples each month. If the cost seems too high, investigate what resources are available in your community to buy or rent a double-electric pump.

Does it matter what kind of breast pump I use?

Yes. If you are establishing a milk supply in the first week or two, you need to stimulate the breast as effectively as a healthy newborn baby would. Most drugstore-variety breast pumps do not have the suction strength or cycling rhythm to empty the breast effectively. Your birth hospital can recommend a hospital-grade breast pump made by a company specializing in breast pumps that will allow you to double pump to maximize your milk supply. If you only need to pump occasionally for a night out once your milk supply is well established, a drugstore manual or small electric breast pump may be all you need.

How often and for how long should I pump?

To establish and maintain a breast milk supply, you need to simulate how a baby breastfeeds. Most newborns breastfeed 8 to 12 times a day in the initial weeks as the milk supply is established. Develop a pumping regimen of a minimum of seven to eight pumping sessions a day, with no more than one 6-hour stretch from the beginning of one pumping session to the next pumping session. Because prolactin levels tend to be higher at night, try to pump at least once during the night.

Pumping sessions should be approximately 2 to 3 hours apart, but this does not have to be rigid. You can have 2 hours between some sessions, 3 or 3½ hours between others. You may also have some pumping sessions an hour apart if you have difficulty fitting in your pumping sessions during the 24 hours. Babies certainly want to feed every hour on occasion.

As a general rule, pump for 10 to 15 minutes each breast. Your total pumping time will be 10 to 15 minutes if you are pumping both breasts at the same time and 20 to 30 minutes total if you are pumping each breast individually. Because milk production increases with more complete emptying of the breasts, pump until the milk stops flowing and then for another 1 to 2 minutes.

Track your 24-hour volumes. If you are producing milk adequately, continue to monitor. If you are not producing a 24-hour supply of milk for your baby, seek help from a lactation consultant or other health-care professional.

✳ How to Hand-Express Milk

Prepare

1. Wash your hands with warm soapy water, rinse and dry with a clean towel.

2. Encourage letdown by applying warm compresses for 5 minutes or by gently touching the nipple or areola for 1 to 2 minutes. Once you and your breasts are used to hand expression, this will not be necessary.

3. Gently massage your breast to help move the milk down toward the nipple. Two ways are shown here. You can use one method or both.

a. Use your fingertips to massage all around the breast in small circles, working from the outer edge of the breast toward the nipple.

b. Cup your breast with one hand on each side of the breast and gently compress as you move from the edge of the breast toward the nipple. Rotate your hands so you reach all parts of your breast.

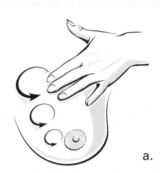

a.

Express

1. Place your finger and thumb at the edge of the areola as a general guideline and press back toward the chest wall. You should be able to draw an imaginary straight line between your thumb, the nipple and your finger.

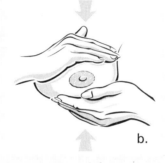

b.

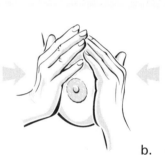

b.

Modified from the original image
© Childbirth Graphics®,
www.ChildbirthGraphics.com.

2. Compress your thumb and finger together at the edge of the areola. This movement involves a slight rolling motion forward with a return to the original position. This milking action mimics the action of the tongue to remove milk. If you are not able to express with your placement at the edge of the areola, you may need to experiment, moving a little farther outside the areola (if you have a small areola) or a little closer toward the nipple (if you have a large areola).

3. Move your finger and thumb around the areola, removing milk from different parts of the breast. This will take about 10 to 15 minutes for each breast. You may want to express your breasts alternately for 5-minute intervals.

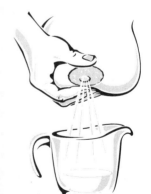

Collect

1. Collect hand-expressed milk in a well-washed and rinsed cup or bowl. A measuring cup works well.

✳ Expressed Milk Requirements

How much milk do you need to express for a feeding? Here are some general guidelines, which may vary according to your baby's age and weight.

Age	Amount per feeding (oz)	Amount per feeding (mL)
Birth to 1 week	1–2	30–60
1 to 2 weeks	2–3	60–90
2 weeks to 2 months	2–5	60–150
2 to 4 months	4–6	120–180
4 to 12 months	5–8	150–240

Expressing by Hand

Even though you may prefer to use a breast pump, it is useful to know how to hand-express. You always have your hands with you. Many women become very adept at hand-expressing and may be able to empty their breasts faster than with a pump, but this method takes a little practice. It may help to have a health-care provider, lactation consultant or another mother demonstrate the technique.

✳ How to Freeze Expressed Breast Milk

The following guidelines will enable you to freeze your breast milk safely. Check hospital policies if you have a sick or premature infant.

1. Wash your hands with warm soapy water, rinse and dry on a clean towel before expressing or preparing milk.

2. Freeze your milk in clean glass or hard plastic containers — or freezer-grade plastic bags manufactured for this purpose. The containers can be washed on the top shelf of a dishwasher or washed with hot soapy water, rinsed well and air-dried. Try not to touch the inside of the containers or lids.

3. Leave 1 inch (2.5 cm) of headspace at the top of the container to allow for the expansion of the milk as it freezes.

4. Store milk in amounts needed for a feeding, but also some 1- and 2-ounce (30 to 60 mL) portions if your baby wants more for a feeding. To freeze handy 1-ounce (30 mL) snack size cubes of breast milk, wash an ice cube tray on the top rack of a dishwasher. Pour fresh expressed breast milk into the cubes and freeze. When frozen, pop the cubes out and put in a freezer-grade ziplock bag. Thaw cubes in a clean cup or bowl as necessary.

5. Label the milk clearly with the date, and use the milk in the order it was pumped.

6. Once a bottle of milk is refrigerated and cold, add other refrigerated milk if you wish, but don't add warm pumped milk to a previously refrigerated or frozen bottle of milk.

✳ Safe Handling of Expressed Breast Milk

To ensure expressed milk is safe for your healthy term baby, follow these handling practices for various storage locations. Check hospital policies if you have a sick or premature infant.

Counter: Covered, on the counter at a standard room temperature of 66°F (19°C) to 79°F (26°C), breast milk can stand for 6 hours before being refrigerated. If the room temperature increases, the milk should be refrigerated sooner.

Refrigerator: In a refrigerator, breast milk can be stored for up to 5 days. Place the milk at the back of the refrigerator, where the temperature is the coolest.

Refrigerator Freezer: In the freezer compartment within a refrigerator, breast milk can be stored for 2 weeks. In the back of a separate freezer in a refrigerator, breast milk can be kept for approximately 3 months. If your freezer can't keep ice cream frozen, it will not keep breast milk frozen either.

Chest Freezer: In a separate manual-defrost chest freezer set at 0°F (19°C), breast milk can be stored for 6 to 12 months. (**Note:** Frozen breast milk should not be placed on the floor of a self-defrosting freezer because the heating coil could begin to thaw the milk as it cycles.)

✳ How to Thaw and Reheat Breast Milk

1. Thaw frozen milk overnight in the refrigerator, run under warm water or place in a container of warm water until thawed.

2. Reheat fresh refrigerated milk under warm running water or in a container of warm water, replacing the water as it cools. Breast milk needs to be heated to body temperature to reactivate the antibodies.

3. Do not heat breast milk in a microwave because it can produce hot spots, which could burn your baby's mouth. Likewise, do not heat milk on the stove. Microwaving and boiling milk can destroy the infection-fighting properties of breast milk.

4. Gently shake the container to redistribute the fat. You will notice that the milk separates into layers. The lighter fat layer rises to the top. Frozen milk may have different-colored layers, depending on what the mother has eaten.

5. Once thawed, use the breast milk within 24 hours.

6. Do not refreeze breast milk once it has thawed.

7. Discard any milk your baby does not finish at a feeding.

✳ Breast Milk Banks

Because of illness or separation from their babies, some mothers are unable to provide breast milk for their own infants at the breast or by expressing. They may wish to use donor milk. Donor milk banking is recommended by the American Academy of Pediatrics, and a new statement in support of donor milk banking is currently under review by the Canadian Paediatric Society.

Breast milk banks accept donations from rigidly screened mothers who may be breastfeeding their own babies or, tragically, from mothers who might have lost a baby to illness or stillbirth and wish to share the gift of their milk with medically fragile infants who would benefit from the milk.

Because breast milk, as a human body fluid, can transfer viruses, donor milk needs to be pasteurized, or heat-treated by accepted standards, to ensure the sterility of the milk before it is dispensed by a doctor's prescription to a sick or premature baby. Although some live cellular components of the breast milk are destroyed in the process of pasteurization, most immunity components are only minimally affected.

If you have good milk production and feel that you would like to donate some of your breast milk, check with your birth hospital to find out if there is a donor milk bank near you.

✱ *Can I breastfeed my adopted baby?*

Yes, you can. Although you may never have been pregnant, your breasts will begin to produce milk with the proper stimulation using an electric double-breast pump a few weeks before you receive your baby. Often you will not make enough milk to meet your new baby's nutritional requirements entirely, but there are manufactured lactation devices that make it quite easy to give supplemental donor milk or infant formula at the breast. Talk to your health-care provider to see if there are any medications that can assist in your milk production.

Introducing Solid Foods while Breastfeeding

The World Health Organization (WHO) recommends exclusive breastfeeding for the first 6 months before introducing solid foods, as stated in their *Global Strategy of Exclusive Breastfeeding*. This recommendation was adopted by Health Canada in *Nutrition for Healthy Term Infants* and by American health-care agencies. The WHO and many national organizations, including the American Academy of Pediatrics, the American Dietetic Association, Health Canada, the Canadian Paediatric Society and the Dietitians of Canada, recommend that after solid foods are introduced at 6 months, breastfeeding continue to at least 1 year or beyond. Solid foods are seen as complementary food sources, with specific nutrients, chiefly iron and zinc, needed for the older infant's healthy growth and development being supplied by the solid food.

 For how many months should I exclusively breastfeed my baby?

Because breastfeeding is the ultimate food choice for infants, some women consider extending exclusive breastfeeding beyond the recommended 6 months, thinking, "Why not carry on as long as possible?" However, waiting 8 to 9 months before introducing solid foods is not recommended. Research shows that if infants are not introduced to some textured food by the age of 7 to 9 months, they may have trouble accepting solid food later on.

Iron-Rich and Fortified Foods

Infants born at full term and breastfed have sufficient iron stores to last until 6 months of age. (The iron found in breast milk is in a perfect form and easily absorbed by the infant). After this time, if an infant continues to exclusively breastfeed, medical experts do not know for certain how long breast milk will supply adequate iron content. Low iron stores can affect cognitive function. The brain needs the oxygen delivered by blood for normal function, and enzymes in the brain and central nervous system depend on iron to function normally.

To ensure against iron deficiency and prevent any long-lasting effects on cognitive development, at 6 months of age a food high in iron content, such as an iron-fortified cereal or meat, should be introduced. Foods that contain plant-based non-heme iron should be served with vitamin C–containing foods, such as oranges and mangoes, to increase the absorption of this form of iron. Recent studies indicate that infants who continue to breastfeed beyond 6 months of age and take in complementary foods with iron have normal iron stores and can avoid iron deficiency, despite the seemingly low but very well-utilized iron supplied by breast milk.

Iron-Enriched Cereals

Most commercially prepared infant cereals are now fortified with iron. While some mothers may choose to make their own cereal, homemade versions may not contain an adequate supply of iron. Mothers may need to consider adding another iron source.

Start by introducing a single-grain cereal, such as rice cereal (which is non-gluten-containing and least allergenic), allowing about 2 to 3 days before trying another new cereal so you can identify any food that your baby is not tolerating or reacting to adversely, as shown in the development of hives, rashes, sudden vomiting or diarrhea. Mix it to match the consistency of applesauce before offering it on a spoon or your finger. You can mix cereal with water or your own breast milk for added nutrition. Some cereals have added cow's milk formula, so for those infants with a cow's milk allergy, these need to be avoided.

Iron-Rich Meat

Meat and meat products are high in iron content and are a good source of zinc. If meat is the first food offered, either homemade or commercially prepared varieties are acceptable. Offer one variety at a time to see if it is well tolerated. The consistency of applesauce is again recommended. Puréed or mashed fish, poultry, cooked egg yolks (not the white), legumes and tofu provide added iron and protein to the diet, as well as other important minerals.

Fruit and Vegetable Sources of Vitamin C

Vitamin C, found in fruits and vegetables, assists in the absorption of iron in the intestines. Fruits and vegetables also provide carbohydrates, fiber and vitamin A, as well as many phytochemicals and minerals.

Fruits and vegetables can be offered as a first solid food. Their flavors may be slightly more appealing than meats and the different colors may be more interesting as your baby starts to explore the tastes of solids. There is no need to offer vegetables before fruits, although some people think that offering fruits before vegetables will result in their baby disliking the taste of vegetables. The opposite can also be true.

If you are preparing your own fruit and vegetables, choose the varieties that are freshest and in season. Mash or purée.

Food Intake

As breast milk is gradually replaced by solid foods, many mothers wonder if their babies are eating enough to remain healthy. Although it is easy for dietitians to say to a mother, "Let your child show you when he is full — just read his cues," it is comforting to have guidelines on how much their baby can be expected to eat as solids are introduced. Remember, every baby is different, and just because your baby eats more or less, it does not mean that you should force-feed more or offer less, especially if your child shows clearly that he wants more or less. Do watch for cues, such as interest in food or lack of interest. Try to feed when you and your baby are relaxed and not hurried, stressed or tired. Keep the television and radio off. Use this dedicated time for added communication and "talking."

Formula

Choosing a milk source other than breast milk after 6 months is not recommended, but for many women this is the only choice due to their lifestyle. A baby may appear to be

Solid Food Intake Guidelines (6 to 12 months)

The amount of solids taken in depends, in part, on the amount of breast milk or formula consumed by your baby. Babies will take varying amounts of food. As babies get older, the portion of total energy taken in from breast milk decreases as it is replaced by solid foods. Below is an example of how much babies may eat.

6 to 9 months (per day)

- Breastfeed on demand: 32 to 18 oz (960 to 540 mL). Higher amount for younger infants, lower amount for older infants.

- Iron-fortified infant cereal (mixed with breast milk): 4 to 8 tbsp (60 to 120 mL)

- Vegetables: 4 to 8 tbsp (60 to 120 mL)

- Fruit: 6 to 8 tbsp (90 to 120 mL)

- Meat, fish or chicken, mashed beans or tofu: 1 to 3 tbsp (15 to 45 mL)

9 to 12 months (per day)

- Breastfeeding on demand: 24 oz (720 mL) decreasing to 18 oz (540 mL). Higher amount for younger infants, lower amount for older infants.

- Cereal (mixed with breast milk), bread, rice or pasta: 8 to 10 tbsp (120 to 150 mL)

- Mashed, minced or diced vegetables: 4 to 10 tbsp (60 to 150 mL)

- Soft or sliced fresh or cooked fruit: 6 to 10 tbsp (90 to 150 mL)

- Mashed minced cooked meat, fish, chicken, tofu, beans, egg yolk: 3 to 4 tbsp (45 to 60 mL)

- Dairy products (cottage cheese, yogurt): 2 to 4 tbsp (30 to 60 mL)

The number and consistency of stools is an indication of how well your baby is digesting solid foods. Solid-food stools may become darker in color and develop a much stronger odor than regular breastfed stools.

What can I do to help prevent my child from becoming overweight or obese?

Approximately 20% to 30% of children in North America and Europe are overweight. Choosing to breastfeed has been shown by a number of studies to help prevent obesity in children. The exact mechanisms are unknown, but it may be that infants are less likely to overfeed while breastfeeding. The components of breast milk may also enable your child's body to learn how to metabolize nutrients appropriately.

Once an infant is old enough to be eating solid foods, recommendations include:

- Offering 2% milk at 2 to 3 years of age instead of whole milk, if weight gain and growth is good.
- Serving fresh cut-up fruits and vegetables as snacks at least 2 to 3 times daily.
- Limiting processed foods with high fat and sugar content.
- Encouraging your child to pay attention to her own satiety cues.
- Ensuring your child has a healthy level of activity daily.

more fussy with formula than with breast milk because formula may not be as easy to digest and may even cause some discomfort. Stools with formula feeding will become more brown in color and will also become more odorous.

Iron-fortified infant formula is recommended until 1 year of age, after which time regular cow's milk (whole) can be introduced. Try to stay with one type of formula so that your baby can adapt to the nutrient content.

Cow's Milk–Based Formula

Cow's milk–based formulas are recommended for infants when mothers choose not to breastfeed or to supplement or discontinue breastfeeding. The iron-fortified formulas are usually recommended to ensure that iron intake is adequate to prevent iron deficiency anemia. Cow's milk–based formulas contain all the nutrients that an infant needs to grow, but they are lacking all the protective factors that breast milk contains.

Cow's milk–based formulas are also available in lactose-free form, meaning that they do not contain the lactose sugar, but still have the cow's milk protein. Lactose-free formulas are sometimes used for infants who have or are recovering from a gastrointestinal illness. These formulas help to reduce stooling and allow diaper rash to heal more quickly, if present.

Soy-Based Formula

Soy formulas do not contain lactose or cow's milk protein. They may be used in the rare case when an infant has lactose intolerance to a cow's milk–based formula or when an infant seems colicky or irritable, in hope of relieving these symptoms. For vegetarian families, soy formulas are often the formula of choice once breastfeeding has been discontinued.

While soy infant formulas meet all of the standards of infant formulas, regular soy milk is not a suitable replacement because this milk is usually too low in energy, iron, calcium and many vitamins. Soy milks are also higher in proteins and minerals that may be harmful to an infant. Soy formulas are not recommended in the case of a cow's milk protein allergy because about 20% to 40% of infants who are allergic to cow's milk protein may be allergic to soy protein as well.

What can I do if my breastfed baby refuses to drink from a bottle or cup?

Babies who have only received breast milk straight from the breast may have a difficult time taking fluids from a bottle or cup when their mother is not available to breastfeed. Some babies increase their nighttime feeding when mothers are unavailable during the day to breastfeed — good for babies, but harder on mothers. Be sure to start this transition by placing expressed milk, not formula, in the bottle or cup so your baby will still smell a familiar food. Removing the stopper in a sippy cup may help to increase chances of an older infant taking milk from the cup. Sometimes spooning the liquid into your baby's mouth may be required until she realizes that the breast will not be offered.

Although this process of trial and error can be stressful, rest assured that your baby will get adequate fluid through solid foods (strained, puréed and mashed foods are about 85% to 90% water). Babies will eventually drink from a bottle and cup.

Specialized Formulas

Some formulas break down specific nutrients for infants with allergies or digestive problems. These are usually much more expensive than regular infant formulas, but are beneficial for infants who really need them. They are generally used in hospital settings or recommended for use at home by your family physician or pediatrician. If babies receive infant formula, they do not need vitamin D supplements beyond the vitamin D added to the formula.

Stooling Patterns with Formula

Stools usually become much firmer when breastfed infants are fed with formula. The stools may also be less frequent and harder, causing the baby to become constipated. While fat in breast milk is easily digested, in formulas it is not as easily digested. Undigested fat can result in harder stools. Infants who are weaned from breastfeeding earlier than 6 months may also experience more spitting up and vomiting with formula.

Homemade Foods

Life is pretty busy with a young baby in the house, even more so if there are siblings to care for. Nevertheless, it is surprisingly easy to find time to prepare homemade food for your baby — and most satisfying as well.

While cooking vegetables for the family, simply add more in the pot and set some aside for preparation for the baby. Most vegetables and fruits require a small amount of water to be added to get to the right consistency of puréed or mashed food. Some cooked vegetables and cooked or fresh fruits can also be mashed to the right consistency. Homemade fruit and vegetable purée can be frozen and stored for about 2 months.

Meat can also be prepared quite easily. Again, choose fresh products and cook thoroughly, adding water or vegetable water (from cooking vegetables) to create the right texture.

Be sure to select fresh produce free from bruises and damage. Bacteria can grow in bruised fruit or vegetables. Practice safe food handling by cleaning the fruits and vegetables well, and make sure the utensils and food preparation surface are clean as well. Keep cutting boards for fruits and vegetables separate from those for meat and poultry.

Introducing Texture

The introduction of more texture in the diet, going from puréed or mashed foods to diced and chopped foods, occurs between about 7 and 12 months or more of age. However, some parents are hesitant to introduce textured foods because they fear their baby may choke. Some wait until they see a few teeth, while others start foods before any appearance of teeth.

Often textures are started when an infant has sampled some table food that a parent is eating, such as a soft cooked green bean, piece of toast or pasta noodle. If there are no signs of choking, and the infant demonstrates by reaching out that he wants more, then he may be ready for textured food.

✳ Textured Foods

- Soft ripe bananas, pears or peaches, without the skin, cut into small ¼- to ½-inch (0.5 to 1 cm) pieces
- Cooked green and wax beans (these are great finger foods)
- Cooked carrots, sliced lengthwise
- Beef or chicken meatballs
- Firm tofu, sliced in ¼- to ½-inch pieces (0.5 to 1 cm)
- Cooked pasta, cut into smaller, shorter lengths of about 1 inch (2.5 cm)

Early Dental Care

Introducing solid food at 6 months of age and the appearance of your baby's first teeth often coincide. A baby's first tooth can come in anywhere from 3 months to 14 months, but it usually occurs around 6 to 8 months of age. The front bottom teeth usually come in first, followed by the front top teeth. Once that first tooth comes in, start cleaning right away. Simply wipe the tooth daily with a clean cloth or use a soft baby toothbrush. Do not use toothpaste. Even though these are not the permanent teeth, first teeth should be taken care of so that the permanent teeth have a better chance of coming in and staying healthy.

✳ Tips for Preventing Choking

- Parents and caregivers should take a first-aid course delivered by an experienced professional so they are prepared to deal with choking.
- Child should be sitting when eating.
- Child should show readiness to try new textures.
- Always supervise young children when eating.
- Foods should be cut up to appropriate size and shape.
- Do not feed the following foods to children less than 2 years of age:
  - Hard candies, chewing gum, lollipops
  - Peanuts and other nuts
  - Whole carrots
  - Fish with bones
  - Whole raisins
  - Hot dogs
  - Snacks with toothpicks
  - Popcorn
- If choking sounds are heard, the child can be left to cough and spit out the food or you can hold the infant upside down and let gravity help out.
- If you do not hear any choking sounds and your baby is turning red or blue, more aggressive measures must be taken, based on first-aid training.

Breastfeeding likely offers protection of the oral cavity, probably because of its array of protective factors against disease. Nevertheless, residual milk, especially from nighttime feedings, can feed the bacteria that cause damage to tooth enamel. Once those first teeth start to come in, do not let your baby fall asleep without cleaning his tooth or teeth. Otherwise, bacteria normally found in the mouth will use the sugar left from milk or formula to produce an acid that can cause harm to the first teeth.

Fluoride

Fluoride is a mineral necessary to make the outer layer of teeth strong. Tooth decay can occur if not enough fluoride is taken in, which may happen if the main or only source of water is bottled or filtered water that contains little or no fluoride.

The American Dental Association does not recommend the use of fluoride-containing toothpaste until 2 years of age. For younger children, only a smear is recommended by the Canadian Dental Association. Do not use toothpaste for infants. When children are older and can spit out the toothpaste, a pea-sized amount is recommended. Check with your dentist to see when to start using a fluoride-containing toothpaste for your child.

Brushing and Flossing

Parents should brush their children's teeth until about 3 years of age, and then, with supervision, children should be able to start brushing on their own. Toothbrushes should be changed every 2 to 4 months for children.

There is no need to floss your child's teeth until about 4 years of age, when teeth grow close enough together to trap food, but some children may require flossing earlier. Check with your dentist on when to start flossing.

Teething Pain

Sometimes babies experience significant discomfort when they are teething. Stools may become looser during these periods, possibly due to effects on the nervous system, which plays a role in the bowel habits of children. Babies may be hard to comfort.

✳ How to Soothe Painful Teeth

1. Breastfeed more often.

2. Offer a cool soothing ring. These rings can be purchased at your local drugstore.

3. Use a finger brush. Slip this little brush over your finger and massage the gums. These brushes are available at your dentist's office or in drugstores.

4. Consult your health-care providers about what they recommend for pain from teething.

Did You Know ...

Fluorosis

Excessive fluoride intake can cause fluorosis, resulting in harmless white specks on teeth or tooth discoloration. Should this occur, see a dentist to discuss methods of avoiding excess fluoride intake.

Did You Know ...

First Dental Appointment

Both the American and the Canadian Dental Associations recommend that a dental appointment is required within 6 months of the first eruption of a tooth so that measures for preventing early childhood caries can be reviewed.

Weaning Your Baby

Weaning can occur at any time after the breast has been stimulated by feeding or pumping to establish a milk supply. For many mothers, this will occur naturally when the baby has developed skill in eating and drinking with spoons and cups. For some mothers, the weaning process may be upsetting as they grieve the loss of this special bond with their baby.

Weaning can proceed unplanned over several months or can be planned to coincide with the mother's circumstances, such as returning to work. Even in this case, breastfeeding does not need to end abruptly. Some mothers want to keep the best of both worlds and plan a partial wean, continuing to breastfeed mornings, nights and weekends, with a caregiver providing other feedings using an alternative method at other times. If for some reason the mother can no longer breastfeed, abrupt weaning may be necessary.

✱ How to Wean Your Child

Weaning is often a trial-and-error process where the wishes of the mother don't always agree with the baby's desires and vice versa. Training the baby to follow the new feeding routine may take a few days to a few weeks, and may cause some frustration for both mother and baby along the way. Persevere.

1. Separate yourself from your baby at feeding times. If your baby has always been breastfed, she will not likely take any other type of feeding if she can see you, smell you or hear your voice. Your baby will not be happy that her mother is not around for feeding time. Go somewhere where you can't hear your baby cry for you.

2. Start with expressed breast milk in the bottle or cup. The transition to a new feeding device by an alternative caregiver is often easier if the fluid is breast milk because the taste is not strange.

3. Try offering diluted fruit juices. Although even diluted fruit juices are rarely recommended for infants and young children, when you are trying to transition your baby to an alternative feeding method, it may work to offer a new taste. Your baby may enjoy this novelty and won't confuse the diluted juice with breast milk, as she may with cow's milk– or soy-based formula.

4. Rest assured that your baby will not starve. Although your baby may go on strike for a few feedings and express her dismay with lots of crying, she will eventually begin to take other milk or formula from a bottle or cup, regardless of how fast this transition needs to happen. Your baby will soon return to her happy self at feeding times.

PART 2

Better Recipes for Breastfeeding

Nutritional Analysis

The nutrient analyses for the recipes were prepared using Vision Software Technologies Inc., version 5.2, and The Food Processor SQL, version 9.9 (adapted for Canadian foods), ESHA Research, Salem, Oregon. The nutrient databases used are the Canadian Nutrient File 2001b (from Health Canada) and the USDA National Nutrient Database for Standard Reference. This also includes the evaluation of recipe servings as sources of nutrients.

The nutrient analyses were based on:

- imperial measures and weights (except for food typically packaged and used in metric);
- the larger number of servings where there is a range;
- the smaller amount where there is a range;
- the first ingredient listed where there is a choice;
- the exclusion of "optional" ingredients; and
- the exclusion of ingredients with non-specified or "to taste" amounts.

The analyses were done on the regular recipes, not "make-ahead" versions, which might vary slightly in the ingredients used.

The evaluation of recipe servings as sources of nutrients combine U.S. and Canadian regulations. Bearing in mind that the two countries have different reporting standards, the highest standard was always used. As a result, some recipes that would have been identified as an excellent source of a particular nutrient in one country may be listed only as a source or a good source because the standard is higher in the other country.

Breakfasts, Breads and Muffins

**MAKES
2 SERVINGS**

Rushing out in the morning? Divide into 2 sealable containers and leave room to add some banana.

TIP

For variety, try serving this muesli with different types of yogurt and fresh fruit in season. You can omit the honey or reduce the amount you use.

Breakfast Muesli to Go

1 cup	large-flake or quick-cooking oats (not instant)	250 mL
1 cup	low-fat plain yogurt	250 mL
½ cup	2% milk	125 mL
2 tbsp	liquid honey or maple syrup	25 mL
1 cup	assorted berries (fresh or frozen)	250 mL
1	large banana, sliced	1

1. In a plastic container, combine oats, yogurt, milk and honey; gently fold in berries. Add banana before serving or add to sealable container before taking muesli on the go.

NUTRITIONAL ANALYSIS PER SERVING

Energy: 432 kcal	Carbohydrate: 80 g	Calcium: 312 mg	Folate: 21 mcg
Protein: 15 g	Fat: 6 g	Iron: 3.1 mg	Fiber: 8.3 mg

**MAKES
6 SERVINGS**

Here's a lower-fat, higher-fiber version of an old favorite.

TIP

Both the whites and the yolks of eggs provide such valuable nutrients as vitamin A, magnesium, iron and riboflavin, in addition to protein.

French Toast

4	egg whites	4
2 tbsp	skim milk	25 mL
½ tsp	vanilla	2 mL
Pinch	ground nutmeg or cinnamon	Pinch
6	slices whole-wheat bread	6

1. Beat together egg whites, milk, vanilla and nutmeg until frothy. Pour into large flat dish; dip both sides of bread slices into mixture.

2. In a large nonstick or lightly buttered skillet, cook bread over medium heat until brown on one side. Flip and cook other side. Serve immediately.

NUTRITIONAL ANALYSIS PER SERVING

Energy: 75 kcal	Carbohydrate: 12 g	Calcium: 33 mg	Folate: 12 mcg
Protein: 5 g	Fat: 1 g	Iron: 0.8 mg	Fiber: 2.3 g

Individual Salsa Fresca Omelets

Excellent source of:
- Folate

Good source of:
- Iron

Source of:
- Calcium and fiber

Salsa Fresca

1 cup	diced seeded tomatoes	250 mL
1 cup	diced cucumber	250 mL
⅓ cup	chopped red onions	75 mL
¼ cup	chopped fresh cilantro or parsley	50 mL
2 tbsp	lime juice	25 mL
	Salt and freshly ground black pepper to taste	

Omelettes

4	eggs	4
1 tbsp	water	15 mL
	Salt and freshly ground black pepper to taste	
1 tsp	butter or vegetable oil	5 mL

**MAKES
2 SERVINGS**

This is an easy meal for older children or teens to prepare for themselves and the family. The ingredients can easily be doubled to serve 4.

1. *Salsa Fresca:* In a bowl, combine tomatoes, cucumber, red onions, cilantro, lime juice, salt and pepper. Let stand for 10 minutes. Drain well.

2. *Omelets:* In a bowl, beat together eggs, water, salt and pepper. In a small (8-inch/20 cm) nonstick skillet over medium-high heat, melt ½ tsp (2 mL) of the butter. Making 1 omelet at a time, pour half of the egg mixture into pan. As eggs begin to set at edges, use a spatula to gently push cooked portions to the center, tilting pan to allow uncooked egg to flow into empty spaces.

3. When eggs are almost set on the surface but still look moist, fill half the omelet with some of the Salsa Fresca. Slip spatula under unfilled side, fold over filling and slide omelet onto plate. Top with additional Salsa Fresca. Repeat with remaining butter, egg mixture and Salsa Fresca.

Variation

Dress up your omelet with chopped ham and green onions, shredded cheese or diced leftover cooked potatoes.

TIPS

If you don't have time to make the salsa, use a commercially prepared salsa instead. Use about ½ cup (125 mL) salsa per omelette.

The extra 1 cup (250 mL) Salsa Fresca in this recipe can be used as a dip for baked tortilla chips.

NUTRITIONAL ANALYSIS PER SERVING			
Energy: 214 kcal	Carbohydrate: 10 g	Calcium: 87 mg	Folate: 99 mcg
Protein: 14 g	Fat: 13 g	Iron: 3.2 mg	Fiber: 2.1 g

**MAKES
4 SERVINGS**

This is a wonderful meal to make ahead for a special breakfast or brunch.

TIPS

This recipe is a great way to use up stale bread, which actually works better than fresh in this recipe; it absorbs more of the egg and milk mixture, which makes the strata taste creamier.

Frozen broccoli can easily be used in place of fresh broccoli. Place frozen broccoli in a microwave-safe bowl, cover and microwave on High for 2 minutes. Drain, pat dry and proceed with recipe.

All food groups are featured in this delicious dish. To boot, the quantities of milk and cheese make it an excellent source of calcium. It is also an excellent source of B vitamins, and vitamins A and C as well as folic acid. When serving this dish, make the remainder of the day's meals lighter, as it is higher in fat.

Overnight Broccoli and Cheese Strata

• Preheat oven to 350°F (180°C)
• 9-inch (2.5 L) casserole, greased

2 cups	chopped fresh broccoli or asparagus	500 mL
4 cups	cubed whole wheat bread (preferably stale)	1 L
2 cups	shredded Swiss or Cheddar cheese	500 mL
4	eggs	4
2 cups	milk	500 mL
½ to 1 tsp	dry mustard	2 to 5 mL
	Cayenne pepper to taste (optional)	

1. In a pot of boiling water, cook broccoli just until tender-crisp; drain and pat dry. Set aside.

2. Place bread cubes in casserole dish. Add cheese and broccoli; gently toss together.

3. In a bowl, beat together eggs, milk, mustard and, if using, cayenne; pour evenly over bread mixture. Cover and refrigerate for 2 hours or overnight.

4. Bake in preheated oven for 50 to 60 minutes or until golden brown and just set in center. Let stand for 3 to 4 minutes before serving.

NUTRITIONAL ANALYSIS PER SERVING

Energy: 425 kcal	Carbohydrate: 22 g	Calcium: 622 mg	Folate: 78 mcg
Protein: 28 g	Fat: 26 g	Iron: 2.6 mg	Fiber: 2.9 mg

Zucchini Frittata

- Preheat broiler

2 cups	sliced zucchini	500 mL
1	small onion, minced	1
1 tbsp	butter or margarine	15 mL
1½ tsp	olive oil	7 mL
6	eggs, beaten	6
1 tbsp	chopped fresh parsley	15 mL
1 tsp	ground fennel (see Tip, at right)	5 mL
½ tsp	ground dried rosemary	2 mL
½ tsp	salt	2 mL
¼ tsp	freshly ground black pepper	1 mL
2 tbsp	shredded Cheddar cheese	25 mL

1. In a large ovenproof skillet over medium-high heat, cook zucchini and onion in butter and olive oil for about 5 minutes or until tender.

2. In a bowl, combine eggs, parsley, fennel, rosemary, salt and pepper; pour over vegetables. Cook over medium heat, without stirring, until bottom of mixture has set but top is still soft. Sprinkle cheese on top. Place under preheated broiler for about 3 minutes or until cheese is melted and top is brown.

Good source of:
- Folate

Source of:
- Calcium and iron

MAKES 6 SERVINGS

Zucchini is a sweet summer squash, North American in origin, that has been warmly embraced in Italian cooking. Make this Italian-style omelet when zucchini is in season or vary the recipe using other vegetables — mushrooms, red or green bell peppers and broccoli would also work well.

TIPS

If the handle of your skillet is not ovenproof, wrap it in aluminum foil for protection.

If you don't have ground fennel in your cupboard, use a generous teaspoon (5 mL) of fennel seeds in this recipe. Toast them over medium heat in a dry pan until they release their aroma, then crush finely before adding to the eggs. The flavor will be even better than if you had used the ground spice.

NUTRITIONAL ANALYSIS PER SERVING

Energy: 125 kcal	Carbohydrate: 3 g	Calcium: 59 mg	Folate: 47 mcg
Protein: 7 g	Fat: 9 g	Iron: 1.4 mg	Fiber: 0.6 g

**MAKES
2 SERVINGS**

So quick and easy to prepare, this dish can be enjoyed at breakfast, lunch or supper. The dill adds freshness and appeal.

Delicious Crab Frittata

4	eggs	4
2 tbsp	mayonnaise	25 mL
Dash	hot pepper sauce	Dash
1	can (4 oz/120 g) crabmeat, drained	1
1	green onion, chopped	1
1 tbsp	chopped fresh dill	15 mL
½ cup	shredded Cheddar cheese	125 mL
1 tbsp	butter	15 mL

1. In a bowl, whisk together eggs, mayonnaise and hot sauce. Whisk in crabmeat, green onion, dill and cheese.

2. In a large skillet, melt butter over medium heat. Pour in egg mixture and cook, using a spatula to pull uncooked egg away from the sides into the middle, until set, about 5 minutes.

NUTRITIONAL ANALYSIS PER SERVING

Energy: 237 kcal	Carbohydrate: 1 g	Calcium: 173 mg	Folate: 36 mcg
Protein: 11 g	Fat: 21 g	Iron: 1.2 mg	Fiber: Trace

Three-Grain Bread

- Preheat oven to 350°F (180°C)
- Two 9- by 5-inch (2 L) loaf pans, greased

½ cup	butter or margarine, softened	125 mL
½ cup	packed brown sugar	125 mL
2	large eggs	2
2 cups	whole wheat flour	500 mL
2 cups	all-purpose flour	500 mL
1 cup	dark rye flour	250 mL
1 cup	quick-cooking rolled oats	250 mL
2 tsp	baking soda	10 mL
1 tsp	salt	5 mL
2½ cups	buttermilk	625 mL

MAKES 2 LOAVES

Think bread making is too time-consuming? Try this easy-to-make bread. It's hearty and ideal for serving with lunch, dinner or as a snack.

TIP

If out of buttermilk, substitute 2 cups (500 mL) 2% milk mixed with 2 tbsp (25 mL) lemon juice or vinegar.

1. In a large bowl, cream butter and brown sugar until light; beat in eggs. Combine whole wheat, all-purpose and dark rye flours, oats, baking soda and salt. Add to creamed mixture alternately with buttermilk, making 3 additions of dry ingredients and 2 of buttermilk. Divide between prepared pans.

2. Bake in preheated oven for 55 to 60 minutes or until wooden skewer inserted in center comes out clean. Cool in pans for 10 minutes, then remove from pans and cool on rack. Store in airtight container.

NUTRITIONAL ANALYSIS PER SERVING (1 OF 24 SLICES)

Energy: 178 kcal	Carbohydrate: 28 g	Calcium: 51 mg	Folate: 15 mcg
Protein: 5 g	Fat: 5 g	Iron: 1.4 mg	Fiber: 1.9 g

MAKES 1 LOAF

This tasty and nutritious quick bread freezes well. Keep some in the freezer for unexpected guests.

TIP

Freeze this and other quick breads in individually wrapped single slices. Pop them into lunch bags. They will be defrosted by the time lunch comes around.

Apricot Bran Bread

- Preheat oven to 350°F (180°C)
- 8- by 4-inch (1.5 L) loaf pan, nonstick or lightly greased

2 cups	bran cereal flakes	500 mL
½ cup	all-purpose flour	125 mL
½ cup	whole wheat flour	125 mL
½ cup	packed brown sugar	125 mL
2 tsp	baking powder	10 mL
½ tsp	salt	2 mL
½ tsp	ground nutmeg	2 mL
¾ cup	chopped dried apricots	175 mL
1 tsp	grated orange zest	5 mL
1	egg, lightly beaten	1
½ cup	skim milk	125 mL
½ cup	orange juice	125 mL
¼ cup	vegetable oil	50 mL

1. Crush cereal to make ¾ cup (175 mL) crumbs. In a large bowl, combine cereal, flours, sugar, baking powder, salt, nutmeg, apricots and orange zest.

2. In a second bowl, beat together egg, milk, orange juice and oil; stir into dry ingredients until well combined. Pour into nonstick or prepared pan. Bake in preheated oven for about 55 minutes or until tester inserted in center comes out clean. Cool for 10 minutes before removing from pan. Cool completely on wire rack.

NUTRITIONAL ANALYSIS PER SERVING (1 OF 14 SLICES)

Energy: 148 kcal	Carbohydrate: 27 g	Calcium: 36 mg	Folate: 15 mcg
Protein: 3 g	Fat: 4 g	Iron: 2.0 mg	Fiber: 0.9 g

Banana Nut Bread

- Preheat oven to 325°F (160°C)
- 9-by 5-inch (2 L) loaf pan, greased

1¾ cups	all-purpose flour	425 mL
1 tsp	baking soda	5 mL
½ tsp	salt	2 mL
2	eggs	2
1 cup	mashed ripe bananas (about 3 ripe)	250 mL
⅓ cup	vegetable oil	75 mL
½ cup	liquid honey	125 mL
⅓ cup	packed brown sugar	75 mL
½ cup	chopped walnuts	125 mL

1. In a bowl, sift together flour, baking soda and salt.
2. In another bowl, beat eggs. Stir in bananas, oil, honey and brown sugar.
3. Stir dry ingredients into banana mixture until combined. Fold in walnuts.
4. Pour batter into prepared loaf pan. Bake in preheated oven for 1¼ hours or until cake tester inserted in center comes out clean. Let pan cool on rack for 15 minutes. Run knife around edge; turn out loaf and let cool on rack.

Good source of:
- Folate

Source of:
- Iron

MAKES 1 LOAF

Everyone has a recipe for banana bread in their files. I've included my best. It's a simple bread that just relies on the flavor of banana and walnuts.

TIPS

Lining the bottom of baking pan with waxed or parchment paper ensures you'll never have trouble removing the bread from the pan.

Left with ripe bananas on your counter but have no time to bake a bread? Simply freeze whole bananas with the peel, then leave at room temperature to defrost. Or peel and mash bananas; pack into containers and freeze for up to 2 months. Defrost at room temperature. Frozen banana purée may darken slightly but will not affect the delicious baked results.

NUTRITIONAL ANALYSIS PER SERVING (1 OF 12 SLICES)

Energy: 247 kcal	Carbohydrate: 38 g	Calcium: 17 mg	Folate: 46 mcg
Protein: 4 g	Fat: 9 g	Iron: 1.3 mg	Fiber: 1.2 mg

MAKES 1 LOAF

Here's a lemony-flavored loaf that stays moist for days — if it lasts that long.

TIP

I like to double this recipe so that I have an extra loaf handy in the freezer. Wrap in plastic wrap, then in foil and freeze for up to 1 month.

Lemon Yogurt Loaf

- Preheat oven to 350°F (180°C)
- 9-by 5-inch (2 L) loaf pan, greased

1¾ cups	all-purpose flour	425 mL
1 tsp	baking powder	5 mL
½ tsp	baking soda	2 mL
¼ tsp	salt	1 mL
2	eggs	2
¾ cup	granulated sugar	175 mL
¾ cup	plain yogurt	175 mL
⅓ cup	vegetable oil	75 mL
1 tbsp	grated lemon zest	15 mL

Topping

⅓ cup	fresh lemon juice	75 mL
⅓ cup	granulated sugar	75 mL

1. In a bowl, combine flour, baking powder, baking soda and salt. In another large bowl, beat eggs. Stir in sugar, yogurt, oil and lemon zest. Fold in flour mixture to make a smooth batter.

2. Spoon into prepared pan; bake in preheated oven for 50 to 60 minutes or until cake tester inserted in center comes out clean. Place pan on rack.

3. *Topping:* In a small saucepan, heat lemon juice and sugar; bring to a boil. Cook, stirring, until sugar is dissolved. (Alternatively, place in a glass bowl and microwave at High for 1 minute, stirring once.) Pour over hot loaf in pan; let cool completely before turning out of pan.

Variation

Lemon Poppy Seed Loaf: Stir 2 tbsp (25 mL) poppy seeds into flour mixture before combining with yogurt mixture.

NUTRITIONAL ANALYSIS PER SERVING (1 OF 12 SLICES)

Energy: 203 kcal	Carbohydrate: 33 g	Calcium: 18 mg	Folate: 38 mcg
Protein: 3 g	Fat: 7 g	Iron: 1.0 mg	Fiber: 0.6 mg

Orange Apricot Oatmeal Scones

- Preheat oven to 375°F (190°C)
- Baking sheet, greased

2 cups	all-purpose flour	500 mL
1 1/2 cups	quick-cooking rolled oats	375 mL
1/4 cup	granulated sugar	50 mL
1 tbsp	baking powder	15 mL
2 tsp	grated orange zest	10 mL
1/2 tsp	baking soda	2 mL
1/4 tsp	salt	1 mL
6 tbsp	butter	90 mL
1/2 cup	chopped dried apricots	125 mL
1 cup	buttermilk or sour milk (see Tip, at right)	250 mL
	Milk	

1. In a bowl, combine flour, oats, all but 1 tsp (5 mL) of the sugar, baking powder, orange zest, baking soda and salt. Using a fork or pastry blender, cut in butter until mixture resembles coarse crumbs. Stir in apricots. Add buttermilk; stir until mixture is just combined.

2. On a lightly floured surface, knead dough gently 4 or 5 times. Divide into 3 pieces. Shape each piece into a round about 1 inch (2.5 cm) thick. Transfer to baking sheet.

3. Cut each round into quarters. Brush tops with milk; sprinkle with reserved sugar. Bake in preheated oven for 20 to 25 minutes or until lightly browned.

Variation

For a change, substitute 1/2 cup (125 mL) dates, raisins, currants or dried cranberries for the apricots.

Source of:
- Iron and fiber

MAKES 12 SERVINGS

These tasty scones are delicious with a relaxing cup of tea. The oats and apricots add fiber to the recipe.

TIP

Sour milk can be used instead of buttermilk. To prepare, combine 2 tsp (10 mL) lemon juice or vinegar with 1 cup (250 mL) milk and let stand for 5 minutes.

NUTRITIONAL ANALYSIS PER SERVING (1 SCONE)

Energy: 209 kcal	Carbohydrate: 32 g	Calcium: 48 mg	Folate: 10 mcg
Protein: 5 g	Fat: 7 g	Iron: 1.5 mg	Fiber: 2.5 g

Bran Flaxseed Muffins

MAKES 15 MUFFINS

These muffins are packed with healthy energy, for a great start to the day. The fiber provided by these muffins will help women who suffer from hemorrhoids or who had stitches after delivery.

- Preheat oven to 350°F (180°C)
- Two 12-cup muffin tins, greased or paper-lined

1½ cups	unbleached all-purpose flour	375 mL
1 cup	packed brown sugar	250 mL
¾ cup	ground flaxseeds	175 mL
¾ cup	oat bran	175 mL
2 tsp	ground cinnamon	10 mL
1 tsp	baking soda	5 mL
½ tsp	baking powder	2 mL
½ tsp	salt	2 mL
2	eggs, beaten	2
¾ cup	milk	175 mL
1 tsp	vanilla	5 mL
2	apples, peeled and shredded	2
1½ cups	shredded carrots	375 mL

1. In a large bowl, combine, flour, brown sugar, flaxseeds, oat bran, cinnamon, baking soda, baking powder and salt.

2. In a small bowl, combine eggs, milk and vanilla. Stir into dry ingredients just until moistened. Stir in apples and carrots. Fill 15 of the muffin cups three-quarters full, filling the empty cups with water.

3. Bake in preheated oven for 15 to 20 minutes, or until muffins pull away from the sides of the pan. Serve warm.

NUTRITIONAL ANALYSIS PER SERVING (1 MUFFIN)

Energy: 174 kcal	Carbohydrate: 31 g	Calcium: 58 mg	Folate: 16 mcg
Protein: 5 g	Fat: 4 g	Iron: 1.9 mg	Fiber: 3.3 g

Carrot Bran Muffins

- Preheat oven to 400°F (200°C)
- 12-cup muffin tin, greased or paper-lined

1¼ cups	whole wheat flour	300 mL
1¼ cups	high-fiber bran cereal	300 mL
1 tsp	baking powder	5 mL
1 tsp	baking soda	5 mL
1 tsp	ground cinnamon	5 mL
½ tsp	ground nutmeg	2 mL
½ tsp	salt	2 mL
2	eggs	2
1 cup	grated carrots	250 mL
¾ cup	buttermilk	175 mL
⅓ cup	packed brown sugar	75 mL
¼ cup	vegetable oil	50 mL
½ cup	raisins	125 mL

1. In a large bowl, combine flour, cereal, baking powder, baking soda, cinnamon, nutmeg and salt.

2. In a separate bowl, beat eggs thoroughly; blend in carrots, buttermilk, brown sugar and vegetable oil. Add to dry ingredients, stirring just until moistened. Stir in raisins.

3. Spoon batter into muffin cups, filling about three-quarters full. Bake in preheated oven for about 20 minutes or until tops of muffins spring back when lightly touched.

Good source of:
- Iron

Source of:
- Folate and fiber

MAKES 12 MUFFINS

Two favorites, carrot and bran, are combined in this tasty muffin. A great start to any day!

TIP

When making these muffins, keep wet and dry ingredients separate until you're ready to mix, then mix just enough to blend the two components. This produces a coarse crumb that is just fine for these muffins.

NUTRITIONAL ANALYSIS PER SERVING (1 MUFFIN)			
Energy: 164 kcal	Carbohydrate: 28 g	Calcium: 51 mg	Folate: 22 mcg
Protein: 5 g	Fat: 5 g	Iron: 2.2 mg	Fiber: 3.2 g

Cornmeal Muffins

MAKES 24 MUFFINS

Keep a supply of these muffins frozen in airtight containers until needed for breakfast, lunch or snacks. Defrost in the microwave for breakfast or pop into a lunch bag directly from the freezer; they'll defrost by the time lunch rolls around.

TIP

Sour milk can be used instead of buttermilk. To prepare, combine 3 tbsp (45 mL) lemon juice or vinegar with 4 cups (1 L) milk and let stand for 5 minutes.

• Preheat oven to 375°F (190°C)
• Two 12-cup muffin tins, greased or paper-lined

4 cups	all-purpose flour	1 L
2 cups	cornmeal	500 mL
¾ cup	granulated sugar	175 mL
2 tbsp	baking powder	25 mL
2 tsp	baking soda	10 mL
½ tsp	salt	2 mL
4 cups	buttermilk or sour milk (see Tip, at left)	1 L
½ cup	vegetable oil	125 mL
3	eggs	3

1. In a bowl, combine flour, cornmeal, all but 2 tsp (10 mL) of the sugar, baking powder, baking soda and salt.

2. In a separate bowl, whisk together buttermilk, oil and eggs. Add to dry ingredients; stir just until combined.

3. Spoon into muffin cups. Sprinkle with remaining sugar. Bake in preheated oven for 18 to 22 minutes or until firm to the touch.

NUTRITIONAL ANALYSIS PER SERVING (1 MUFFIN)			
Energy: 212 kcal	Carbohydrate: 33 g	Calcium: 66 mg	Folate: 13 mcg
Protein: 5 g	Fat: 6 g	Iron: 1.2 mg	Fiber: 0.7 g

Blueberry Cornmeal Muffins

Source of:
• Iron and folate

MAKES 12 MUFFINS

When it comes to celebrating the pleasures of summer fruits, nothing beats juicy blueberries. They are especially welcome when teamed with lemon in these deliciously moist muffins.

- Preheat oven to 400°F (200°C)
- 12-cup muffin pan, well-greased or paper-lined

1 1/2 cups	all-purpose flour	375 mL
1/3 cup	cornmeal	75 mL
1/2 cup	granulated sugar	125 mL
2 1/2 tsp	baking powder	12 mL
1/4 tsp	salt	1 mL
1	egg	1
3/4 cup	milk	175 mL
1/4 cup	butter, melted	50 mL
1 tsp	grated lemon zest	5 mL
1 cup	fresh or frozen blueberries	250 mL

1. In a bowl, stir together flour, cornmeal, sugar, baking powder and salt.

2. In another bowl, beat egg. Stir in milk, melted butter and lemon zest. Combine with dry ingredients until just mixed. Gently fold in blueberries.

3. Spoon into prepared muffin cups so they are three-quarters full.

4. Bake in preheated oven for 20 to 24 minutes or until top is firm to the touch and lightly browned. Remove from pans and let muffins cool on rack.

TIP

To minimize the problem of frozen blueberries tinting the batter blue, place berries in a sieve and quickly rinse under cold water to get rid of any ice crystals. Blot dry with paper towels. Place berries in a bowl and toss with 2 tbsp (25 mL) of the muffin flour mixture. Use immediately; fold into batter with a few quick strokes.

NUTRITIONAL ANALYSIS PER SERVING

Energy: 148 kcal	Carbohydrate: 25 g	Calcium: 31 mg	Folate: 38 mcg
Protein: 3 g	Fat: 5 g	Iron: 1.0 mg	Fiber: 1.1 mg

**MAKES
20 MUFFINS**

These muffins, which are so moist you won't need to add butter, are chock-full of fruit. They are best eaten warm from the oven. If you must store them, do so in the freezer and thaw as needed.

TIPS

Since these muffins freeze well, they are particularly convenient for brown baggers. Pop a frozen muffin into a lunch bag. By the time lunch rolls around, it will be defrosted and ready to eat.

The wheat germ in these muffins, although high in fat, provides vitamin E, an antioxidant, which promotes health. Wheat germ, once opened, should be stored in the refrigerator because of its high fat content.

Fruit and Oatmeal Muffins

- Preheat oven to 400°F (200°C)
- Two 12-cup muffin tins, greased or paper-lined

2½ cups	all-purpose flour	625 mL
1½ cups	quick-cooking rolled oats	375 mL
1 cup	wheat germ	250 mL
¾ cup	granulated sugar	175 mL
2 tbsp	baking powder	25 mL
½ tsp	salt	2 mL
1 cup	raisins	250 mL
1	medium apple (unpeeled), chopped	1
⅓ cup	shelled sunflower seeds	75 mL
2	eggs	2
1 cup	mashed ripe bananas	250 mL
¾ cup	skim milk	175 mL
2 tbsp	grated orange zest	25 mL
½ cup	orange juice	125 mL
⅓ cup	vegetable oil	75 mL

1. In a large bowl, combine flour, oats, wheat germ, sugar, baking powder and salt; stir in raisins, apple and sunflower seeds.

2. In another bowl, whisk eggs lightly; blend in bananas, milk, orange zest and juice, and oil. Pour into dry ingredients, stirring just until moistened.

3. Spoon about ⅓ cup (75 mL) batter into each greased or paper-lined muffin cup. Bake in preheated oven for about 20 minutes or until firm to the touch. Cool in pans for 5 minutes. Remove from tins and cool on rack. Store in airtight container in freezer.

NUTRITIONAL ANALYSIS PER SERVING (1 MUFFIN)

Energy: 228 kcal	Carbohydrate: 38 g	Calcium: 47 mg	Folate: 32 mcg
Protein: 6 g	Fat: 7 g	Iron: 2.2 mg	Fiber: 2.2 g

Appetizers and Dips

**MAKES
6 SERVINGS**

This easy snack or appetizer is fast to assemble and is great when fresh tomatoes and herbs are in season. We used cherry or grape tomatoes because they taste great year-round.

TIP

You can use larger tomatoes, if desired. Three medium tomatoes or 5 Roma (plum) tomatoes will make about the same amount of chopped.

Easy Tomato Basil Bruschetta

- Preheat broiler
- Baking sheet

6	slices light rye bread	6
2 tbsp	extra-virgin olive oil, divided	25 mL
18	cherry or grape tomatoes, coarsely chopped	18
5	leaves fresh basil, chopped	5
2	large roasted red bell peppers, drained and coarsely chopped	2
1	clove garlic, minced	1
2 tbsp	freshly grated Parmesan cheese	25 mL
2 tsp	hot pepper sauce (optional)	10 mL
1 tsp	freshly ground black pepper	5 mL
1/2 tsp	salt	2 mL
1/4 cup	feta cheese (optional)	50 mL

1. Arrange bread on baking sheet. Brush lightly with 1 tbsp (15 mL) of the olive oil. Toast under preheated broiler for 3 minutes or until light brown.

2. In a medium bowl, toss cherry tomatoes, basil, red peppers, garlic, Parmesan, the remaining olive oil, hot pepper sauce (if using), pepper and salt. Distribute evenly on top of bread. Sprinkle with feta cheese, if using.

3. Broil until heated through, about 5 minutes. Cut each slice of bread in half diagonally.

NUTRITIONAL ANALYSIS PER SERVING			
Energy: 175 kcal	Carbohydrate: 22 g	Calcium: 92 mg	Folate: 50 mcg
Protein: 5 g	Fat: 8 g	Iron: 1.5 mg	Fiber: 3.4 mg

Bruschetta with Basil and Oregano

MAKES 4 TO 6 SERVINGS OR 12 SLICES

- Preheat broiler
- Baking sheet

2	small tomatoes, diced	2
2 tbsp	olive oil	25 mL
1 tsp	crushed garlic	5 mL
2 tbsp	chopped fresh basil (or 1 tsp/5 mL dried)	25 mL
1 tbsp	chopped fresh oregano (or 1/2 tsp/2 mL dried)	15 mL
1 tbsp	chopped green onion	15 mL
12	slices (1/2 inch/1 cm thick) French bread	12
1 tbsp	freshly grated Parmesan cheese	15 mL

1. In small bowl, combine tomatoes, oil, garlic, basil, oregano and onion. Let stand for at least 20 minutes.

2. Toast bread on baking sheet under broiler, turning once, until brown on both sides. Divide tomato mixture over bread; sprinkle with cheese. Broil for 2 minutes or until heated through.

Variation

Vary the bruschetta by adding 3 tbsp (45 mL) finely diced yellow or red pepper or red onion to mixture. Or sprinkle 2 tbsp (25 mL) diced sun-dried tomatoes over slices just before broiling.

Make Ahead

Prepare tomato mixture early in day and marinate to allow flavors to blend well. Bake just before serving.

NUTRITIONAL ANALYSIS PER SERVING			
Energy: 132 kcal	Carbohydrate: 19 g	Calcium: 29 mg	Folate: 14 mcg
Protein: 3 g	Fat: 5 g	Iron: 0.9 mg	Fiber: 0.9 g

MAKES 4 TO 6 SERVINGS OR 24 HORS D'OEUVRES

TIPS

Substitute fresh coriander for the parsley for a change.

This recipe can also be made with fresh clams.

Serve as a salad over lettuce.

Make Ahead

Prepare and refrigerate mixture early in day to allow flavors to blend. Spoon into shells a couple of hours prior to serving and keep chilled.

Fresh Mussels with Tomato Salsa

24	mussels	24
½ cup	water or wine	125 mL
¾ cup	finely chopped onions, divided	175 mL
1½ tsp	crushed garlic, divided	7 mL
1 cup	coarsely chopped tomato	250 mL
4 tsp	chopped fresh basil (or ½ tsp/2 mL dried)	20 mL
2 tbsp	chopped fresh parsley	25 mL
2 tsp	olive oil	10 mL
¼ tsp	chili powder	1 mL
	Salt and pepper	

1. Scrub mussels under cold running water; remove any beards. Discard any mussels that do not close when tapped.

2. In saucepan, combine mussels, water, ¼ cup (50 mL) of the onions and 1 tsp (5 mL) of the garlic; cover and steam just until mussels open, approximately 5 minutes. Discard any that do not open. Let cool, then remove mussels from shells, reserving half of shell. Place mussels in bowl.

3. In food processor, combine remaining ½ cup (125 mL) onions and ½ tsp (2 mL) garlic, tomatoes, basil, parsley, oil, chili powder, and salt and pepper to taste; process using on/off motion just until chunky. Do not purée. Add to mussels and stir to mix. Refrigerate until chilled.

4. Divide mussel mixture evenly among reserved shells and arrange on serving plate.

NUTRITIONAL ANALYSIS PER SERVING			
Energy: 83 kcal	Carbohydrate: 6 g	Calcium: 30 mg	Folate: 36 mcg
Protein: 8 g	Fat: 3 g	Iron: 3.0 mg	Fiber: 1.0 g

Crab Celery Sticks

1	can (4.2 oz/120 g) crabmeat, well drained	1
¼ cup	sliced green onions	50 mL
¼ tsp	crushed garlic	1 mL
3 tbsp	chopped fresh dill (or 1 tsp/5 mL dried dillweed)	45 mL
1 tbsp	lemon juice	15 mL
¼ cup	chopped celery	50 mL
¼ cup	chopped sweet red or green pepper	50 mL
2 tbsp	2% yogurt	25 mL
¼ cup	light mayonnaise	50 mL
	Salt and pepper	
24	pieces (2 inch/5 cm) celery stalks	24
	Paprika	

1. In food processor, combine crabmeat, green onions, garlic, dill, lemon juice, chopped celery, red pepper, yogurt and mayonnaise. Using on/off motion, process just until combined but still chunky. Season with salt and pepper to taste.

2. Stuff each celery stalk evenly with mixture. Sprinkle with paprika to taste.

MAKES 4 TO 6 SERVINGS OR 24 HORS D'OEUVRES

TIPS

Serve as a dip with vegetables or broiled on top of pitas or English muffins.

For a less expensive version, use imitation crab, often called surimi.

Make Ahead

Make and refrigerate filling early in day. Stir well and pour off any excess liquid before filling celery.

NUTRITIONAL ANALYSIS PER SERVING

Energy: 49 kcal	Carbohydrate: 2 g	Calcium: 18 mg	Folate: 42 mcg
Protein: 4 g	Fat: 3 g	Iron: 0.4 mg	Fiber: 0.3 g

Double Salmon and Dill Pâté

MAKES
8 SERVINGS

TIPS

Leaving in the bones from the canned salmon increases the calcium content.

Leftover cooked salmon can also be used instead of canned.

Also tastes great as a spread on French bread or served with vegetables.

Make Ahead

Prepare up to a day ahead and keep refrigerated.

1 cup	5% ricotta cheese	250 mL
1	can (7½ oz/213 g) salmon, drained and skin removed	1
¼ cup	chopped green onions (about 2 medium)	50 mL
3 tbsp	chopped fresh dill (or 1 tsp/5 mL dried dillweed)	45 mL
2 tbsp	lemon juice	25 mL
4 oz	smoked salmon, cut into thin shreds	125 g

1. Place ricotta, canned salmon, green onions, dill and lemon juice in bowl of food processor; process for 20 seconds or until smooth.
2. Transfer mixture to serving bowl and fold in shredded smoked salmon. Serve with crackers.

NUTRITIONAL ANALYSIS PER SERVING

Energy: 96 kcal	Carbohydrate: 2 g	Calcium: 88 mg	Folate: 7 mcg
Protein: 13 g	Fat: 4 g	Iron: 0.5 mg	Fiber: 0.1 mg

Avocado Tomato Salsa

MAKES
8 SERVINGS

TIPS

Serve with crackers or tortilla crisps.

For an authentic, intense flavor, use ½ tsp (2 mL) finely diced chili pepper or more chili powder.

Make Ahead

Prepare up to 4 hours ahead; stir before serving.

2 cups	finely chopped plum tomatoes	500 mL
½ cup	finely chopped ripe but firm avocado (about ½ avocado)	125 mL
⅓ cup	chopped fresh coriander	75 mL
¼ cup	chopped green onions (about 2 medium)	50 mL
1 tbsp	olive oil	15 mL
1 tbsp	lime or lemon juice	15 mL
1 tsp	minced garlic	5 mL
⅛ tsp	chili powder	1 mL

1. In serving bowl, combine tomatoes, avocado, coriander, green onions, olive oil, lime juice, garlic and chili powder; let marinate 1 hour before serving.

NUTRITIONAL ANALYSIS PER SERVING

Energy: 46 kcal	Carbohydrate: 3 g	Calcium: 7 mg	Folate: 13 mcg
Protein: 1 g	Fat: 4 g	Iron: 0.4 mg	Fiber: 1.0 g

Lightened-Up Guacamole and Chips

• Preheat oven to 350°F (180°C)

2	ripe avocados, peeled and mashed	2
1	tomato, chopped (optional)	1
1	clove garlic, minced (or ½ tsp/2 mL garlic powder)	1
½ cup	fat-free plain yogurt	125 mL
⅓ cup	tomato salsa (mild, medium or hot)	75 mL
2 tbsp	chopped green onion (optional)	25 mL
2 tsp	freshly squeezed lemon juice	10 mL
1 tsp	ground cumin (or to taste)	5 mL
1 tsp	chili powder (or to taste)	5 mL
8 to 10	10-inch (25 cm) multigrain or whole wheat tortillas	8 to 10

1. In a large bowl, combine avocados, tomato (if using), garlic, yogurt, salsa, green onion (if using), lemon juice, cumin and chili powder.

2. In batches, place tortillas directly on the middle rack of preheated oven and toast, turning once, for 10 to 15 minutes or until golden brown and starting to crisp (check periodically to make sure they are not getting too brown). Let cool on a wire rack, then break into dipping-size pieces.

3. Serve guacamole in a dish, surrounded by toasted tortilla chips.

MAKES 10 SERVINGS

This recipe was an instant hit with the tasting panel for its great flavor, and it has less fat than commercial guacamole and chips. Kids love it.

TIPS

The tortilla chips will keep for up to 2 weeks in an airtight plastic bag at room temperature.

Use the baked tortillas as an inexpensive replacement for store-bought crispy flat breads.

NUTRITIONAL ANALYSIS PER SERVING

| Energy: 236 kcal | Carbohydrate: 49 g | Calcium: 46 mg | Folate: 46 mcg |
| Protein: 8 g | Fat: 7 g | Iron: 2.2 mg | Fiber: 6.6 mg |

**MAKES
8 SERVINGS**

*This combination is
great as a side dish or
over salad.*

TIP

You could also purée the
ingredients in a blender or
food processor and serve
as a dip.

Avocado and Chickpea Melody

1	large avocado, chopped	1
1	can (19 oz/540 mL) chickpeas	1
¼ cup	salsa	50 mL
	Juice of 1 lemon	

1. In a large bowl, combine avocado, chickpeas, salsa and lemon juice. Cover and refrigerate for at least 1 hour, until chilled, or for up to 3 days.

NUTRITIONAL ANALYSIS PER SERVING

Energy: 122 kcal	Carbohydrate: 17 g	Calcium: 26 mg	Folate: 61 mcg
Protein: 4 g	Fat: 5 g	Iron: 1.3 mg	Fiber: 3.1 mg

Good source of:
• Iron and folate

Source of:
• Calcium and fiber

**MAKES
6 TO 8 SERVINGS**

Tofu and Chickpea Garlic Dip

1 cup	canned chickpeas, rinsed and drained	250 mL
8 oz	soft (silken) tofu, drained	250 g
2 tbsp	tahini	25 mL
2 tbsp	freshly squeezed lemon juice	25 mL
1 tsp	minced garlic	5 mL
¼ cup	chopped fresh dill (or 1 tsp/5 mL dried)	50 mL
¼ cup	chopped green onions	50 mL
¼ cup	chopped green olives	50 mL
¼ cup	chopped red bell peppers	50 mL
¼ tsp	freshly ground black pepper	1 mL

1. In a food processor, combine chickpeas, tofu, tahini, lemon juice and garlic; purée. Stir in dill, green onions, olives, red peppers and pepper.
2. Chill. Serve with vegetables, crackers or bread.

NUTRITIONAL ANALYSIS PER SERVING

Energy: 88 kcal	Carbohydrate: 8 g	Calcium: 68 mg	Folate: 45 mcg
Protein: 5 g	Fat: 5 g	Iron: 2.7 mg	Fiber: 2.2 g

Hummus

¼ cup	water	50 mL
1 cup	drained canned chickpeas	250 mL
¾ tsp	crushed garlic	4 mL
2 tbsp	lemon juice	25 mL
4 tsp	olive oil	20 mL
¼ cup	tahini	50 mL
1 tbsp	chopped fresh parsley	15 mL

1. In food processor, combine water, chickpeas, garlic, lemon juice, oil and tahini; process until creamy and smooth.
2. Transfer to serving dish; sprinkle with parsley.

NUTRITIONAL ANALYSIS PER SERVING

Energy: 133 kcal	Carbohydrate: 10 g	Calcium: 58 mg	Folate: 58 mcg
Protein: 4 g	Fat: 9 g	Iron: 1.7 mg	Fiber: 3 g

Good source of:
• Folate

Source of:
• Calcium, iron and fiber

MAKES 4 TO 6 SERVINGS OR 1 CUP (250 ML)

Tahini is a Middle Eastern condiment found in the specialty section of some supermarkets. If it's not available, use smooth peanut butter.

Roasted Garlic Sweet Pepper Strips

• Preheat oven to 400°F (200°C)

4	large sweet peppers (combination of green, red and yellow)	4
2 tbsp	olive oil	25 mL
1½ tsp	crushed garlic	7 mL
1 tbsp	grated Parmesan cheese	15 mL

1. On baking sheet, bake whole peppers for 15 to 20 minutes, turning occasionally, or until blistered and blackened. Place in paper bag; seal and let stand for 10 minutes.
2. Peel off charred skin from peppers; cut off tops and bottoms. Remove seeds and ribs; cut into 1-inch (2.5 cm) wide strips and place on serving platter.
3. Mix oil with garlic; brush over peppers. Sprinkle with cheese.

NUTRITIONAL ANALYSIS PER SERVING

Energy: 76 kcal	Carbohydrate: 4 g	Calcium: 24 mg	Folate: 13 mcg
Protein: 1 g	Fat: 6 g	Iron: 1 mg	Fiber: 1.4 g

Source of:
• Iron and folate

MAKES 4 SERVINGS

When shopping, be critical of the foods you put in your cart. Stick to the freshest and healthiest foods possible. Keep the sweet and salty treats out of your cart — if they're not in the house, you're less likely to eat them.

**MAKES
8 SERVINGS**

Serve with crackers or crusty bread, or as a side dish.

TIP

To make quick work of mincing the garlic, use a garlic press.

Eggplant Salsa

- Preheat oven to 350°F (180°C)
- Baking sheet, sprayed with vegetable cooking spray

1	large eggplant, halved lengthwise	1
2 tbsp	water	25 mL
1	red bell pepper, finely chopped	1
1	small onion, minced	1
4	cloves garlic, minced	4
1	large tomato, finely chopped	1
3 tbsp	freshly squeezed lemon juice	45 mL
2 tbsp	chopped fresh chives	25 mL
1 tbsp	dried basil	15 mL

1. Place eggplant halves cut side up on prepared baking sheet and bake for 1 hour, until tender. Let cool.

2. In a skillet, heat water over medium-high heat. Sauté red pepper, onion and garlic until onions are translucent, about 5 minutes. Transfer to a bowl and let cool.

3. Scrape eggplant flesh from skin, chop and add to cooled vegetables. Stir in tomato, lemon juice, chives and basil. Cover and refrigerate for at least 1 hour, until chilled, or for up to 3 days.

NUTRITIONAL ANALYSIS PER SERVING			
Energy: 36 kcal	Carbohydrate: 8 g	Calcium: 50 mg	Folate: 18 mcg
Protein: 2 g	Fat: Trace	Iron: 1.2 mg	Fiber: 2.0 g

Soups

Asparagus and Leek Soup

MAKES 4 TO 6 SERVINGS

Choose the greenest asparagus, with straight, firm stalks. The tips should be tightly closed and firm.

Make Ahead

Make and refrigerate up to a day before and serve cold or reheat gently before serving, adding more stock if too thick.

¾ lb	asparagus	375 g
1½ tsp	vegetable oil	7 mL
1 tsp	crushed garlic	5 mL
1 cup	chopped onion	250 mL
2	leeks, sliced	2
3½ cups	chicken stock	875 mL
1 cup	diced peeled potato	250 mL
	Salt and pepper	
2 tbsp	freshly grated Parmesan cheese	25 mL

1. Trim asparagus; cut stalks into pieces and set tips aside.

2. In large nonstick saucepan, heat oil; sauté garlic, onion, leeks and asparagus stalks just until softened, approximately 10 minutes.

3. Add stock and potato; reduce heat, cover and simmer for 20 to 25 minutes or until vegetables are tender. Purée in food processor until smooth. Taste and adjust seasoning with salt and pepper. Return to saucepan.

4. Steam or microwave reserved asparagus tips just until tender; add to soup. Serve sprinkled with Parmesan cheese.

NUTRITIONAL ANALYSIS PER SERVING

Energy: 140 kcal	Carbohydrate: 20 g	Calcium: 83 mg	Folate: 117 mcg
Protein: 8 g	Fat: 4 g	Iron: 1.9 mg	Fiber: 3 g

Broccoli and Sweet Potato Soup

1 tbsp	canola oil	15 mL
2	large onions, chopped	2
2	stalks celery, chopped	2
3	carrots, chopped	3
2	potatoes, peeled and chopped	2
2	sweet potatoes, peeled and chopped	2
7 cups	vegetable stock	1.75 L
1	bunch broccoli, broken into florets, stalks trimmed, peeled and sliced	1
½ cup	chopped fresh parsley	125 mL
2 tbsp	chopped fresh basil or dill	25 mL
1 cup	skim milk	250 mL
1 tsp	margarine or butter	5 mL
	Salt and freshly ground black pepper	

1. In a large soup pot, heat oil over medium heat. Sauté onions and celery for 5 to 7 minutes, or until softened (if necessary, add a little water to prevent burning). Add carrots and sauté, stirring occasionally, for 3 to 4 minutes, or until softened. Add potatoes, sweet potatoes and vegetable stock; bring to a boil. Reduce heat and simmer for 10 to 15 minutes, or until potatoes are slightly tender. Add broccoli and simmer for about 10 minutes, or until vegetables are soft. Stir in parsley and basil.

2. Working in batches, transfer some or all of the soup (depending on the desired texture) to a food processor or blender and purée until smooth. Return to pot and stir in milk, margarine, and salt and pepper to taste; heat through.

Good source of:
- Folate and fiber

Source of:
- Calcium and iron

MAKES 8 SERVINGS

Packed full of goodness, this soup can be served as a starter or as a main meal.

NUTRITIONAL ANALYSIS PER SERVING			
Energy: 148 kcal	Carbohydrate: 26 g	Calcium: 111 mg	Folate: 77 mcg
Protein: 7 g	Fat: 3 g	Iron: 1.4 mg	Fiber: 4.3 mg

**MAKES 4 TO
6 SERVINGS**

*A dollop of light sour
cream on top of each
bowlful gives a great taste
and sophisticated look.*

Make Ahead

Prepare and refrigerate up
to a day before and reheat
gently, adding more stock
if too thick.

Broccoli Lentil Soup

1½ tsp	vegetable oil	7 mL
2 tsp	crushed garlic	10 mL
1	medium onion, chopped	1
1	celery stalk, chopped	1
1	large carrot, chopped	1
4 cups	chicken stock	1 L
2½ cups	chopped broccoli	625 mL
¾ cup	dried green lentils	175 mL
2 tbsp	freshly grated Parmesan cheese	25 mL

1. In large nonstick saucepan, heat oil; sauté garlic, onion, celery and carrot until softened, approximately 5 minutes.
2. Add stock, broccoli and lentils; cover and simmer for 30 minutes, stirring occasionally, or until lentils are tender.
3. Purée in food processor until creamy and smooth. Serve sprinkled with Parmesan.

NUTRITIONAL ANALYSIS PER SERVING

Energy: 183 kcal	Carbohydrate: 25 g	Calcium: 68 mg	Folate: 156 mcg
Protein: 12 g	Fat: 4 g	Iron: 2.6 mg	Fiber: 8.8 g

**MAKES 4 TO
6 SERVINGS**

*Great soup in just under
30 minutes. Fresh basil
is excellent as a garnish.*

Make Ahead

Prepare up to 2 days in
advance or freeze for up to
3 weeks. Add more stock if
necessary when reheating.

Corn, Tomato and Zucchini Soup

2 tsp	vegetable oil	10 mL
1 tsp	minced garlic	5 mL
3 cups	diced zucchini	750 mL
1½ cups	chopped onions	375 mL
3 cups	basic vegetable stock	750 mL
1	can (19 oz/540 mL) whole tomatoes	1
1¼ cups	frozen or canned corn, drained	300 mL
2 tsp	dried basil	10 mL

1. In a nonstick saucepan sprayed with vegetable spray, heat oil over medium-high heat. Add garlic, zucchini and onions; cook for 5 minutes or until softened.
2. Stir in stock, tomatoes, corn and basil. Bring to a boil, reduce heat to low and simmer 20 minutes, breaking up whole tomatoes with the back of a spoon.

NUTRITIONAL ANALYSIS PER SERVING

Energy: 106 kcal	Carbohydrate: 19 g	Calcium: 61 mg	Folate: 42 mcg
Protein: 3 g	Fat: 3 g	Iron: 1.4 mg	Fiber: 4.0 g

Carrot Soup with Raita

Raita

1 cup	low-fat plain yogurt	250 mL
2/3 cup	grated English cucumber	150 mL
1/4 cup	minced red onion	50 mL
1 tbsp	lemon juice	15 mL
1 tsp	ground cumin	5 mL

Soup

1 tbsp	olive oil	15 mL
1	medium onion, chopped	1
4 cups	coarsely chopped carrots	1 L
5 cups	vegetable or chicken broth	1.25 L
1/2 tsp	salt	2 mL
1/4 tsp	freshly ground black pepper	1 mL

1. *Raita:* In a small bowl, mix together yogurt, cucumber, onion, lemon juice and cumin; chill until serving time.

2. *Soup:* In a saucepan, heat oil over medium heat; cook onion, stirring, for 2 to 3 minutes or until softened. Add carrots; cook, stirring, for 1 to 2 minutes. Add broth; bring to a boil. Reduce heat and simmer, uncovered, for 25 to 30 minutes or until carrots are tender.

3. In a blender or food processor, purée soup in batches until smooth. Strain, if desired. Return to saucepan and heat until hot; add salt and pepper. Serve soup in bowls with 2 spoonfuls of raita on top.

MAKES 5 SERVINGS

The sweetness of harvest-fresh carrots permeates this light-tasting soup. The raita suggests exotic India.

TIP

Raita, a sauce made from yogurt and cucumber, is often used as an accompaniment to curry to balance the heat. It is a staple of Indian cuisine. Here, it adds a flavorful and exotic touch to a classically simple soup.

NUTRITIONAL ANALYSIS PER SERVING

Energy: 130 kcal	Carbohydrate: 19 g	Calcium: 134 mg	Folate: 31 mcg
Protein: 6 g	Fat: 4 g	Iron: 0.7 mg	Fiber: 3.6 mg

**MAKES
12 SERVINGS**

This soup is a fresh-tasting, delicious blend of healthy vegetables. It's a great way to introduce parsnips to those who have never tried this carrot-like vegetable.

TIP

For a little color, you can add a chopped carrot to the soup with the parsnips.

Make Ahead

This soup freezes well for up to 3 months.

Parsnip Soup

2 tbsp	olive oil	25 mL
1	stalk celery, diced	1
½	Spanish onion, diced	½
1 to 2	cloves garlic, minced	1 to 2
6	parsnips, peeled and cut into chunks	6
2	large potatoes, peeled and diced	2
8 cups	chicken or vegetable stock	2 L
	Salt and freshly ground black pepper	
	Chopped fresh chives and/or dill	

1. In a large soup pot, heat oil over medium-high heat. Sauté celery and onion until onion is translucent, about 5 minutes. Add garlic to taste and sauté for 2 minutes. Add parsnips, potatoes and chicken stock; bring to a boil. Reduce heat and simmer for 35 minutes, until parsnips are tender.

2. Working in batches, transfer soup to a food processor or blender and purée until smooth. Season with salt and pepper to taste. Garnish with chives and/or dill.

NUTRITIONAL ANALYSIS PER SERVING			
Energy: 132 kcal	Carbohydrate: 18 g	Calcium: 27 mg	Folate: 45 mcg
Protein: 5 g	Fat: 4 g	Iron: 1.0 mg	Fiber: 0.6 g

Red and Yellow Bell Pepper Soup

• Preheat oven to broil

2	red peppers	2
2	yellow peppers	2
2 tsp	vegetable oil	10 mL
2 tsp	minced garlic	10 mL
1½ cups	chopped onions	375 mL
1¼ cups	chopped carrots	300 mL
½ cup	chopped celery	125 mL
4 cups	chicken or vegetable stock	1 L
1½ cups	diced, peeled potatoes	375 mL
	Freshly ground black pepper to taste	
¼ cup	chopped fresh coriander, dill or basil	50 mL

1. Roast the peppers under the broiler for 15 to 20 minutes, turning several times until charred on all sides. Place in a bowl covered tightly with plastic wrap; let stand until cool enough to handle. Remove skin, stem and seeds.

2. In a nonstick saucepan sprayed with vegetable spray, heat oil over medium heat. Add garlic, onion, carrots and celery; cook for 8 minutes or until vegetables are softened, stirring occasionally. Add stock and potatoes; bring to a boil. Reduce heat to low; cover, and let cook for 20 to 25 minutes or until carrots and potatoes are tender.

3. Put the red peppers in food processor and process until smooth. Add half of the soup mixture to the red pepper purée and process until smooth. Season with pepper and pour into serving bowl. Rinse out food processor. Put yellow peppers in food processor and process until smooth; add remaining soup to yellow pepper purée and process until smooth. Season with pepper and pour into another serving bowl. To serve, ladle some of the red pepper soup into one side of individual bowl, at the same time ladling some of the yellow pepper soup into the other side of the bowl. Add coriander to soup and serve.

MAKES 6 SERVINGS

Roasted peppers in a jar (packed in water) can replace fresh peppers. Use about 4 oz (125 g) peppers in a jar for each fresh pepper required.

TIPS

If desired, coriander can be added before puréeing for a more intense flavor.

Orange peppers can be used instead of red or yellow.

Make Ahead

Roast peppers earlier in the day and set aside.

Prepare both soups earlier in day, and keep them separate until serving.

NUTRITIONAL ANALYSIS PER SERVING

Energy: 146 kcal	Carbohydrate: 22 g	Calcium: 36 mg	Folate: 29 mcg
Protein: 6 g	Fat: 4 g	Iron: 1.6 mg	Fiber: 3.5 g

**MAKES
6 SERVINGS**

A dollop of light sour cream enhances each soup bowl.

Make Ahead

Prepare and refrigerate early in day, then serve cold or reheat gently.

Fresh Tomato Dill Soup

1 tbsp	olive oil	15 mL
1 tsp	crushed garlic	5 mL
1	medium carrot, chopped	1
1	celery stalk, chopped	1
1 cup	chopped onion	250 mL
2 cups	chicken stock	500 mL
5 cups	chopped ripe tomatoes	1.25 L
3 tbsp	tomato paste	45 mL
2 tsp	granulated sugar	10 mL
3 tbsp	chopped fresh dill	45 mL

1. In large nonstick saucepan, heat oil; sauté garlic, carrot, celery and onion until softened, approximately 5 minutes.

2. Add stock, tomatoes and tomato paste; reduce heat, cover and simmer for 20 minutes, stirring occasionally.

3. Purée in food processor until smooth. Add sugar and dill; mix well.

NUTRITIONAL ANALYSIS PER SERVING			
Energy: 112 kcal	Carbohydrate: 17 g	Calcium: 58 mg	Folate: 29 mcg
Protein: 5 g	Fat: 4 g	Iron: 2.1 mg	Fiber: 3.0 g

White, Red and Black Bean Soup

2 tsp	vegetable oil	10 mL
2 tsp	minced garlic	10 mL
⅔ cup	chopped onions	150 mL
¾ cup	chopped carrots	175 mL
⅓ cup	chopped celery	75 mL
3¾ cups	chicken or vegetable stock	925 mL
1¼ cups	canned black beans, drained	300 mL
1¼ cups	canned red kidney beans, drained	300 mL
1¼ cups	canned white kidney beans, drained	300 mL
1¼ tsp	dried basil	6 mL
½ tsp	dried oregano	2 mL
¼ cup	chopped fresh basil or parsley	50 mL

1. In saucepan sprayed with vegetable spray, heat oil over medium heat; add garlic, onions, carrots and celery and cook for 5 minutes or until onions are softened. Add chicken stock and 1 cup (250 mL) each of the black, red and white kidney beans; add basil and oregano. Bring to a boil. Cover, reduce heat to low and let simmer for 15 minutes or until carrots are tender.

2. Transfer soup to blender or food processor and purée. Return puréed soup to saucepan and stir in remaining ¼ cup (50 mL) each black, red and white kidney beans. Cook gently for 5 minutes or until heated through. Serve garnished with basil.

Excellent source of:
• Fiber

Good source of:
• Folate

Source of:
• Iron

MAKES 6 SERVINGS

TIPS

Any other combination of cooked beans will work well.

If cooking your own beans, use 1 cup (250 mL) of dry to make 3 cups (750 mL) cooked.

Other dried herbs can replace basil and oregano. Try bay leaves and rosemary.

Make Ahead

Prepare and refrigerate up to a day ahead. Reheat gently before serving, adding more stock if too thick.

NUTRITIONAL ANALYSIS PER SERVING

| Energy: 179 kcal | Carbohydrate: 31 g | Calcium: 43 mg | Folate: 50 mcg |
| Protein: 11 g | Fat: 2 g | Iron: 1.0 mg | Fiber: 10.0 mg |

**MAKES 8 TO
10 SERVINGS
AS A STARTER OR
4 TO 6 SERVINGS
AS A MAIN COURSE**

I love the combination of flavors in this unusual soup. The red lentils partially dissolve while cooking, creating a creamy texture and the coconut milk creates an intriguing, almost nutty note. Serve as a starter or add an Indian bread and salad for a delicious light meal.

TIPS

For an enhanced cumin flavor, toast the cumin seeds and coarsely crush before using in this recipe.

If you don't have fresh chili peppers, stir in your favorite hot pepper sauce, to taste, just before serving.

Make ahead

This soup can be partially prepared the night before it is cooked. Complete Steps 1 and 2. Cover and refrigerate overnight. The next day, continue cooking as directed in Step 3.

Red Lentil and Carrot Soup with Coconut

• Large (minimum 5 quart) slow cooker

2 cups	red lentils	500 mL
1 tbsp	vegetable oil	15 mL
2	onions, finely chopped	2
2	large carrots, peeled, cut in half lengthwise and thinly sliced	2
4	cloves garlic, minced	4
2 tsp	turmeric	10 mL
2 tsp	cumin seeds (see Tip, at left)	10 mL
1 tsp	salt	5 mL
½ tsp	cracked black peppercorns	2 mL
1	can (28 oz/796 mL) tomatoes, including juice	1
6 cups	vegetable stock	1.5 L
1	can (14 oz/398 mL) coconut milk	1
1 tbsp	freshly squeezed lemon juice	15 mL
1	long red chili pepper or 2 Thai chilies, finely chopped (see Tip, at left)	1
	Thin slices lemon (optional)	
	Finely chopped cilantro (optional)	

1. In a colander, rinse lentils thoroughly under cold running water. Set aside.

2. In a skillet, heat oil over medium heat. Add onions and carrots and cook, stirring, until softened, about 5 minutes. Add garlic, turmeric, cumin seeds, salt and peppercorns and cook, stirring, for 1 minute. Add tomatoes with juice and bring to a boil, breaking up with the back of a spoon. Stir in reserved lentils and stock.

3. Transfer mixture to slow cooker stoneware. Cover and cook on Low for 8 to 10 hours or on High for 4 to 5 hours, until carrots are tender and mixture is bubbling. Stir in coconut milk, lemon juice and chili pepper and cook on High for 20 to 30 minutes, until heated through.

4. When ready to serve, ladle into bowls and top with lemon slices and cilantro, if using.

NUTRITIONAL ANALYSIS PER SERVING

Energy: 344 kcal	Carbohydrate: 42 g	Calcium: 58 mg	Folate: 123 mcg
Protein: 15 g	Fat: 15 g	Iron: 3.0 mg	Fiber: 6.0 g

Red Lentil Soup with Cheese Tortellini

¾ cup	chopped onions	175 mL
2 tsp	minced garlic	10 mL
4 cups	vegetable or chicken stock	1 L
1½ cups	chopped peeled sweet potatoes	375 mL
1 cup	chopped red bell peppers	250 mL
½ cup	chopped carrots	125 mL
½ cup	red lentils	125 mL
1 tsp	dried basil	5 mL
4 oz	fresh or frozen cheese tortellini	125 g

1. In a nonstick saucepan sprayed with vegetable spray, cook onions and garlic over medium heat for 5 minutes or until golden. Add stock, sweet potatoes, red peppers, carrots, red lentils and basil; bring to a boil. Reduce heat to low; cook, covered, for 15 minutes or until lentils and vegetables are tender.

2. In a food processor or blender, purée soup in batches. Return to saucepan over medium-high heat; bring to a boil. Add tortellini; reduce heat to simmer. Cook for 5 minutes or until tortellini are tender.

Excellent source of:
- Fiber

Good source of:
- Iron and folate

Source of:
- Calcium

MAKES 4 SERVINGS

This soup is perfect for the whole family. Because it's puréed, children can't identify specific vegetables they might otherwise object to eating!

NUTRITIONAL ANALYSIS PER SERVING

Energy: 290 kcal	Carbohydrate: 53 g	Calcium: 115 mg	Folate: 47 mcg
Protein: 15 g	Fat: 3 g	Iron: 2.2 mg	Fiber: 6.1 mg

**MAKES 2 TO
4 SERVINGS**

TIPS

Little square packs of instant ramen noodles with various flavorings are available almost everywhere. With a little effort, they can be quickly transformed into a special meal.

This recipe works well with vegetable, chicken and seafood flavorings.

The spinach can be replaced with kale, broccoli or cabbage.

Ramen Noodle Soup with Red Snapper, Spinach and Garlic

8 oz	red snapper fillets, or any other firm white fish	250 g
Broth		
4 cups	water	1 L
1 tsp	minced garlic	5 mL
2	packages ramen soup noodles, with seasoning	2
4 oz	fresh spinach, finely chopped	125 g
1 tsp	chopped cilantro	5 mL
1 tsp	sesame oil	5 mL
	Hot sauce to taste	

1. Remove any skin or bones from fish. Cut into ½-inch (1 cm) cubes and set aside.

2. In a large pot, bring water to a boil. Add fish and garlic and return to a boil. Add noodles, reduce heat and simmer for 3 minutes or until noodles are soft. Add seasoning packet, spinach, cilantro, sesame oil and hot sauce; stir gently. Ladle soup into bowls and serve immediately.

NUTRITIONAL ANALYSIS PER SERVING			
Energy: 238 kcal	Carbohydrate: 32 g	Calcium: 40 mg	Folate: 2 mcg
Protein: 17 g	Fat: 5 g	Iron: 1.2 mg	Fiber: 4.5 mg

Salads

**MAKES
4 SERVINGS**

Greek's signature salad sings when you use the ripest tomatoes and really good olive oil, along with imported Greek feta and oregano.

TIP

As in all salads, I use the finest extra virgin olive oils for best flavor. Experiment with oils from different countries. Greece, for example, is a major olive producing country and you can find a selection of oils in fine food shops and in some supermarkets that stock various good oils.

Classic Greek Salad

2	ripe tomatoes, halved lengthwise, cut into wedges	2
1	small Vidalia or red onion, halved, cut into wedges	1
1/2	English cucumber, quartered lengthwise and cut into thick slices	1/2
1	red bell pepper, cut into cubes	1
1	yellow or green bell pepper, cut into cubes	1
1/4 cup	olive oil (see Tip, at left)	50 mL
2 tbsp	freshly squeezed lemon juice	25 mL
1 tsp	dried oregano	5 mL
1/4 tsp	salt	1 mL
	Freshly ground black pepper	
2 tbsp	chopped fresh flat-leaf parsley	25 mL
4 oz	feta cheese, cubed	125 g
12	Kalamata olives	12

1. In a salad bowl, combine tomatoes, onion, cucumber and peppers.
2. In a separate bowl, whisk together oil, lemon juice, oregano, salt and pepper. Pour dressing over vegetables and gently toss. Sprinkle with parsley and garnish with feta and olives. Serve immediately.

NUTRITIONAL ANALYSIS PER SERVING			
Energy: 245 kcal	Carbohydrate: 15 g	Calcium: 190 mg	Folate: 37 mcg
Protein: 6 g	Fat: 19 g	Iron: 1.5 mg	Fiber: 2.4 mg

Orange Spinach Salad with Almonds

Good source of:
• Fiber

Source of:
• Calcium, iron and folate

Dressing

¼ cup	olive oil	50 mL
2 tbsp	white wine or rice vinegar	25 mL
1 tbsp	honey mustard	15 mL
1 tsp	dried fines herbes or tarragon leaves	5 mL
1 tsp	grated orange zest	5 mL
¼ tsp	salt	1 mL
¼ tsp	freshly ground black pepper	1 mL

Salad

8 cups	baby spinach	2 L
3	seedless oranges, peeled and sectioned (see Tip, at right)	3
1	large Hass avocado, peeled and diced	1
3	green onions, sliced	3
⅓ cup	slivered almonds, toasted (see Tip, at right)	75 mL

1. *Dressing:* In a bowl, whisk together oil, vinegar, honey mustard, fines herbes, orange zest, salt and pepper.
2. *Salad:* In a large bowl, combine spinach, orange sections, avocado and green onions. Pour dressing over salad and lightly toss. Sprinkle with almonds and serve immediately.

MAKES 6 SERVINGS

This is one of my favorite salads to serve for a brunch. It's a good match with egg-based dishes thanks to the sweetness of the oranges and the dressing.

TIPS

Remove peel and white pith from oranges. Working over medium bowl, cut between membranes to release segments.

To toast almonds: Place nuts on a baking sheet in a 350°F (180°C) oven for 7 to 9 minutes.

NUTRITIONAL ANALYSIS PER SERVING

Energy: 220 kcal	Carbohydrate: 14 g	Calcium: 65 mg	Folate: 32 mcg
Protein: 4 g	Fat: 18 g	Iron: 1.9 mg	Fiber: 5.5 mg

**MAKES
8 SERVINGS**

*Loaded with fiber,
iron and protein, this
is a colorful and tasty
addition to fish or
chicken, but it's also
great as an entrée
on its own.*

Black-Eyed Pea and Roasted Veggie Salad

• Preheat oven to 425°F (220°C)
• 8-inch (2 L) glass baking dish, sprayed with vegetable cooking spray

3	carrots, chopped	3
3	parsnips, peeled and chopped	3
2	sweet potatoes, peeled and diced	2
2	stalks celery, chopped	2
1	red bell pepper, chopped	1
1/4	onion, chopped	1/4
1/4 cup	water	50 mL
1 tbsp	olive oil	15 mL
1	can (14 to 19 oz/398 to 540 mL) black-eyed peas, drained and rinsed	1
1 tbsp	cider vinegar	15 mL
	Salt and freshly ground black pepper	

1. In prepared pan, combine carrots, parsnips, sweet potatoes, celery, red pepper, onion, water and oil. Bake in preheated oven for 45 to 55 minutes, or until parsnips and sweet potatoes are tender.

2. Transfer vegetables to a serving bowl. Stir in peas, vinegar, and salt and pepper to taste. Serve warm or let cool to room temperature.

NUTRITIONAL ANALYSIS PER SERVING			
Energy: 148 kcal	Carbohydrate: 28 g	Calcium: 57 mg	Folate: 62 mcg
Protein: 5 g	Fat: 3 g	Iron: 1.7 mg	Fiber: 6.0 mg

Green Bean and Plum Tomato Salad

**MAKES
6 SERVINGS**

1 lb	young green beans, trimmed	500 g
8	small plum tomatoes (about 1 lb/500 g)	8
2	green onions, sliced	2

Dressing

¼ cup	olive oil	50 mL
4 tsp	red wine vinegar	20 mL
1 tbsp	grainy mustard	15 mL
1	clove garlic, minced	1
½ tsp	granulated sugar	2 mL
¼ tsp	salt	1 mL
¼ tsp	freshly ground black pepper	1 mL
¼ cup	chopped fresh parsley	50 mL

When preparing this dish ahead, I like to keep the blanched green beans, tomatoes and dressing separate and toss them just before serving to prevent the salad from getting soggy.

TIP

Use the terrific mustardy dressing with other favorite vegetable salad mixtures and crisp greens.

1. In a medium saucepan of boiling salted water, cook beans for 3 to 5 minutes or until just tender-crisp. Drain and rinse under cold water to chill; drain well. Pat dry with paper towels or wrap in a clean, dry towel.

2. Cut plum tomatoes in half lengthwise; using a small spoon, scoop out centers. Cut each piece again in half lengthwise; place in a bowl. Just before serving, combine beans, tomatoes and green onions in a serving bowl.

3. *Dressing:* In a small bowl, whisk together oil, vinegar, mustard, garlic, sugar, salt and pepper. Stir in parsley. Pour dressing over salad and toss well.

NUTRITIONAL ANALYSIS PER SERVING			
Energy: 137 kcal	Carbohydrate: 12 g	Calcium: 62 mg	Folate: 26 mcg
Protein: 3 g	Fat: 9 g	Iron: 1.3 mg	Fiber: 3.9 mg

**MAKES
6 SERVINGS**

*Bean salad is another
staple we've grown up
with over the years.
Originally this salad
used canned string
beans, but fresh beans
give it a new lease on
taste, as does the
addition of fiber-packed
chickpeas.*

Bean Salad with Mustard-Dill Dressing

1 lb	green beans	500 g
1	can (19 oz/540 mL) chickpeas, drained and rinsed	1
⅓ cup	chopped red onions	75 mL

Dressing

2 tbsp	olive oil	25 mL
2 tbsp	red wine vinegar	25 mL
1 tbsp	Dijon mustard	15 mL
1 tbsp	granulated sugar	15 mL
¼ tsp	salt	1 mL
¼ tsp	freshly ground black pepper	1 mL
2 tbsp	finely chopped fresh dill	25 mL

1. Trim ends of beans; cut into 1-inch (2.5 cm) lengths. In a large pot of boiling salted water, cook beans for 3 to 5 minutes (start timing when water returns to a boil) or until tender-crisp. Drain; rinse under cold water to chill. Drain well.

2. In a serving bowl, combine green beans, chickpeas and onions.

3. *Dressing:* In a small bowl, whisk together oil, vinegar, mustard, sugar, salt and pepper until smooth. Stir in dill.

4. Pour over beans and toss well. Refrigerate until serving time.

Variation

Instead of chickpeas, you can try canned mixed beans. This includes a combination of chickpeas, red and white kidney beans and black-eyed peas. It's available in supermarkets.

NUTRITIONAL ANALYSIS PER SERVING			
Energy: 161 kcal	Carbohydrate: 22 g	Calcium: 73 mg	Folate: 2 mcg
Protein: 6 g	Fat: 6 g	Iron: 1.8 mg	Fiber: 6.0 mg

Edamame Salad

1	red bell pepper, diced	1
2 cups	cooked edamame beans (removed from pods)	500 mL
2 cups	cooked corn kernels	500 mL
1/3 cup	Asian Vinaigrette (see recipe, below)	75 mL

1. In a large bowl, combine red pepper, edamame, corn and vinaigrette. Cover and refrigerate for at least 1 hour to allow flavors to meld.

Asian Vinaigrette

2	green onions, finely chopped	2
1/2 cup	rice wine vinegar	125 mL
1/4 cup	unsweetened apple juice	50 mL
2 tbsp	sesame oil	25 mL
2 tbsp	reduced-sodium soy sauce	25 mL
1 tbsp	grated gingerroot	15 mL
1 tsp	granulated sugar	5 mL

1. In blender, on high speed, blend green onions, vinegar, apple juice, sesame oil, soy sauce, ginger and sugar until well combined. Makes about 1 cup (250 mL).

Source of:
- Calcium, iron, folate and fiber

MAKES 6 SERVINGS

Edamame, or fresh soybeans, have become very popular recently. This simple but tasty dish is great on its own or as part of a composed salad plate for lunch or dinner.

TIPS

To cook edamame, add 2 cups (500 mL) to 1/2 cup (125 mL) boiling water. Reduce heat, cover and simmer for 4 minutes. Drain well.

This salad will keep for up to 3 days in the refrigerator. The dressing will keep for up to 5 days.

NUTRITIONAL ANALYSIS PER SERVING			
Energy: 201 kcal	Carbohydrate: 29 g	Calcium: 64 mg	Folate: 37 mcg
Protein: 9 g	Fat: 7 g	Iron: 1.7 mg	Fiber: 3.0 mg

Mediterranean Lentil and Rice Salad

MAKES 10 SERVINGS

This salad travels well, making it a great lunchbox choice. It can work on its own or be served with veggie sticks.

TIPS

For 3 cups (750 mL) cooked brown rice, cook 1 cup (250 mL) rice with 2 cups (500 mL) water.

If you serve this as a main course instead of as a side salad, it serves 6.

This salad keeps well for up to 1 week in the refrigerator.

2	roasted red bell peppers, patted dry and julienned	2
1	can (19 oz/540 mL) lentils, drained and rinsed	1
3 cups	cooked brown rice	750 mL
1 cup	chopped fresh Italian (flat-leaf) parsley	250 mL
½ cup	thinly sliced green onions	125 mL
¼ cup	slivered dried apricots	50 mL

Dressing

¼ cup	olive oil	50 mL
2 tbsp	freshly squeezed lemon juice	25 mL
2 tbsp	balsamic vinegar	25 mL
1 tsp	liquid honey	5 mL
1 tsp	ground cumin	5 mL
½ tsp	ground coriander	2 mL
	Salt and freshly ground black pepper	

1. In a large bowl, combine red peppers, lentils, rice, parsley, green onions and apricots.
2. *Dressing:* In a small bowl, whisk together olive oil, lemon juice, vinegar, honey, cumin, coriander, and salt and pepper to taste.
3. Pour dressing over salad and toss to coat.

NUTRITIONAL ANALYSIS PER SERVING			
Energy: 178 kcal	Carbohydrate: 28 g	Calcium: 24 mg	Folate: 23 mcg
Protein: 6 g	Fat: 5 g	Iron: 1.2 mg	Fiber: 6.2 mg

Terrific Thai Chicken Salad

Good source of:
- Iron

Source of:
- Folate

1 lb	boneless skinless chicken breasts	500 g
4 oz	rice vermicelli	125 g
½	medium seedless cucumber, cut into thin 2-inch (5 cm) strips	½
1	large red bell pepper, cut into thin 2-inch (5 cm) strips	1
¼ cup	chopped fresh basil, mint or cilantro	50 mL

Dressing

¼ cup	fish sauce	50 mL
3 tbsp	freshly squeezed lime juice	45 mL
2 tbsp	packed brown sugar	25 mL
1 tbsp	minced fresh gingerroot	15 mL
1	large clove garlic, minced	1
1 tsp	chili paste or hot pepper sauce to taste	5 mL

MAKES 4 SERVINGS

Many supermarkets stock a wide variety of Asian food products, including fish sauce and chili paste. Fish sauce, called nam pla, is a salty brown seasoning that is the backbone of Thai cooking.

TIP

Save the poaching liquid and use in soups and stews.

1. In a large saucepan, bring 2 cups (500 mL) lightly salted water to a boil; reduce heat to medium-low. Add chicken; poach for 10 to 12 minutes or until no longer pink inside. Let cool in poaching liquid. Remove and cut chicken into thin strips. Discard poaching liquid or see Tip, at right.

2. In a bowl, cover vermicelli with hot water; let stand for 3 minutes or until softened. Drain well.

3. In another bowl, combine chicken, vermicelli, cucumber, red pepper and basil.

4. *Dressing:* In a bowl, combine fish sauce, lime juice, brown sugar, ginger, garlic and chili paste. Just before serving, pour over chicken mixture; toss well. Garnish with additional basil.

Variations

Substitute 3 tbsp (45 mL) soy sauce for the fish sauce.

Replace rice vermicelli with the same amount of spaghettini, cooked according to package directions.

NUTRITIONAL ANALYSIS PER SERVING

Energy: 344 kcal	Carbohydrate: 37 g	Calcium: 47 mg	Folate: 27 mcg
Protein: 37 g	Fat: 4 g	Iron: 2.3 mg	Fiber: 1.3 mg

**MAKES
4 SERVINGS**

TIP

To toast almonds:
Heat a dry heavy skillet over medium heat for 30 seconds. Add almonds and cook until they begin to turn golden, about 2 minutes. Immediately remove from heat, as they'll continue cooking until they cool.

Rice Noodle Salad with Sugar Snap Peas, Sweet Peppers and Almonds

8 oz	medium vermicelli (rice stick noodles) or dried fettuccine	250 g
⅔ cup	Nuoc Cham (see recipe, opposite), divided	150 mL
1 tbsp	butter	15 mL
1 tbsp	olive oil	15 mL
3 cups	trimmed sugar snap or snow peas	750 mL
2 tsp	minced garlic	10 mL
2 tbsp	vegetable or chicken stock	25 mL
1 cup	thinly sliced red bell peppers	250 mL
1 cup	thinly sliced yellow bell peppers	250 mL
½ cup	toasted sliced almonds	125 mL
¼ cup	cilantro leaves	50 mL
	Coarsely ground black pepper, to taste	

1. In a heatproof bowl or pot, cover noodles with boiling water and soak for 5 minutes. (If using pasta, prepare according to package directions.) Drain, toss with ⅓ cup (75 mL) of the Nuoc Cham and let cool to room temperature.

2. In a nonstick pan, heat butter and oil over medium-high heat until just smoking. Add peas and stir-fry until well-coated, about 30 seconds. Add garlic and stock. Cover and cook until peas are tender-crisp, about 1 minute. Add peppers and stir-fry until warmed through and liquid is absorbed, about 1 minute. Remove from heat. Add remaining Nuoc Cham and mix well.

3. In a large salad bowl, combine noodles, vegetables, almonds and cilantro; toss. Sprinkle with black pepper to taste and serve.

Nuoc Cham

⅓ cup	sugar (or to taste)	75 mL
1 cup	warm water	250 mL
1 or 2	small red chilies, seeded and minced (or 2 tsp/10 mL dried chili flakes)	1 or 2
2 tbsp	white rice vinegar	25 mL
2 tbsp	freshly squeezed lime juice	25 mL
1 tbsp	minced garlic	15 mL
½ cup	fish sauce	125 mL
1	small carrot, peeled and finely shredded	1

1. In a small bowl, combine sugar and warm water, stirring until sugar is dissolved. Add remaining ingredients, except carrots, and mix well. Let stand for at least 30 minutes to develop flavors.

2. Just before serving the sauce, wrap shredded carrots in a clean towel and squeeze to remove excess moisture; add carrots to sauce. Makes about 2 cups (500 mL).

NUTRITIONAL ANALYSIS PER SERVING

Energy: 565 kcal	Carbohydrate: 92 g	Calcium: 178 mg	Folate: 46 mcg
Protein: 16 g	Fat: 16 g	Iron: 4.6 mg	Fiber: 9.0 mg

**MAKES
4 SERVINGS**

You won't believe how easy it is to make this elegant grilled salmon on a bed of freshly tossed greens. This meal-in-one dish is ideal for a patio supper with friends. The dressing, made quickly in the food processor, does double duty as a marinade for the salmon and a dressing for the salad.

TIP

Cook the salmon on a stovetop grill pan or place on a broiler pan 4 inches (10 cm) below preheated broiler for the same cooking time.

Grilled Salmon and Romaine Salad

• Preheat barbecue grill, greased
• Wooden skewers

Dressing

2 cups	lightly packed fresh parsley	500 mL
¼ cup	freshly squeezed orange juice	50 mL
2 tbsp	olive oil	25 mL
2 tbsp	red wine vinegar	25 mL
1 tbsp	Dijon mustard	15 mL
½ tsp	salt	2 mL
½ tsp	freshly ground black pepper	2 mL
1	clove garlic, minced	1
1 tsp	grated orange zest	5 mL

Salad

1	center-cut piece salmon fillet (1¼ lbs/625 g)	1
8 cups	torn romaine lettuce	2 L
2 cups	halved cherry tomatoes	500 mL
½	medium seedless cucumber, halved lengthwise and sliced	½

1. *Dressing:* In a food processor, combine parsley, orange juice, oil, vinegar, mustard, salt and pepper; process until parsley is very finely chopped. Transfer to a glass measure. Stir in garlic and orange zest.

2. *Salad:* Remove skin from salmon and slice lengthwise into 4 long strips. Thread salmon lengthwise onto skewers. Place in shallow baking dish to hold salmon in an even layer. Spread with ¼ cup (50 mL) of the dressing. Let marinate at room temperature for 15 minutes, turning occasionally.

3. Place salmon on preheated grill over medium-high heat; grill, brushing with dressing, turning once, for about 4 minutes per side or until fish flakes easily.

4. Meanwhile, in a bowl, combine romaine, cherry tomatoes and cucumber. Pour over remaining dressing; toss to lightly coat. Divide salad among serving plates; top with salmon.

NUTRITIONAL ANALYSIS PER SERVING			
Energy: 336 kcal	Carbohydrate: 11 g	Calcium: 119 mg	Folate: 255 mcg
Protein: 35 g	Fat: 17 g	Iron: 4.8 mg	Fiber: 3.2 mg

Meat

MAKES
4 SERVINGS

The mix of vegetables and tender steak with pasta make this dish a real family favorite.

Asian-Flavored Steak and Mushrooms with Pasta

- Preheat broiler

8 oz	angel hair pasta	250 g
2 tbsp	vegetable oil	25 mL
2 tsp	minced garlic	10 mL
1 lb	mushrooms, halved	500 g
2 cups	broccoli florets	500 mL
1 cup	diced tomatoes or halved cherry tomatoes	250 mL
1/4 cup	soy sauce	50 mL
1/4 tsp	hot pepper sauce	1 mL
1 lb	boneless beef sirloin, flank or other grilling steak	500 g
1/2 cup	baby salad greens	125 mL
	Additional soy sauce and hot pepper sauce	

1. Cook pasta as directed on package. Drain, reserving 1/4 cup (50 mL) cooking liquid, and keep warm.

2. Meanwhile, in a large skillet, heat oil over medium heat. Sauté garlic for 30 seconds. Add mushrooms and broccoli; sauté until broccoli is tender-crisp and mushrooms are golden, about 5 minutes. Remove from heat and stir in tomatoes, soy sauce and hot pepper sauce. Add pasta and toss until well combined. Cover and keep warm.

3. Broil steak, turning once, for 3 to 4 minutes per side for medium-rare, or until desired doneness. Remove to cutting board and thinly slice on the diagonal across the grain.

4. Toss steak with pasta mixture. Add reserved pasta cooking liquid as needed and additional soy sauce and hot sauce to taste. Serve garnished with salad greens.

NUTRITIONAL ANALYSIS PER SERVING			
Energy: 530 kcal	Carbohydrate: 56 g	Calcium: 67 mg	Folate: 90 mcg
Protein: 40 g	Fat: 17 g	Iron: 6.0 mg	Fiber: 5.7 g

Sesame Steak

¼ cup	light soy sauce	50 mL
1	clove garlic, minced	1
1	small onion, finely chopped	1
1 tbsp	liquid honey	15 mL
1 tbsp	sesame seeds	15 mL
1 tsp	grated gingerroot	5 mL
1 tsp	freshly ground black pepper	5 mL
1 lb	flank steak	500 g

1. In a shallow nonaluminum pan, mix together soy sauce, garlic, onion, honey, sesame seeds, ginger and pepper. Add steak, turning to coat. Cover and marinate in refrigerator for at least 4 to 6 hours or preferably overnight.

2. Preheat barbecue or broiler; place steak on greased grill or under broiler; cook for 4 to 5 minutes per side for medium-rare. Slice across the grain to serve.

Good source of:
- Iron

Source of:
- Folate

MAKES 4 SERVINGS

Flank steak is a popular cut of beef because it is versatile and extremely flavorful. In this recipe, the steak is marinated in a soy, garlic, ginger and honey sauce. The result is both tender and packed with flavor. Serve with stir-fried vegetables or salad and garlic bread.

TIP

Marinating meat adds flavor while it tenderizes. For convenience, marinate meat in a resealable plastic freezer bag.

NUTRITIONAL ANALYSIS PER SERVING

Energy: 246 kcal	Carbohydrate: 8 g	Calcium: 39 mg	Folate: 16 mcg
Protein: 29 g	Fat: 10 g	Iron: 3.0 mg	Fiber: 1.0 g

MAKES 4 TO 6 SERVINGS

This classic stir-fry marries Asian flavors with beef and vegetables. All you need to add is cooked rice.

TIPS

When preparing food for stir-frying, cut into small pieces of approximately equal size so that they will cook through rapidly and in the same period of time. Have sauce and ingredients prepared and easily accessible before starting to cook.

This Asian-style meal is perfect for a busy weeknight. For a quick and easy dessert that continues the Asian theme, serve sliced melon, such as cantaloupe, sprinkled with gingered sugar (granulated sugar mixed with ground ginger to taste).

Beef with Broccoli

1 lb	sirloin steak, cut into thin strips	500 g
¼ cup	soy sauce	50 mL
2 tbsp	cornstarch, divided	25 mL
1	clove garlic, minced	1
1	thin slice gingerroot, minced	1
2 tbsp	safflower oil, divided	25 mL
2	medium onions, cut into wedges	2
3	large carrots, sliced into coins	3
1	head broccoli, cut into florets	1
1¼ cups	water, divided	300 mL
1 tbsp	oyster sauce	15 mL
1 tsp	granulated sugar	5 mL

1. Place steak in a medium bowl. In a separate bowl, combine soy sauce, 1 tbsp (15 mL) of the cornstarch, garlic and ginger; pour over steak.

2. In a wok or nonstick skillet, heat 1 tbsp (15 mL) of the oil over high heat. Add beef and stir-fry until browned. Set aside.

3. In wok, heat remaining oil over high heat. Add onions and stir-fry for 1 minute. Add carrots, broccoli and 1 cup (250 mL) of the water; cover and steam for 4 minutes.

4. Combine remaining water, oyster sauce, remaining cornstarch and sugar. Stir sauce into wok; cook until smooth and thickened. Return meat to wok. Reheat to serving temperature.

NUTRITIONAL ANALYSIS PER SERVING

Energy: 188 kcal	Carbohydrate: 10 g	Calcium: 46 mg	Folate: 34 mcg
Protein: 20 g	Fat: 7 g	Iron: 2.5 mg	Fiber: 1.7 g

Hoisin Beef and Broccoli Stir-Fry

2 tsp	vegetable oil	10 mL
12 oz	sirloin or inside round steak, cut into 3- by ½-inch (7.5 by 1 cm) strips	375 g
1 tbsp	chopped gingerroot	15 mL
1 tsp	minced garlic	5 mL
3 cups	small broccoli florets	750 mL
⅓ cup	sliced water chestnuts	75 mL
½ tsp	cornstarch	2 mL
⅓ cup	orange juice or beef stock	75 mL
2 tbsp	hoisin sauce	25 mL
½ tsp	sesame oil (optional)	2 mL
	Freshly ground black pepper	
1 tbsp	toasted sesame seeds (optional)	15 mL

1. In a large nonstick skillet, heat oil over medium-high heat; add beef strips and stir-fry for 1 to 2 minutes or until browned. Add ginger, garlic, broccoli and water chestnuts; stir-fry for another 2 to 3 minutes or until broccoli is tender-crisp.

2. In a small bowl or glass measuring cup, whisk together cornstarch, orange juice, hoisin sauce and, if using, sesame oil. Add to skillet; cook, stirring, for 1 to 2 minutes or until thickened and heated through. Season with pepper to taste. If desired, sprinkle with sesame seeds.

MAKES 4 SERVINGS

There are endless variations on the theme of stir-fried beef and broccoli. This one highlights flavorful hoisin sauce, a spicy-sweet condiment made from fermented soybeans. Serve over cooked rice.

TIPS

Hoisin sauce also makes a great glaze for fish fillets or chicken breasts. Look for it in the Asian food section of most supermarkets. Refrigerate after opening.

Using a nonstick skillet helps you cook with very small amounts of oil — and makes cleanup a breeze. Adding a tiny amount of flavored oil, such as sesame oil, provides taste without adding too much fat.

NUTRITIONAL ANALYSIS PER SERVING			
Energy: 200 kcal	Carbohydrate: 9 g	Calcium: 26 mg	Folate: 42 mcg
Protein: 22 g	Fat: 8 g	Iron: 2.7 mg	Fiber: 1.1 g

**MAKES
6 SERVINGS**

Vegetables can be varied in this beef stir-fry — red or white onions, sliced carrots, snow peas, chopped broccoli or cauliflower. Remember that brown rice is not only more flavorful than white, it is also more nutritious.

TIPS

Be sure to use a tomato-based chili sauce in this recipe rather than one made from chili peppers; otherwise the result will be overwhelmingly spicy.

This hearty dish is almost a meal in itself. It is loaded with high-quality protein, B vitamins, iron and fiber.

Ginger Vegetable Beef Medley

1½ cups	brown rice	375 mL
4 cups	boiling water	1 L
¼ cup	safflower oil, divided	50 mL
2	small onions, cut into wedges	2
1	clove garlic, minced	1
½ lb	green beans, diagonally sliced	250 g
1 lb	mushrooms, sliced	500 g
1 cup	sliced water chestnuts	250 mL
2 tsp	chopped gingerroot	10 mL
½ tsp	freshly ground black pepper	2 mL
1½ lb	sirloin or top round steak, cut into thin strips	750 g
3 tbsp	cornstarch	45 mL
2 tsp	ground ginger	10 mL
½ cup	water	125 mL
⅓ cup	chili sauce	75 mL
¼ cup	soy sauce	50 mL

1. In a saucepan, add rice to boiling water. Cover and cook for 45 minutes or until tender and water is absorbed.

2. In a wok or nonstick skillet, heat 2 tbsp (25 mL) of the oil over high heat. Add onions and garlic; stir-fry for 1 minute. Add green beans, mushrooms and water chestnuts. Cover and steam for 4 minutes. Stir in ginger and pepper. Remove mixture and keep warm.

3. Coat beef strips in cornstarch and ground ginger. In wok, stir-fry beef over high heat in remaining oil until brown. Stir in water, chili sauce and soy sauce.

4. Arrange rice on platter; top with vegetable mixture and beef strips.

NUTRITIONAL ANALYSIS PER SERVING			
Energy: 523 kcal	Carbohydrate: 60 g	Calcium: 61 mg	Folate: 65 mcg
Protein: 36 g	Fat: 16 g	Iron: 5.3 mg	Fiber: 5.2 g

Chili Bean Stew

1½ tsp	vegetable oil	7 mL
1 tsp	crushed garlic	5 mL
1 cup	chopped onion	250 mL
8 oz	lean ground beef	250 g
1	can (19 oz/540 mL) tomatoes, crushed	1
2 cups	beef stock	500 mL
1½ cups	diced peeled potatoes	375 mL
¾ cup	drained canned red kidney beans	175 mL
¾ cup	corn niblets	175 mL
2 tbsp	tomato paste	25 mL
1½ tsp	chili powder	7 mL
1½ tsp	dried oregano	7 mL
1½ tsp	dried basil	7 mL
⅓ cup	small shell pasta	75 mL

1. In large nonstick saucepan, heat oil; sauté garlic and onion until softened, approximately 5 minutes.

2. Add beef and cook, stirring to break up chunks, until no longer pink; pour off any fat.

3. Add tomatoes, stock, potatoes, kidney beans, corn, tomato paste, chili powder, oregano and basil. Cover and reduce heat; simmer for 40 minutes, stirring occasionally.

4. Add pasta; cook until firm to the bite, approximately 10 minutes.

Excellent source of:
• Fiber

Good source of:
• Iron and folate

Source of:
• Calcium

MAKES 4 TO 6 SERVINGS

TIP

Ground chicken or veal can substitute for beef, and other cooked beans can be used instead of kidney beans.

Make Ahead

Make and refrigerate up to a day before. Reheat gently, adding more stock if too thick.

NUTRITIONAL ANALYSIS PER SERVING

Energy: 224 kcal	Carbohydrate: 34 g	Calcium: 64 mg	Folate: 60 mcg
Protein: 16 g	Fat: 4 g	Iron: 3.0 mg	Fiber: 7.1 mg

**MAKES
8 SERVINGS**

This marvelously moist dish (which you can make the day before) is excellent served as part of a cold buffet with salads and bread.

TIPS

If making this dish ahead of time, refrigerate the veal in a clean container within 2 hours of cooking.

Using vegetables, herbs and lemon to flavor the meat in this recipe increases the taste without increasing the fat content.

Braised Roasted Veal

- Preheat oven to 475°F (240°C)
- Roasting pan

2 lb	veal leg (top portion)	1 kg
½ tsp	crumbled dried rosemary	2 mL
½ tsp	dried thyme	2 mL
Pinch	dried tarragon	Pinch
1	stalk celery, chopped	1
1	medium onion, chopped	1
1	medium carrot, diced	1
⅓ cup	water	75 mL
¼ cup	vinegar	50 mL
¼ cup	white wine	50 mL
1 tsp	grated lemon zest	5 mL
1 tbsp	lemon juice	15 mL

1. Place veal in roasting pan; sprinkle with rosemary, thyme and tarragon. Place celery, onion and carrot around veal. Roast in preheated oven for 10 minutes.

2. Reduce temperature to 375°F (190°C). Add water, vinegar, wine, lemon zest and juice. Cover and roast for 1 hour. Remove from pan and cool. Chill. Slice to serve.

NUTRITIONAL ANALYSIS PER SERVING			
Energy: 210 kcal	Carbohydrate: 3 g	Calcium: 25 mg	Folate: 11 mcg
Protein: 25 g	Fat: 10 g	Iron: 4.0 mg	Fiber: 0.5 g

Pork Tenderloin with Roasted Potatoes

- Preheat oven to 375°F (190°C)
- 11- by 7-inch (2 L) baking dish, greased

1	12-oz (375 g) pork tenderloin	1
2 tsp	orange marmalade	10 mL
2 tsp	Dijon mustard	10 mL
1 tsp	vegetable oil, divided	5 mL
2 cups	potatoes, cut into 1-inch (2.5 cm) pieces	500 mL
1 tbsp	lemon juice	15 mL
1 tsp	crumbled dried rosemary	5 mL

1. Pat pork tenderloin dry; place in center of baking dish.

2. In a small bowl, combine marmalade, mustard and ½ tsp (2 mL) of the oil; brush over pork.

3. In a medium bowl, toss potatoes with remaining oil; arrange around pork in baking dish. Sprinkle potatoes with lemon juice. Sprinkle pork and potatoes with rosemary. Bake in preheated oven for 40 to 45 minutes or until pork is just slightly pink at center and potatoes are tender. Cut pork into ½-inch (1 cm) slices before serving.

Good source of:
- Iron

Source of:
- Folate and fiber

MAKES 3 SERVINGS

This dish takes only 10 minutes to prepare. And because it cooks in 1 baking dish, cleanup is a snap!

TIPS

If you need to feed more than 3 people, just buy another pork tenderloin and double the remaining ingredients.

Serve with green beans, applesauce, whole-grain rolls and a glass of cold milk. To boost your vitamin A intake, replace 1 cup (250 mL) white potatoes with sweet potatoes.

NUTRITIONAL ANALYSIS PER SERVING			
Energy: 259 kcal	Carbohydrate: 24 g	Calcium: 27 mg	Folate: 20 mcg
Protein: 29 g	Fat: 5 g	Iron: 2.7 mg	Fiber: 3.0 g

MAKES 5 SERVINGS

Teriyaki is a Japanese soy-based sauce that is usually used to glaze fish or meat that is grilled or stir-fried. Here, it is used as a marinade and combines with fruit, vegetables and almonds to create a uniquely flavored dish.

TIPS

Vary the vegetables in this stir-fry — add sliced red or white onions, sliced carrots, snow peas, broccoli or cauliflower florets or chopped green or red pepper, as desired. Cut pieces about the same size to ensure even cooking.

Stir-fried vegetables retain their crunchy texture and bright colors. They also retain more nutrients because of the fast cooking time. This dish, which delivers a healthy dose of iron, contains foods from all the food groups, except for Milk Products. Complete the meal with a dairy-rich dessert such as a baked custard.

Pork Teriyaki

1 lb	pork tenderloin, cut into thin strips	500 g
¼ cup	teriyaki sauce	50 mL
1 cup	water	250 mL
½ cup	dried apricots, halved	125 mL
2½ cups	pineapple or orange juice	625 mL
1¼ cups	white rice	300 mL
1 tbsp	vegetable oil	15 mL
1	medium onion, chopped	1
1	medium red bell pepper, chopped	1
1	small yellow bell pepper, chopped	1
¼ cup	slivered almonds	50 mL

1. Marinate pork in teriyaki sauce for several hours in refrigerator.

2. Bring water and apricots to a boil in a small saucepan. Cook for about 20 minutes or until tender. Remove apricots, reserving liquid. Add pineapple juice to saucepan; return to boil. Add rice and cook for about 15 minutes or until rice is tender and liquid is absorbed.

3. In a large skillet over medium-high heat, stir-fry pork in hot oil for about 5 minutes or until browned. Add onion and peppers; stir-fry for 5 minutes. Stir in apricots and almonds. Serve over rice.

NUTRITIONAL ANALYSIS PER SERVING

Energy: 350 kcal	Carbohydrate: 43 g	Calcium: 65 mg	Folate: 53 mcg
Protein: 25 g	Fat: 9 g	Iron: 3.2 mg	Fiber: 2.7 g

Grilled Lamb Chops with Sautéed Peppers and Zucchini

MAKES 4 SERVINGS

Try this impressive dish for your next dinner party. Your guests need never know how easy it is to make!

TIPS

For extra-easy cleanup, line the broiler pan with foil.

If weather permits, grill chops on the barbecue; you'll improve their flavor — and enjoy some time outdoors!

To cook the vegetables on the grill, place vegetables and sauce in a heavy-duty foil packet and barbecue for about 10 minutes, turning once.

• Preheat broiler or barbecue

¼ cup	balsamic or red wine vinegar	50 mL
2 tbsp	olive oil, divided	25 mL
1 tbsp	Dijon mustard	15 mL
1 tsp	dried thyme	5 mL
1 tsp	minced garlic	5 mL
Pinch	freshly ground black pepper	Pinch
8 to 12	bone-in, center-cut loin lamb chops, trimmed of fat (about 1½ lb/750 g in total)	8 to 12
1½ cups	sliced zucchini	375 mL
1½ cups	julienned red bell peppers	375 mL
1 cup	sliced sweet onion	250 mL

1. In a large bowl, blend together vinegar, 1 tbsp (15 mL) of the oil, mustard, thyme, garlic and pepper. Transfer 2 to 3 tbsp (25 to 45 mL) of the mixture to a small bowl; set aside.

2. Place chops on broiling pan or grill; spoon reserved vinaigrette on top. Cook, turning once, for 8 to 10 minutes or until cooked to desired doneness.

3. Meanwhile, in a large nonstick skillet, heat remaining 1 tbsp (15 mL) oil over medium-high heat. Add zucchini, peppers and onion; stir-fry for 6 to 8 minutes or until tender-crisp. Add remaining vinaigrette to pan; cook, stirring, for 1 to 2 minutes or until heated through.

NUTRITIONAL ANALYSIS PER SERVING

Energy: 460 kcal	Carbohydrate: 10 g	Calcium: 55 mg	Folate: 27 mcg
Protein: 38 g	Fat: 30 g	Iron: 4.9 mg	Fiber: 2.5 g

**MAKES
6 SERVINGS**

This complete one-pot meal is a lifesaver when you have only about 45 minutes to make and eat dinner before heading out to evening activities. Dice the vegetables ahead of time to save an extra 10 minutes.

Mediterranean Lamb Curry Couscous

	Vegetable cooking spray	
1 lb	ground lamb	500 g
1 cup	finely diced onion	250 mL
1 cup	finely diced celery	250 mL
1 cup	finely diced carrot	250 mL
1 cup	finely diced broccoli (fresh or frozen)	250 mL
1 tsp	curry powder	5 mL
1 tsp	garlic powder	5 mL
1 tsp	dried parsley	5 mL
1 tsp	ground turmeric (optional)	5 mL
1 tsp	fancy molasses or liquid honey	5 mL
1¼ cups	water	300 mL
⅔ cup	whole wheat couscous	150 mL

1. Heat a large skillet over medium heat. Spray with vegetable cooking spray. Cook ground lamb, breaking up clumps, until evenly browned, about 15 minutes. Transfer to a colander and rinse under hot running water to remove excess fat. Drain well. Rinse out skillet.

2. Reheat skillet over medium heat. Spray with vegetable cooking spray. Sauté onion, celery, carrot and broccoli for 5 minutes. Add curry powder, garlic powder, parsley, turmeric (if using) and molasses. Stir in water, cover and bring to a boil. Return lamb to skillet and cook for 5 minutes. Stir in couscous. Cover, remove from heat and let stand for 5 minutes. Fluff with a fork.

Variations

If your family does not like curry seasoning, omit the curry powder and turmeric and add salt and pepper to taste.

Substitute ground chicken, turkey or beef for the lamb.

NUTRITIONAL ANALYSIS PER SERVING			
Energy: 292 kcal	Carbohydrate: 17 g	Calcium: 46 mg	Folate: 39 mcg
Protein: 15 g	Fat: 18 g	Iron: 2.1 mg	Fiber: 3.3 mg

Chicken

MAKES 6 SERVINGS

This tasty combination of noodles, cheese, chicken and vegetables in a creamy sauce is comfort food. Make this casserole the day before you intend to serve it and reheat for even better flavor.

TIP

Substitute Swiss cheese for the Cheddar if you prefer.

Chicken and Broccoli Bake

- Preheat oven to 350°F (180°C)
- Oblong baking dish, lightly greased

6	chicken breast halves, skinned and boned	6
1	green onion, finely chopped	1
3 tbsp	butter or margarine	45 mL
2 tsp	lemon juice	10 mL
3 tbsp	all-purpose flour	45 mL
2 cups	2% milk	500 mL
1 tbsp	chopped fresh parsley	15 mL
½ tsp	salt	2 mL
¼ tsp	dried basil	1 mL
Pinch	freshly ground black pepper	Pinch
1 cup	shredded Cheddar cheese, divided	250 mL
1 cup	egg noodles	250 mL
2	medium tomatoes, sliced	2
2 cups	chopped broccoli, blanched	500 mL

1. In a large skillet over medium-high heat, cook chicken and green onion in butter on one side until golden brown. Turn chicken to brown other side; sprinkle with lemon juice. Remove chicken. Whisk flour into pan juices; cook, stirring, for 2 minutes. Gradually whisk in milk, stirring constantly until smooth and thickened. Stir in seasonings and half of the cheese.

2. In a large pot of boiling water, cook noodles according to package directions or until tender but firm; drain well. Place cooked noodles in lightly greased oblong baking dish. Top with half of the sauce. Arrange tomato slices, broccoli and chicken on top of noodles. Cover with remaining sauce. Sprinkle with remaining cheese. Bake, uncovered, in preheated oven for about 30 minutes or until bubbling hot.

NUTRITIONAL ANALYSIS PER SERVING			
Energy: 320 kcal	Carbohydrate: 18 g	Calcium: 284 mg	Folate: 41 mcg
Protein: 27 g	Fat: 16 g	Iron: 1.6 mg	Fiber: 1.7 g

Chicken with Red Pepper and Onions

Source of:
• Iron and folate

**MAKES
4 SERVINGS**

- Preheat oven to 400°F (200°C)
- Baking dish, sprayed with nonstick vegetable spray

4	chicken breasts or legs	4
	All-purpose flour for dusting	

Sauce

1 tbsp	margarine	15 mL
1½ tsp	crushed garlic	7 mL
¾ cup	diced onion	175 mL
1½ cups	diced red bell peppers	375 mL
1 tbsp	all-purpose flour	15 mL
1⅓ cups	chicken stock	325 mL
	Parsley sprigs	

1. Dust chicken with flour. In large nonstick skillet sprayed with nonstick vegetable spray, brown chicken on both sides, approximately 10 minutes. Place in baking dish; cover and bake for 20 to 30 minutes or until no longer pink inside and juices run clear when chicken is pierced.

2. *Sauce:* Meanwhile, in small saucepan, melt margarine; sauté garlic, onion and red peppers for 5 minutes or until softened. Add flour and cook, stirring, for 1 minute. Add stock and cook, stirring, just until thickened, approximately 3 minutes.

3. Place chicken on serving dish; pour sauce over top. Garnish with parsley. Remove skin before eating.

TIPS

When using margarine, choose a soft (non-hydrogenated) version to limit consumption of trans fats.

This red pepper sauce can also be puréed.

NUTRITIONAL ANALYSIS PER SERVING

Energy: 275 kcal	Carbohydrate: 9 g	Calcium: 25 mg	Folate: 24 mcg
Protein: 21 g	Fat: 17 g	Iron: 1.8 mg	Fiber: 1.2 g

**MAKES
6 SERVINGS**

*Say "salsa" and you
probably think of
tomatoes, onions and
peppers. But this salsa
uses dried fruit —
raisins, apricots and
pears — for a delicious
change with a
Mediterranean flair.*

TIPS

For variety, try poaching
the chicken instead of
grilling. It can also be
served cold.

Like most salsas, this one
can be prepared ahead of
time. Leftovers make a
great accompaniment to
grilled meats.

Grilled Chicken Breast with Dried Fruit Salsa

Dried Fruit Salsa

1	medium red bell pepper, diced	1
⅓ cup	raisins or diced pitted prunes	75 mL
⅓ cup	diced dried apricots	75 mL
⅓ cup	diced dried pears	75 mL
¼ cup	diced red onion	50 mL
¼ cup	coarsely chopped fresh cilantro	50 mL
⅓ cup	lime juice	75 mL
1 tbsp	olive oil	15 mL
¼ tsp	each salt and freshly ground black pepper	1 mL

Chicken

6	boneless skinless chicken breasts (3 oz/90 g each)	6

1. *Dried Fruit Salsa:* In a glass bowl, combine red pepper, raisins, apricot, pears, onion, cilantro, lime juice, oil, salt and pepper. Cover and chill for at least 1 hour.

2. Preheat barbecue or grill. Grill or broil chicken for 4 to 5 minutes per side or until no longer pink inside. Serve topped with salsa.

NUTRITIONAL ANALYSIS PER SERVING			
Energy: 197 kcal	Carbohydrate: 20 g	Calcium: 28 mg	Folate: 12 mcg
Protein: 22 g	Fat: 4 g	Iron: 1.7 mg	Fiber: 1.9 g

Grilled Chicken with Curry Sauce

Source of:
• Calcium and iron

MAKES 4 SERVINGS

Here is an easy "fusion" recipe that combines a variety of toothsome flavors from around the world.

TIP

Sauce used to marinate raw meat, poultry or seafood should not be used on cooked foods as it may contain harmful bacteria. Boil leftover marinade or prepare extra for basting cooked food. Wash and sanitize your brush or use separate brushes when marinating raw and cooked foods.

Chicken

4	boneless skinless chicken breasts (about 1 lb/500 g)	4
2 tsp	grated lemon or lime zest	10 mL
1/3 cup	lemon or lime juice	75 mL
2 tbsp	chopped fresh basil (or 2 tsp/10 mL dried)	25 mL
4 tsp	Dijon mustard	20 mL
2 tsp	chopped fresh thyme (or 1/4 tsp/1 mL dried)	5 mL
	Black pepper	

Curry Sauce

1/4 cup	light mayonnaise	50 mL
1/4 cup	low-fat plain yogurt	50 mL
1 tsp	grated lime zest	5 mL
1 tbsp	lime juice	15 mL
1/2 tsp	curry powder	2 mL

1. *Chicken:* Place chicken in single layer in glass dish. Combine lemon zest and juice, basil, mustard, thyme, and pepper to taste; pour over chicken. Cover and refrigerate for 3 to 12 hours, turning chicken occasionally.

2. Preheat barbecue or grill. Remove chicken from marinade. Grill for 6 to 8 minutes per side or until no longer pink inside.

3. *Curry Sauce:* In a bowl, combine mayonnaise, yogurt, lime zest and juice, and curry powder. Serve with chicken.

NUTRITIONAL ANALYSIS PER SERVING

Energy: 162 kcal	Carbohydrate: 5 g	Calcium: 65 mg	Folate: 8 mcg
Protein: 24 g	Fat: 5 g	Iron: 1.3 mg	Fiber: 0.4 g

**MAKES
4 SERVINGS**

TIPS

You can substitute other vegetables, such as asparagus, broccoli or bean sprouts, for the snow peas.

Tender beef or veal can replace the chicken.

Chicken, Red Pepper and Snow Pea Stir-Fry

Sauce

½ cup	chicken stock	125 mL
1 tbsp	soy sauce	15 mL
1 tbsp	hoisin sauce	15 mL
2 tsp	cornstarch	10 mL
1 tsp	minced gingerroot	5 mL
8 oz	boneless skinless chicken breasts, cubed	250 g
	All-purpose flour for dusting	
1 tbsp	vegetable oil	15 mL
1 tsp	sesame oil	5 mL
1 tsp	crushed garlic	5 mL
1 cup	thinly sliced sweet red pepper	250 mL
1 cup	sliced water chestnuts	250 mL
1 cup	snow peas, cut in half	250 mL
¼ cup	cashews, coarsely chopped	50 mL
1	large green onion, chopped	1

1. *Sauce:* In small bowl, mix together stock, soy sauce, hoisin sauce, cornstarch and ginger; set aside.

2. Dust chicken cubes with flour. In nonstick skillet, heat vegetable and sesame oils; sauté garlic, chicken, red pepper, water chestnuts and snow peas over high heat just until vegetables are tender-crisp, approximately 2 minutes.

3. Add sauce to skillet; cook for 2 minutes or just until chicken is no longer pink inside and sauce has thickened. Garnish with cashews and green onions.

NUTRITIONAL ANALYSIS PER SERVING

Energy: 261 kcal	Carbohydrate: 25 g	Calcium: 41 mg	Folate: 32 mcg
Protein: 20 g	Fat: 10 g	Iron: 2.4 mg	Fiber: 3.0 g

Chicken with Black Bean Sauce and Sautéed Mushrooms

- Preheat oven to 400°F (200°C)
- Baking dish

2 tsp	vegetable oil	10 mL
4	chicken legs	4
1/3 cup	all-purpose flour	75 mL
2½ cups	sliced mushrooms	625 mL

Sauce

1 cup	chicken stock	250 mL
3 tbsp	honey	45 mL
3 tbsp	black bean sauce	45 mL
1 tbsp	soy sauce	15 mL
1 tbsp	rice wine vinegar	15 mL
1 tbsp	sesame oil	15 mL
1 tbsp	cornstarch	15 mL
2 tsp	minced garlic	10 mL
1 tsp	minced gingerroot	5 mL
½ cup	chopped green onions (about 4 medium)	125 mL

TIPS

Try using oyster mushrooms instead of regular button mushrooms.

Of the two kinds of bottled black bean sauce available — whole black bean sauce and puréed black bean garlic sauce — the whole bean sauce is lower in sodium.

Make Ahead

Prepare sauce and mushrooms earlier in the day. Add more stock if sauce is too thick.

1. In large nonstick skillet sprayed with vegetable spray, heat oil over high heat. Dust chicken pieces with flour; cook for 8 minutes, turning often, or until well browned on all sides. Transfer to baking dish. Bake for 30 to 40 minutes or until juices run clear when pierced at thickest point. Pour off fat and place on serving platter and keep covered.

2. In a nonstick skillet sprayed with vegetable spray, sauté mushrooms until just cooked (approximately 4 minutes). Drain any excess liquid and set aside.

3. Meanwhile, in saucepan whisk together stock, honey, black bean sauce, soy sauce, vinegar, sesame oil, cornstarch, garlic and ginger until smooth; cook over medium heat for 5 minutes, or until slightly thickened. Add mushrooms and pour over baked chicken. Garnish with green onions. Remove skin before eating.

NUTRITIONAL ANALYSIS PER SERVING

| Energy: 347 kcal | Carbohydrate: 29 g | Calcium: 35 mg | Folate: 55 mcg |
| Protein: 31 g | Fat: 12 g | Iron: 2.7 mg | Fiber: 1.5 mg |

**MAKES
6 SERVINGS**

To get more mono- and polyunsaturated fat in your diet, use olive, canola, safflower, corn, soybean or sunflower oils for cooking.

TIPS

This is delicious served cold.

This is a simple-looking chicken dish, but unbelievably tasty. Great for leftovers.

Increase garlic and ginger to taste.

Make Ahead

Prepare up to a day ahead and serve at room temperature.

Chinese Chicken with Garlic Ginger Sauce

3 lb	whole chicken	1.5 kg
Sauce		
1/3 cup	chicken stock	75 mL
1/4 cup	chopped green onions (about 2 medium)	50 mL
3 tbsp	vegetable oil	45 mL
4 tsp	soy sauce	20 mL
1 tsp	minced garlic	5 mL
1 tsp	minced gingerroot	5 mL

1. Remove neck and giblets from chicken and discard. Place chicken in large saucepan and add water to cover. Cover saucepan and bring to a boil over high heat. Reduce heat to low and simmer, covered, for 45 minutes, or until juices run clear from chicken leg when pierced.

2. Meanwhile, whisk together stock, green onions, oil, soya sauce, garlic and ginger in a small bowl.

3. Remove chicken from pot and let cool slightly. Remove skin; cut into serving pieces. Serve with dipping sauce.

NUTRITIONAL ANALYSIS PER SERVING			
Energy: 556 kcal	Carbohydrate: 1 g	Calcium: 28 mg	Folate: 15 mcg
Protein: 43 g	Fat: 41 g	Iron: 2.1 mg	Fiber: 0.1 g

Exotic Ginger Cumin Chicken

Source of:
• Iron and folate

MAKES 8 SERVINGS

Here's another curry-style chicken dish you can make using ingredients you're likely to have on hand.

1 tbsp	vegetable oil, divided	15 mL
2 lb	boneless skinless chicken breasts, cut into bite-size pieces	1 kg
2 tsp	minced garlic	10 mL
½ cup	chopped onion	125 mL
1 tbsp	finely chopped gingerroot (or ½ tsp/2 mL ground ginger)	15 mL
¼ to ½ tsp	cayenne pepper	1 to 2 mL
1 tsp	ground coriander	5 mL
1 tsp	ground cumin	5 mL
1 tsp	ground turmeric	5 mL
½ cup	chicken stock	125 mL
1	can (19 oz/540 mL) stewed tomatoes	1
2 tbsp	tomato paste	25 mL
2 tsp	granulated sugar	10 mL
½ tsp	salt	2 mL
¾ cup	low-fat plain yogurt	175 mL
2 tbsp	chopped fresh cilantro (optional)	25 mL

TIPS

Try using canola oil in this and other recipes calling for vegetable oil. Canola oil is high in monounsaturated fat. It is inexpensive and widely available. And because of its neutral flavor, it is an excellent all-purpose oil for baking, cooking and salad dressings.

Serve this flavorful chicken dish over basmati rice, a long-grain rice grown in India that is aged before it is husked.

1. In a large saucepan or Dutch oven, heat 2 tsp (10 mL) of the oil over medium-high heat. Add half of the chicken and cook for 2 to 3 minutes or until brown. Remove from pan and set aside. Repeat with remaining chicken.

2. Add remaining oil to pan; add garlic, onion and ginger. Reduce heat to medium and cook, stirring constantly, for 4 to 5 minutes or until softened but not brown. Stir in cayenne, coriander, cumin and turmeric; sauté for 1 minute or until fragrant.

3. Stir in stock, tomatoes, tomato paste, sugar and salt; return chicken to pan. Bring to a boil; reduce heat and simmer for 5 minutes or until chicken is no longer pink inside.

4. Stir in yogurt and cilantro, if using; simmer over very low heat for 1 to 2 minutes.

NUTRITIONAL ANALYSIS PER SERVING

Energy: 192 kcal	Carbohydrate: 10 g	Calcium: 9 mg	Folate: 15 mcg
Protein: 29 g	Fat: 4 g	Iron: 1.8 mg	Fiber: 1.1 g

MAKES 4 TO 6 SERVINGS AS AN APPETIZER

A great way to start a dinner party — especially on the seventh day of the Chinese New Year, when it's everyone's birthday. The deep-fried bean thread noodles are light and crispy and add visual drama as a garnish, especially when drizzled with colorful herb or chili oils.

Chopped Chicken in Lettuce Wrap with Crispy Glass Noodles

6	large dried Chinese mushrooms or other dried mushrooms	6
Marinade		
½ tsp	salt	2 mL
½ tsp	pepper	2 mL
1 tbsp	dry sherry	15 mL
1½ tsp	cornstarch	7 mL
1 lb	boneless skinless chicken breasts, cut in ¼-inch (5 mm) dice	500 g
2 oz	bean thread noodles	50 g
1 cup	vegetable oil	250 mL
1	small onion, diced	1
1 cup	diced carrots	250 mL
1 cup	diced celery	250 mL
1	can (6 oz/150 g) sliced water chestnuts, diced	1
¼ cup	chicken stock	50 mL
2 tsp	soy sauce	10 mL
1 tbsp	hoisin sauce	15 mL
2 tsp	sesame oil	10 mL
2 tbsp	chopped cilantro	25 mL
12 leaves	iceberg lettuce	12 leaves

1. In a heatproof bowl or pot, cover mushrooms with boiling water and soak for 15 minutes. Drain. Cut off stems and dice caps finely. Set aside.

2. In a bowl, combine ingredients for marinade. Add chicken; mix well to coat. Set aside for 20 minutes.

3. In a nonstick wok or skillet, heat oil over medium-high heat until a piece of noodle dropped into the oil puffs up, turns white and floats to the top instantly. Fry noodles in batches. Drain on paper towel and keep warm. Reserve 1 tbsp (15 mL) oil.

4. In same skillet, heat reserved oil over high heat for 30 seconds. Add onion and chicken and stir-fry for 1 minute. Reduce heat to medium-high; add mushrooms, carrots and celery and stir-fry for 1 minute. Add water chestnuts, chicken stock, soy sauce, hoisin sauce and sesame oil. Cook until vegetables are just tender and liquid is absorbed, about 1 minute. Remove from heat, add cilantro and mix.

5. *To serve:* Using kitchen shears or a pair of scissors, cut fried noodles into 1-inch (2.5 cm) strands. Line a large platter with noodles and top with chicken mixture. Arrange lettuce leaves and a small dish of extra hoisin sauce on another platter. Pass both platters around and invite diners to assemble their own wraps by placing a large spoonful of the chicken-noodle mixture and hoisin sauce on a lettuce leaf. Eat open, or rolled up.

NUTRITIONAL ANALYSIS PER SERVING

Energy: 529 kcal	Carbohydrate: 18 g	Calcium: 39 mg	Folate: 24 mcg
Protein: 24 g	Fat: 41 g	Iron: 1.3 mg	Fiber: 2.8 mg

MAKES
4 SERVINGS

TIP

Shred cabbage by cutting into thin strips, starting at the tip of the leaves. If using a green cabbage, cut the head in quarters, remove core and shred.

Shanghai Noodles with Shredded Chicken, Chinese Cabbage and a Spicy Sesame Sauce

1 lb	fresh Shanghai noodles or 8 oz (250 g) dried spaghetti	500 g
1 tbsp	vegetable oil, plus oil for coating noodles	15 mL
8 oz	boneless skinless chicken breasts	250 g
2 tbsp	cornstarch	25 mL
1 tsp	minced gingerroot	5 mL
3 cups	shredded Chinese cabbage or green cabbage	750 mL
1 tsp	minced garlic	5 mL
2 tbsp	water	25 mL
1 tbsp	dark soy sauce	15 mL
1 tbsp	chopped fresh cilantro	15 mL
1 tsp	chili paste (or to taste)	5 mL
1 tsp	sesame oil	5 mL
1 tbsp	toasted sesame seeds, plus extra seeds for garnish	15 mL
	Sliced green onion for garnish	

1. In a heatproof bowl or pot, cover noodles with boiling water and soak for 5 minutes. (If using pasta, prepare according to package directions.) Drain, toss with a little oil and set aside.

2. On a cutting board, cut chicken into thin slices and then cut each slice into thin strips. Dredge strips in cornstarch, shaking off excess starch. Set aside.

3. In a nonstick wok or skillet, heat oil over medium-high heat for 30 seconds. Add ginger and cook until it starts to sizzle. Add chicken and sauté until brown, about 4 to 5 minutes. Add cabbage and garlic and stir-fry until cabbage is wilted. Add water and noodles; toss to coat. Cook, covered, over low heat for 2 minutes. Add soy sauce, cilantro, chili paste, sesame oil and sesame seeds; toss well. Garnish with green onion and additional sesame seeds. Serve immediately.

NUTRITIONAL ANALYSIS PER SERVING			
Energy: 415 kcal	Carbohydrate: 54 g	Calcium: 163 mg	Folate: 69 mcg
Protein: 29 g	Fat: 9 g	Iron: 3.1 mg	Fiber: 3.9 mg

Chicken and Eggplant Parmesan

- Preheat oven to 425°F (220°C)
- Baking sheet, sprayed with vegetable spray

1	whole egg	1
1	egg white	1
1 tbsp	water or milk	15 mL
2/3 cup	seasoned bread crumbs	150 mL
3 tbsp	chopped fresh parsley (or 2 tsp/10 mL dried)	45 mL
1 tbsp	freshly grated Parmesan cheese	15 mL
4	crosswise slices of eggplant, skin on, approximately 1/2 inch (1 cm) thick	4
1 lb	boneless skinless chicken breasts (about 4)	500 g
2 tsp	vegetable oil	10 mL
1 tsp	minced garlic	5 mL
1/2 cup	tomato pasta sauce	125 mL
1/2 cup	grated mozzarella cheese	125 mL

1. In small bowl, whisk together whole egg, egg white and water. On plate, stir together bread crumbs, parsley and Parmesan. Dip eggplant slices in egg wash, then coat with bread crumb mixture. Place on prepared pan and bake for 20 minutes, or until tender, turning once.

2. Meanwhile, pound chicken breasts between sheets of waxed paper to 1/4-inch (5 mm) thickness. Dip chicken in remaining egg wash, then coat with remaining bread crumb mixture. Heat oil and garlic in nonstick skillet sprayed with vegetable spray and cook for 4 minutes or until golden brown, turning once.

3. Spread 1 tbsp (15 mL) of tomato sauce on each eggplant slice. Place one chicken breast on top of each eggplant slice. Spread another 1 tbsp (15 mL) of tomato sauce on top of each chicken piece. Sprinkle with cheese and bake for 5 minutes or until cheese melts.

Excellent source of:
- Fiber

Good source of:
- Calcium, iron and folate

MAKES 4 SERVINGS

Choose lean meat, fish and poultry with skins removed over high-fat deli meats, bacon and sausages.

TIPS

Turkey, veal or pork scallopini can replace chicken.

A stronger cheese, such as Swiss, can replace mozzarella.

A great dish to reheat the next day.

NUTRITIONAL ANALYSIS PER SERVING

Energy: 328 kcal	Carbohydrate: 31 g	Calcium: 205 mg	Folate: 71 mcg
Protein: 31 g	Fat: 10 g	Iron: 3.5 mg	Fiber: 6.6 mg

MAKES 4 TO 6 SERVINGS

TIPS

Serve over baked potatoes, in tortillas or tacos, or over rice or pasta.

Diced pork, beef or turkey can replace chicken.

Other varieties of canned beans can be used.

Make Ahead

Make and refrigerate up to a day ahead. Reheat gently, adding more stock if too thick.

Chicken Bean Chili

1½ tsp	vegetable oil	7 mL
1 cup	diced carrots	250 mL
1 cup	chopped onions	250 mL
1 tsp	crushed garlic	5 mL
1	can (19 oz/540 mL) tomatoes, crushed	1
2 cups	chicken stock	500 mL
2 tsp	chili powder	10 mL
1½ tsp	dried basil	7 mL
1 tsp	dried oregano	5 mL
2 tbsp	tomato paste	25 mL
¾ cup	canned white kidney beans, drained	175 mL
¾ cup	canned black beans, drained	175 mL
¾ cup	corn niblets	175 mL
8 oz	boneless skinless chicken breasts	250 g

1. In large nonstick saucepan, heat oil; sauté carrots, onions and garlic until softened, approximately 5 minutes.

2. Add tomatoes, stock, chili powder, basil, oregano, tomato paste, beans and corn. Simmer uncovered for 30 to 40 minutes, stirring occasionally.

3. Meanwhile, in small nonstick skillet sprayed with vegetable spray, sauté chicken until just cooked, approximately 3 minutes. Set aside.

4. When chili mixture is cooked, add sautéed chicken. Mix well and serve chili alone in bowl, wrapped in tortillas or on top of a baked potato sprinkled with cheese.

NUTRITIONAL ANALYSIS PER SERVING			
Energy: 167 kcal	Carbohydrate: 25 g	Calcium: 70 mg	Folate: 22 mcg
Protein: 15 g	Fat: 2 g	Iron: 2.7 mg	Fiber: 6.2 mg

Crunchy Cheese Chicken Fingers

- Preheat oven to 400°F (200°C)
- Baking sheet, sprayed with vegetable spray

1 lb	skinless boneless chicken breasts, cut into 1-inch (2 cm) strips	500 g
1½ cups	Cheerios breakfast cereal	375 mL
2 tbsp	freshly grated Parmesan cheese	25 mL
½ tsp	chili powder	2 mL
½ tsp	dried basil	2 mL
½ tsp	dried oregano	2 mL
1 tsp	minced garlic	5 mL
1	egg	1
2 tbsp	milk or water	25 mL

1. Put Cheerios, Parmesan, chili powder, basil, oregano and garlic in food processor; process until Cheerios are fine crumbs. Place on plate.

2. In small bowl, whisk together egg and milk. Dip each chicken strip in egg wash, then roll in crumbs; place on prepared baking sheet. Bake for 10 to 15 minutes until browned and chicken is cooked through.

MAKES 4 SERVINGS

TIPS

For a change — and less fat — substitute firm fish fillets (such as haddock, halibut or cod) for chicken.

Try other dried spices of your choice.

Bread crumbs or bran- or corn flakes cereal can replace Cheerios.

NUTRITIONAL ANALYSIS PER SERVING			
Energy: 248 kcal	Carbohydrate: 10 g	Calcium: 119 mg	Folate: 89 mcg
Protein: 37 g	Fat: 6 g	Iron: 5.5 mg	Fiber: 1.6 mg

**MAKES
8 SERVINGS**

Asian chili sauce is a fiery concoction of chili peppers, garlic, sugar and rice vinegar. It's really hot! So if you've got a sensitive palate, use it sparingly. This sauce also makes a good substitute in recipes that call for hot chili peppers.

TIPS

If your kids don't like rice, serve this dish over 1 lb (500 g) of spaghetti.

You can omit onions.

If you like pineapple, add 1 cup (250 mL) pineapple cubes (canned or fresh) at the end of the cooking time.

Make Ahead

Make up to 2 days ahead and reheat. Can be frozen for up to 6 weeks. Great for leftovers.

Sweet-and-Sour Chicken Meatballs over Rice

Meatballs

12 oz	ground chicken	375 g
¼ cup	finely chopped onions	50 mL
2 tbsp	ketchup	25 mL
2 tbsp	bread crumbs	25 mL
1	egg	1
2 tsp	olive oil	10 mL
2 tsp	minced garlic	10 mL
⅓ cup	chopped onions	75 mL
2 cups	tomato juice	500 mL
2 cups	pineapple juice	500 mL
½ cup	chili sauce	125 mL
2 cups	white rice	500 mL

1. In bowl, combine chicken, onions, ketchup, bread crumbs and egg; mix well. Form each 1 tbsp (15 mL) into a meatball and place on plate; set aside.

2. In large saucepan, heat oil over medium heat. Add garlic and onions and cook just until softened, approximately 3 minutes. Add tomato and pineapple juices, chili sauce and meatballs. Cover and simmer, uncovered, for 30 to 40 minutes, just until meatballs are tender.

3. Meanwhile, bring 4 cups (1 L) of water to a boil. Stir in rice, reduce heat, cover and simmer for 20 minutes or until liquid is absorbed. Remove from heat and let stand for 5 minutes, covered. Serve meatballs and sauce over rice.

NUTRITIONAL ANALYSIS PER SERVING			
Energy: 334 kcal	Carbohydrate: 52 g	Calcium: 58 mg	Folate: 75 mcg
Protein: 14 g	Fat: 8 g	Iron: 2.8 mg	Fiber: 1.9 mg

Fish and Seafood

**MAKES
4 SERVINGS**

*These are fairly
substantial burgers,
so serve them with
something light. For
young children, half
a burger will probably
be enough.*

TIP

Dipping the fish in an egg
mixture before covering
with the coating helps the
crumb mixture to stick.

Crunchy Fish Burgers

- Preheat oven to 375°F (190°C)
- Baking sheet, greased

Crunchy Coating

1 cup	crushed corn flakes cereal	250 mL
½ tsp	garlic powder	2 mL
½ tsp	dry mustard	2 mL
¼ tsp	freshly ground black pepper	1 mL

Burgers

1	egg	1
1 tbsp	water	15 mL
1 lb	fresh or frozen fish fillets (sole, perch or halibut), patted dry	500 g

Zippy Tartar Sauce

¼ cup	sweet pickle or dill pickle relish	50 mL
2 tbsp	light mayonnaise	25 mL
¼ tsp	horseradish	1 mL
4	6-inch (15 cm) submarine-type buns, halved	4
4	lettuce leaves	4
2	medium tomatoes, sliced	2

1. *Crunchy Coating:* In a heavy plastic bag, combine crumbs, garlic powder, mustard and pepper.

2. *Burgers:* In a shallow bowl, lightly beat together egg and water; set aside. Dip fish fillets in egg mixture and transfer, 1 piece at a time, to plastic bag; shake gently to coat. Place on baking sheet. Bake in preheated oven for 10 to 15 minutes or until fish is opaque and flakes easily when tested with fork.

3. *Zippy Tartar Sauce:* In a small bowl, blend together relish, mayonnaise and horseradish.

4. *Assembly:* Spread buns with tartar sauce; add fish fillets and top with lettuce and tomato.

NUTRITIONAL ANALYSIS PER SERVING			
Energy: 351 kcal	Carbohydrate: 43 g	Calcium: 53 g	Folate: 38 mcg
Protein: 31 g	Fat: 6 g	Iron: 3.2 mg	Fiber: 1.1 g

Basil and Tomato Fillets

2 tbsp	olive oil, divided	25 mL
1 lb	whitefish, tuna or salmon	500 g
	Salt and freshly ground black pepper	
½ cup	chopped firm tomatoes	125 mL
2 tbsp	chopped fresh basil leaves	25 mL

1. In a nonstick skillet over medium-high heat, heat 1 tbsp (15 mL) oil. Season fish lightly with salt and pepper. Add to skillet.

2. Combine tomatoes, basil and remaining oil. Top fish with spoonfuls of the mixture. Cover skillet tightly and cook on medium-high heat for 10 minutes or until fish is opaque and flakes easily when tested with a fork.

NUTRITIONAL ANALYSIS PER SERVING

| Energy: 207 kcal | Carbohydrate: 1 g | Calcium: 34 mg | Folate: 8 mcg |
| Protein: 22 g | Fat: 12 g | Iron: 0.5 mg | Fiber: 0.3 mg |

Good source of:
• Protein

**MAKES
4 SERVINGS**

Tomato and basil are natural partners. Add fish for a fresh, delicious meal.

Yogurt-Lime Fish Fillets

• Preheat oven to 450°F (230°C)
• Shallow oblong pan, greased

1¼ lbs	fish fillets	625 g
1	lime	1
¼ cup	plain yogurt	50 mL
1 tsp	ground cumin	5 mL
	Salt and freshly ground black pepper	

1. Place fish in prepared baking pan.

2. Grate ½ tsp (2 mL) zest from lime and squeeze out 2 tbsp (25 mL) juice, reserving extra for another use. Place zest and juice in a small bowl. Stir in yogurt, cumin and salt and pepper. Spoon over fish.

3. Bake for 10 minutes per inch (2.5 cm) of thickness or until fish is opaque and flakes easily when tested with a fork.

NUTRITIONAL ANALYSIS PER SERVING

| Energy: 226 kcal | Carbohydrate: 3 g | Calcium: 76 mg | Folate: 6 mcg |
| Protein: 31 g | Fat: 10 g | Iron: 1.0 mg | Fiber: 0.5 mg |

Source of:
• Calcium and iron

**MAKES
4 SERVINGS**

Take any fish fillet, such as salmon, whitefish, sole or turbot, add this easy sauce, and you will quickly have an elegant dinner for guests.

**MAKES
4 SERVINGS**

Any firm fish, such as swordfish, salmon, halibut or whitefish, will do for this recipe.

Ginger-Lime Fish Fillets

• Preheat broiler
• Broiler pan, lightly greased

2	limes	2
2 tbsp	grated gingerroot	25 mL
2 tbsp	liquid honey	25 mL
	Salt and freshly ground black pepper	
4	fish fillets (about ¾ inch/2 cm thick)	4

1. Grate 1 tsp (5 mL) zest from lime and squeeze out ½ cup (125 mL) juice, reserving any extra for another use. Place zest and juice in a shallow dish. Whisk in ginger, honey, and salt and pepper to taste.

2. Dip fish into lime mixture. Place on prepared broiling pan. Broil for 10 minutes or until fish is opaque and flakes easily when tested with a fork.

3. Meanwhile, in a small saucepan over medium heat, bring remaining lime mixture to a boil. Cook until reduced by half. Drizzle warm sauce over fish and serve.

NUTRITIONAL ANALYSIS PER SERVING			
Energy: 304 kcal	Carbohydrate: 13 g	Calcium: 62 mg	Folate: 9 mcg
Protein: 37 g	Fat: 11 g	Iron: 0.9 mg	Fiber: 1.0 mg

Oriental Fish Fillets

4	green onions, sliced diagonally	4
2	cloves garlic, minced	2
1 tbsp	canola oil	15 mL
4	fish fillets (turbot, cod, haddock or halibut)	4
1 tbsp	finely chopped gingerroot	15 mL
½ cup	dry sherry	125 mL
2 tbsp	soy sauce	25 mL
¼ cup	coarsely chopped fresh cilantro	50 mL

1. In a heavy skillet over high heat, cook green onions and garlic in hot oil for about 2 minutes. Remove onion mixture and add fish to skillet.

2. Combine onion mixture, ginger, sherry and soy sauce; pour over fish. Sprinkle with cilantro. Cook, covered, over medium heat for about 5 minutes or until fish flakes easily when tested with fork. Transfer fillets to preheated platter. Cook sauce over high heat until reduced and slightly thickened. Pour sauce over fish and serve.

MAKES 4 SERVINGS

In this recipe, the oriental flavors of gingerroot, soy sauce and cilantro give ordinary fish fillets a new lease on life.

TIPS

Don't confuse cilantro with parsley. They look similar, but they are different. Cilantro is the parsley-like leaf on the coriander plant. Cilantro leaves are more tender than parsley and have a zesty, almost bitter, flavor that lingers on the tongue.

To continue the oriental theme, serve this tasty fish with plain rice. Add some crisp stir-fried vegetables for added vitamins as well as fiber.

NUTRITIONAL ANALYSIS PER SERVING

Energy: 171 kcal	Carbohydrate: 4 g	Calcium: 36 mg	Folate: 15 mcg
Protein: 21 g	Fat: 4 g	Iron: 1.0 mg	Fiber: 0.2 g

**MAKES
4 SERVINGS**

Nothing could be easier than this citrus-flavored fish dish, which is ready in less than 15 minutes. Use snapper, sole or any firm white fish if halibut isn't available.

TIP

You can use frozen fish for this recipe, if desired. To cook from its frozen state, double the cooking time to 20 minutes per inch (2.5 cm) of thickness, measuring the fish from its thickest point.

South Side Halibut

• Preheat oven to 400°F (200°C)
• Baking dish

1	clove garlic, minced	1
1/3 cup	finely chopped onion	75 mL
1 tsp	vegetable oil	5 mL
2 tbsp	chopped fresh parsley	25 mL
1/2 tsp	grated orange zest	2 mL
1/8 tsp	black pepper	0.5 mL
1/4 cup	orange juice	50 mL
1 tbsp	lemon juice	15 mL
4	halibut steaks (4 oz/125 g each) or 1 lb (500 g) halibut or Pacific snapper fillets	4

1. In a small skillet, sauté garlic and onion in oil over medium heat until tender. Remove from heat; stir in parsley, orange zest and pepper. Combine orange juice and lemon juice.

2. Arrange fish in baking dish. Spread onion mixture over fish; pour juice over top. Cover tightly with foil. Bake in preheated oven for 8 to 10 minutes or until fish flakes easily when tested with fork.

NUTRITIONAL ANALYSIS PER SERVING			
Energy: 149 kcal	Carbohydrate: 3 g	Calcium: 25 mg	Folate: 27 mcg
Protein: 26 g	Fat: 3 g	Iron: 1.0 mg	Fiber: 0.3 g

Salmon Oasis

Source of:
• Iron, folate and fiber

- Preheat broiler
- Baking sheet, ungreased

4	whole wheat English muffins	4
1	can (7½ oz/213 g) salmon, drained	1
¼ cup	light mayonnaise	50 mL
2 tbsp	finely chopped green onion	25 mL
2 tsp	lemon juice	10 mL
½ tsp	curry powder	2 mL
¼ tsp	freshly ground black pepper	1 mL
8	green bell pepper strips	8
¾ cup	shredded part-skim mozzarella cheese	175 mL
	Paprika to taste	

1. Split muffins in half and toast.
2. Combine salmon, mayonnaise, onion, lemon juice, curry powder and pepper. Spread on muffin halves; top with green pepper and cheese. Sprinkle with paprika. Place on ungreased baking sheet. Broil for about 3 minutes or just until cheese melts.

MAKES 4 SERVINGS

This tasty combination of English muffins and salmon with a hint of zest makes a satisfying and delicious lunch.

NUTRITIONAL ANALYSIS PER SERVING			
Energy: 193 kcal	Carbohydrate: 15 g	Calcium: 31 mg	Folate: 21 mcg
Protein: 15 g	Fat: 8 g	Iron: 1.1 mg	Fiber: 2.2 g

**MAKES
6 SERVINGS**

Salmon has such a marvelous flavor that little else is needed in the way of seasoning. This simple herb-oil mixture makes it easy.

TIP

Whole salmon is best kept in the coldest part of the refrigerator at a temperature of less than 40°F (4°C), lightly covered with a damp towel. Store steaks, fillets and portions wrapped individually in sealed plastic bags, covered with ice.

Herb-Roasted Salmon

- Preheat oven to 450°F (230°C)
- Shallow oblong pan, greased

1	large salmon fillet (about 2 lbs/1 kg)	1
1 tbsp	olive oil	15 mL
2 tbsp	chopped fresh chives	25 mL
1 tbsp	chopped fresh tarragon or 1 tsp (5 mL) dried	15 mL
	Salt and freshly ground black pepper	

1. Place fish skin side down in prepared pan.
2. In a small bowl, combine oil, chives and tarragon. Rub half into flesh of salmon.
3. Bake for 10 minutes per inch (2.5 cm) of thickness or until fish is opaque and flakes easily when tested with a fork.
4. To serve, cut salmon in half crosswise. Lift flesh from skin with a spatula. Transfer to a platter. Discard skin, and then drizzle fish with remaining herbs and oil. Season lightly with salt and pepper.

NUTRITIONAL ANALYSIS PER SERVING			
Energy: 235 kcal	Carbohydrate: Trace	Calcium: 21 mg	Folate: 39 mcg
Protein: 30 g	Fat: 12 g	Iron: 1.2 mg	Fiber: Trace

Salmon with Spinach

- Preheat oven to 450°F (230°C)
- Shallow oblong pan, greased

1	package (10 oz/300 g) frozen chopped spinach, thawed	1
1 tbsp	grated gingerroot	15 mL
2	large white mushrooms, thickly sliced	2
	Salt and freshly ground black pepper	
4	salmon steaks or fillets (see Variations, below)	4

1. In a sieve, drain spinach, pressing with a spoon to remove excess liquid. Discard liquid. Spread spinach in bottom of prepared pan in a shape resembling the size of the fish. Arrange ginger and mushrooms evenly over spinach. Season lightly with salt and pepper. Add fish. Sprinkle lightly with salt and pepper.

2. Cover pan loosely with a tent of foil. Bake for 15 minutes or until fish is opaque and flakes easily when tested with a fork.

Variations

As well as salmon, any white or firm-fleshed fish will do. These are turbot, swordfish, halibut or tuna. For ease of serving fish fillets, cut them into serving-size pieces before baking.

Crusty Layered Salmon: Sprinkle toasted sesame seeds over the fish before baking to give it a crusty crunch.

MAKES 4 SERVINGS

Salmon will remain moist using this cooking procedure. Layer spinach and mushrooms, then top with salmon. Bake on high heat for the recommended 10 minutes per inch (2.5 cm) of thickness of the fish. Due to the extra thickness of fish and vegetables, you may need a few extra minutes of baking time.

NUTRITIONAL ANALYSIS PER SERVING			
Energy: 569 kcal	Carbohydrate: 5 g	Calcium: 156 mg	Folate: 178 mcg
Protein: 79 g	Fat: 25 g	Iron: 4.2 mg	Fiber: 2.4 mg

**MAKES
8 SERVINGS**

In this elegant recipe, salmon is smothered with seasoning, green onion and minced garlic, then poached in the oven on spinach leaves. Serve with a medley of fresh vegetables, if desired.

TIP

When buying spinach, look for crisp, unblemished and fresh-smelling leaves. Spinach that has passed its peak has an acrid and unpleasant taste. Spinach that hasn't been prewashed (the kind that comes in a cellophane bag) is very sandy, so wash loose spinach leaves well in a container of tepid water, then rinse thoroughly in a colander before using.

Smothered Salmon with Spinach

- Preheat oven to 325°F (160°C)
- 13- by 9-inch (3 L) baking dish

12	large spinach leaves	12
2 lb	whole salmon	1 kg
1 tbsp	chopped fresh dill (or 1 tsp/5 mL dried dillweed)	15 mL
½ tsp	salt	2 mL
½ tsp	freshly ground black pepper	2 mL
1 cup	cold water	250 mL
1½ tsp	margarine, melted	7 mL
1	bunch green onions, sliced (about ⅔ cup/150 mL)	1
1	clove garlic, minced	1

1. Arrange spinach leaves on bottom of baking dish. Top with salmon; sprinkle with dill, salt and pepper. Pour water and margarine over salmon. Top with green onions and garlic. Cover tightly with foil.

2. Bake in preheated oven for 25 to 30 minutes or until salmon flakes easily when tested with fork, basting twice. Arrange salmon with spinach on serving platter with pan juices.

NUTRITIONAL ANALYSIS PER SERVING

Energy: 259 kcal	Carbohydrate: 1 g	Calcium: 113 mg	Folate: 60 mcg
Protein: 26 g	Fat: 16 g	Iron: 1.5 mg	Fiber: 0.5 g

Salmon with Spicy Mayo Sauce

- Preheat oven to 400°F (200°C)
- 13-by 9-inch (3 L) baking dish, sprayed with vegetable cooking spray

1	lime	1
¼ cup	mayonnaise	50 mL
1 tsp	dried oregano	5 mL
1 tsp	ground cumin	5 mL
1 tsp	salt	5 mL
1 tsp	hot pepper sauce	5 mL
1½ lb	boneless skinless salmon fillet	750 g
2 tbsp	chopped fresh basil	25 mL

1. Squeeze juice from the lime into a small bowl. Stir in mayonnaise, oregano, cumin, salt and hot pepper sauce.

2. Place salmon in prepared baking dish and spread spicy mayo sauce over top.

3. Bake in the center of the preheated oven for about 15 minutes or until salmon is opaque and flakes easily with a fork.

Source of:
- Calcium, iron and folate

MAKES 4 SERVINGS

Serve with Thai rice or rice noodles.

NUTRITIONAL ANALYSIS PER SERVING

Energy: 224 kcal	Carbohydrate: 2 g	Calcium: 124 mg	Folate: 26 mcg
Protein: 19 g	Fat: 15 g	Iron: 1.3 mg	Fiber: 0.1 g

**MAKES
4 SERVINGS**

This dish is easy to prepare and has wonderful flavor. It's great served with Thai rice and cooked spinach.

Salmon with Asian Sauce

- Preheat oven to 425°F (220°C)

1½ lb	boneless skinless salmon fillet	750 g
4	green onions, chopped	4
¼ cup	chicken stock	50 mL
2 tbsp	orange juice	25 mL
1 tbsp	sesame oil	15 mL
1 tbsp	soy sauce	15 mL
2 tsp	grated gingerroot	10 mL

1. Place salmon fillet on a sheet of foil large enough to enclose it.
2. In a small bowl, combine onion, chicken stock, orange juice, sesame oil, soy sauce and ginger. Spread evenly over salmon. Fold foil over salmon.
3. Bake in preheated oven for about 14 minutes or until salmon is opaque and flakes easily with a fork.

NUTRITIONAL ANALYSIS PER SERVING			
Energy: 374 kcal	Carbohydrate: 3 g	Calcium: 246 mg	Folate: 24 mcg
Protein: 37 g	Fat: 23 g	Iron: 2.7 mg	Fiber: 1.0 g

Broad Egg Noodles with Salmon, Red Pepper, Orange and Ginger Cream

1 lb	fresh broad egg noodles or fresh fettuccine	500 g
	Vegetable oil for coating noodles	
1 cup	whipping (35%) cream	250 mL
1 cup	white wine	250 mL
1 tbsp	minced gingerroot	15 mL
1 tbsp	orange zest	15 mL
	Juice of 1 orange	1
2	red bell peppers, seeded and sliced	2
8 oz	salmon, cut into 1/2-inch (1 cm) cubes	250 g
	Salt and freshly ground black pepper to taste	
1 tbsp	cornstarch, dissolved in 2 tbsp (25 mL) water	15 mL
2 cups	washed chopped Chinese mustard greens or spinach, packed down	500 mL

1. In a large pot of boiling salted water, cook noodles until al dente, about 5 or 6 minutes. (If using pasta, prepare according to the package instructions.) Drain, toss with a little vegetable oil and set aside.

2. In a nonstick wok or skillet combine cream, wine, ginger, and orange zest and juice. Bring to a boil. Reduce heat to medium. Add peppers and simmer until soft, about 5 to 8 minutes.

3. Add salmon to pan and season with salt and pepper. Add dissolved cornstarch and stir until sauce thickens. Reduce heat to low and simmer for 3 to 4 minutes. Add mustard greens and noodles, toss well and serve immediately.

Source of:
- Iron, folate and fiber

MAKES 4 SERVINGS

Salmon is an amazing fish — flavorful, healthy and used in many different cuisines. Here it's part of a sophisticated noodle dish.

TIP

Toss in the salmon just before serving to preserve its silky texture and avoid overcooking.

NUTRITIONAL ANALYSIS PER SERVING

Energy: 440 kcal	Carbohydrate: 56 g	Calcium: 49 mg	Folate: 20 mcg
Protein: 15 g	Fat: 17 g	Iron: 1.7 mg	Fiber: 2.7 mg

**MAKES
4 SERVINGS**

This delicious crunchy coating seals in the flavor and works for almost any type of fish, particularly cod, halibut and trout.

TIP

The salsa is delicious — for extra bite, lace it with some chili sauce.

Cornmeal-Crusted Snapper with Tomato Ginger Lemon Salsa

Salsa

2	large ripe tomatoes, diced	2
1 tbsp	minced gingerroot	15 mL
2	green onions, thinly sliced	2
	Zest and juice of one lemon	
1 tsp	liquid honey	5 mL
	Salt and freshly ground black pepper to taste	

Fish

1 cup	yellow cornmeal	250 mL
2 tbsp	freshly grated Parmesan cheese	25 mL
1 lb	boneless skinless snapper fillets, or any firm white fish, cut into 4 equal pieces	500 g
	Salt and freshly ground black pepper to taste	
2 tbsp	vegetable oil	25 mL

1. In a small bowl, combine tomatoes, ginger, green onions, lemon zest, lemon juice and honey; mix well. Season with salt and pepper. Set aside.

2. On a plate, combine cornmeal and Parmesan cheese. Season fish with salt and pepper; dredge in cornmeal mixture until well coated.

3. In a nonstick skillet, heat oil over medium heat for 30 seconds. Add fish and fry until golden brown, about 5 minutes per side. Serve with salsa.

NUTRITIONAL ANALYSIS PER SERVING

Energy: 372 kcal	Carbohydrate: 33 g	Calcium: 94 mg	Folate: 28 mcg
Protein: 27 g	Fat: 14 g	Iron: 1.2 mg	Fiber: 3.4 mg

Pan-Roasted Tilapia

- Preheat oven to 400°F (200°C)

1½ lbs	fish fillets (tilapia, snapper or cod)	750 g
½ tsp	coarse salt	2 mL
¼ tsp	freshly ground black pepper	1 mL
¼ cup	all-purpose flour	50 mL
2 tbsp	vegetable oil, divided	25 mL
2 tbsp	finely chopped onions	25 mL
2 tsp	minced gingerroot	10 mL
1 tsp	finely chopped jalapeño pepper	5 mL
1 tsp	minced garlic	5 mL
2 tbsp	black bean sauce	25 mL
2 tbsp	chicken stock	25 mL
1	large tomato, cut into 1-inch (2.5 cm) cubes	1
Pinch	granulated sugar	Pinch
3 or 4	sprigs cilantro	3 or 4

1. With a sharp knife, score fish fillets in a crisscross pattern. Rub with salt and pepper. (If using a whole fish, make sure it's scaled and cleaned; score each side as above and rub with salt and pepper, inside and out.) Place flour in a plastic bag; add fish and toss until well coated.

2. Heat a heavy ovenproof skillet over high heat for 1 minute. Add 1 tbsp (15 mL) oil and heat until just smoking. Fry fish on each side until golden, about 1 minute per side. Place pan in oven (or transfer to a baking dish) and roast for 5 minutes (10 minutes if using a whole fish) or until fish flakes easily.

3. In a nonstick wok or skillet, heat remaining oil for 30 seconds. Add onions, ginger and jalapeño; sauté for 30 seconds. Add garlic and black bean sauce; cook, stirring, another 30 seconds. Stir in chicken stock; bring to a boil. Add tomatoes; cook, stirring, for 2 minutes. Adjust flavoring with a pinch of sugar, or to taste.

4. *To serve:* Transfer fish to a warm platter; cover evenly with sauce and garnish with cilantro.

MAKES 4 SERVINGS

Traditionally, the Chinese prefer buying fish whole and live whenever possible, as this is the ultimate standard of freshness. Unfortunately, demand and availability has driven up the prices of many wild species to the point where their use has become a luxury. Farmed tilapia is available live in Asian fish markets and is reasonably priced. If possible, buy a whole fish; otherwise, tilapia fillets or those of other firm-fleshed white fish make suitable substitutes.

NUTRITIONAL ANALYSIS PER SERVING

Energy: 261 kcal	Carbohydrate: 9 g	Calcium: 43 mg	Folate: 38 mcg
Protein: 35 g	Fat: 9 g	Iron: 1.3 mg	Fiber: 1.0 mg

**MAKES
4 SERVINGS**

In this simple but delicious dish, thin rice stick noodles are combined with a distinctly West Coast combination of crab, tomatoes and basil. Although best with fresh crab, a can of snow crab, lightly rinsed in water to reduce the salt, will do just fine.

Rice Stick Noodles with Crab in a Basil-Tomato Sauce

8 oz	thin vermicelli (thin rice stick noodles) or spaghettini	250 g
1 tbsp	extra-virgin olive oil, plus oil for coating noodles	15 mL
1	can (19 oz/398 mL) tomatoes, including juice	1
1	onion, diced	1
1 tsp	minced garlic	5 mL
4 oz	fresh or canned crabmeat	125 g
2 tbsp	finely chopped basil (or ½ tsp/1 mL dried)	25 mL
	Salt and freshly ground black pepper to taste	

1. In a heatproof bowl or pot, cover noodles with boiling water and soak for 3 minutes. (If using pasta, prepare according to package instructions.) Drain, toss with a little olive oil and set aside.

2. In a medium-sized bowl, crush tomatoes with a fork (or process on and off in a food processor) until they are in bite-sized pieces.

3. In a nonstick wok or skillet, heat oil over medium-high heat for 30 seconds. Add onions and garlic and cook, stirring often, until onions have softened and are just beginning to color, about 5 minutes. Add tomatoes and their juice. Increase heat and cook until liquid is reduced and sauce is slightly thickened, about 5 minutes.

4. Reduce heat to a gentle simmer, add the crab, stir, and cook for 2 to 3 minutes. Add basil and noodles and mix well to distribute the sauce. Season with salt and pepper; serve immediately.

NUTRITIONAL ANALYSIS PER SERVING			
Energy: 328 kcal	Carbohydrate: 61 g	Calcium: 117 mg	Folate: 15 mcg
Protein: 11 g	Fat: 4 g	Iron: 3.6 mg	Fiber: 3.4 mg

Shrimp and Mussels with Couscous

1 tbsp	olive oil	15 mL
1 cup	sliced leeks (green and white parts)	250 mL
½ cup	diced carrots	125 mL
1	can (19 oz/540 mL) stewed tomatoes	1
1 tsp	minced garlic	5 mL
1 cup	green bell pepper strips	250 mL
1 lb	fresh mussels, cleaned and debearded	500 g
1½ cups	quick-cooking couscous	375 mL
12	large cooked shrimp	12

1. In a large saucepan or Dutch oven, heat oil over medium-high heat. Add leeks and sauté for 2 to 3 minutes. Add carrots, tomatoes and garlic; bring to a boil. Cover, reduce heat and simmer for 10 minutes.

2. Add green pepper strips and mussels; cook, covered, for about 5 minutes or until mussels have opened. Discard any mussels that haven't opened.

3. Meanwhile, cook couscous according to package directions.

4. Add shrimp to mussel mixture; cook for 2 minutes or until heated through. Serve over couscous.

Excellent source of:
- Iron and fiber

Good source of:
- Calcium and folate

MAKES 4 SERVINGS

Here's a dish that is as delicious as it is easy to prepare! The couscous makes a great accompaniment — and it's ready in minutes.

TIPS

Mussels should be rinsed in several changes of cold water to rid them of any grit. If still intact, the beard from the outer mussel shells should be removed by scrubbing with a hard brush prior to cooking. Inspect mussels before cooking and discard any with shells that are broken or any that do not close when tapped: these are not safe to eat. Likewise, discard any that have not opened after cooking.

Enjoy adding different varieties of grains to your diet. Couscous is made from hard durum semolina wheat. It is popular in Middle Eastern cooking, particularly in Moroccan cuisine, where it is traditionally served with a stew known as tagine. It is widely available in supermarkets, health food stores and specialty food shops.

NUTRITIONAL ANALYSIS PER SERVING

Energy: 491 kcal	Carbohydrate: 73 g	Calcium: 222 mg	Folate: 51 mcg
Protein: 33 g	Fat: 7 g	Iron: 7.6 mg	Fiber: 6.6 g

**MAKES
4 SERVINGS AS
A MAIN COURSE
OR 6 SERVINGS
AS A STARTER**

This dish is a wonderful mixture of Indonesian spices and mussels in a complex tomato broth. Try cooking it in a Chinese sand hotpot and serve from the container along with a loaf of crusty sourdough bread.

Mussels in a Spiced Tomato Broth with Bean Thread Noodles

2 oz	bean thread noodles or angel hair pasta	50 g
Broth		
1 tbsp	vegetable oil	15 mL
1	onion, finely diced	1
1 tbsp	minced garlic	15 mL
1 tbsp	minced ginger root	15 mL
1 tsp	coriander seeds	5 mL
1 tsp	anise seeds	5 mL
1 tsp	mustard seeds	5 mL
1	cinnamon stick (or 1 tsp/5 mL ground cinnamon)	1
1	stalk lemongrass, coarsely chopped, or 1 tbsp (15 mL) lemon zest	1
4 cups	tomato juice	1 L
2 cups	chicken or vegetable stock or clam juice	500 mL
	Hot pepper sauce to taste	
	Salt and freshly ground black pepper to taste	
2 lbs	fresh mussels	1 kg
	Chopped cilantro to taste	

1. In a heatproof bowl or pot, cover noodles with boiling water and soak for 3 minutes. Drain. (If using pasta, prepare according to package directions, drain and coat with a little oil.) Set aside.

2. *Broth:* In a large pot, heat oil over medium-high heat for 30 seconds. Add onion and cook until it softens and begins to change color. Add garlic and ginger; sauté for 1 minute. Add coriander, anise and mustard seeds; toss while heating through to release flavors.

3. Add cinnamon, lemongrass, tomato juice and stock or clam juice; bring mixture to a boil. Reduce heat and simmer for 15 minutes. Season to taste with hot pepper sauce, salt and pepper. If possible, allow mixture to stand for 30 minutes to develop flavor. Strain broth through a fine-mesh strainer and return to pot.

4. Bring broth back to a boil. Add mussels and noodles; cook until the mussels open. (Discard any that don't open.) Remove from heat and transfer to warm bowls. Sprinkle with chopped cilantro and serve.

NUTRITIONAL ANALYSIS PER SERVING

Energy: 350 kcal	Carbohydrate: 37 g	Calcium: 113 mg	Folate: 154 mcg
Protein: 31 g	Fat: 9 g	Iron: 11.5 mg	Fiber: 3.2 mg

**MAKES
4 SERVINGS**

*This easy shrimp filling
is absolutely delicious!*

Seafood Quesadillas

8	medium flour tortillas	8
½ cup	shredded Monterey Jack cheese	125 mL
1	can (4 oz/113 g) salad shrimp, drained and mashed (see Variations, below)	1
¼ cup	salsa, mild, medium or hot	50 mL

1. Place 4 tortillas on a flat surface.
2. In a bowl, combine cheese, shrimp and salsa. Divide mixture equally over each tortilla, spreading to the edge. Top with remaining 4 tortillas. Press edges gently to seal.
3. Heat a nonstick skillet over medium-high heat. One at a time, cook tortillas, turning once, until browned and cheese is melted. Remove from pan. Continue with remaining tortillas. Using a pizza cutter or a sharp knife, cut each tortilla into quarters and serve.

Variations

Any canned seafood, such as salmon, tuna, lobster or crabmeat, can replace the shrimp.

NUTRITIONAL ANALYSIS PER SERVING

| Energy: 294 kcal | Carbohydrate: 34 g | Calcium: 138 mg | Folate: 76 mcg |
| Protein: 13 g | Fat: 11 g | Iron: 2.5 mg | Fiber: 2.0 mg |

Vegetarian Main Courses

**MAKES
6 SERVINGS**

Quinoa (pronounced keen-wa) is a seed-like grain, available from health food stores, that originates from the Andes Mountains in South America. Here, its slightly crunchy texture and nutty flavor add a new twist to a conventional stir-fry.

TIPS

Quinoa is rich in plant fat and, like seeds and nuts, it spoils easily. Store in an airtight glass container no longer than a month, or in the refrigerator or freezer.

Although on their own plant sources of protein do not contain the complete array of amino acids that your body needs, vegetarians can ensure a full complement of protein every day by combining grains such as quinoa and couscous with legumes such as kidney beans and lentils.

Vegetable Quinoa

1 cup	quinoa	250 mL
1 cup	boiling water	250 mL
¼ cup	diced tomatoes	50 mL
¼ cup	carrot strips	50 mL
¼ cup	chopped broccoli	50 mL
¼ cup	cauliflower florets	50 mL
¼ cup	diced zucchini	50 mL
2 tbsp	sunflower oil	25 mL
1 tbsp	soy sauce	15 mL

1. Rinse quinoa under cold water until water runs clear. In a medium saucepan, add quinoa to boiling water; cover and simmer for about 15 minutes or until tender. (Watch carefully to prevent sticking.)

2. In a skillet over medium-high heat, stir-fry tomatoes, carrot, broccoli, cauliflower and zucchini in oil for about 4 minutes. Stir vegetables and soy sauce into quinoa and serve immediately.

NUTRITIONAL ANALYSIS PER SERVING

Energy: 148 kcal	Carbohydrate: 21 g	Calcium: 23 mg	Folate: 21 mcg
Protein: 4 g	Fat: 6 g	Iron: 2.8 mg	Fiber: 2 g

Greens and Grains Gratin

- Preheat oven to 350°F (180°C)

⅓ cup	bulgur	75 mL
⅓ cup	millet (or more bulgur)	75 mL
1⅓ cup	boiling water	325 mL
1	bunch greens (such as spinach, collard greens, Swiss chard)	1
4 tsp	olive oil, divided	20 mL
6	cloves garlic, minced	6
	Salt and freshly ground black pepper	
2 cups	shredded old Cheddar cheese, divided	500 mL
¼ cup	dry bread crumbs	50 mL
¼ cup	finely chopped nuts (such as almonds)	50 mL
2 tbsp	minced fresh flat-leaf parsley	25 mL

1. In a heatproof bowl, combine bulgur and millet. Pour in boiling water, cover and let stand for 15 minutes. Drain off any excess water.

2. Meanwhile, clean greens and tear into small pieces.

3. In ovenproof skillet, heat 1 tbsp (15 mL) of the olive oil over medium-low heat. Sauté garlic until golden, about 2 minutes. Add grains and greens; sauté until grains are slightly browned and greens are wilted, about 5 minutes. Season to taste with salt and pepper. Remove from heat. Transfer half of the mixture to a bowl and set aside.

4. Spread the remaining mixture in the bottom of the skillet. Top with 1 cup (250 mL) of the cheese. Spread reserved half of mixture over cheese.

5. In a small bowl, combine the remaining 1 tsp (5 mL) oil, the remaining 1 cup (250 mL) cheese, bread crumbs, nuts and parsley. Spread evenly over grains mixture.

6. Bake in preheated oven for 30 minutes or until cheese is bubbly and top is golden brown.

MAKES 6 SERVINGS

Get glowing reviews for greens! This hearty dish makes a delicious meal when served with a baked potato, or stands out as a superb side dish.

TIP

The gratin can be made ahead through Step 4; cover and refrigerate for up to 8 hours. You may need to increase the baking time by 10 minutes, but check it after 30 minutes.

NUTRITIONAL ANALYSIS PER SERVING			
Energy: 303 kcal	Carbohydrate: 20 g	Calcium: 309 mg	Folate: 27 mcg
Protein: 14 g	Fat: 19 g	Iron: 1.6 mg	Fiber: 2.8 mg

**MAKES
4 SERVINGS**

Serve this simple gratin with sliced tomatoes in vinaigrette or roasted red peppers tossed in extra-virgin olive oil for a tasty meal.

TIP

To clean leeks: Fill sink full of lukewarm water. Split leeks in half lengthwise and submerge in water, swishing them around to remove all traces of dirt. Transfer to a colander and rinse under cold water.

Leek, Potato and Mushroom Gratin

- Large (minimum 5 quart) slow cooker, greased

2 tbsp	butter, divided	25 mL
8 oz	shiitake mushrooms, stems removed, caps thinly sliced	250 g
2	medium potatoes, peeled and thinly sliced	2
3	leeks, white part only, cleaned and thinly sliced (see Tip, at left)	3
1 tbsp	minced garlic	15 mL
1 tsp	dried thyme	5 mL
1 tsp	salt	5 mL
	Freshly ground black pepper, to taste	
1 tbsp	all-purpose flour	15 mL
1½ cups	vegetable stock	375 mL

Topping

1 cup	bread crumbs	250 mL
½ cup	freshly grated Parmesan cheese (optional)	125 mL
1 tsp	paprika	5 mL
¼ tsp	salt	1 mL
	Freshly ground black pepper, to taste	
2 tbsp	melted butter	25 mL

1. In a skillet, melt 1 tbsp (15 mL) butter over medium heat. Add mushrooms and cook, stirring, just until they begin to release their liquid. Remove from heat. Spread potatoes in layers evenly over bottom of prepared slow cooker. Spread mushrooms evenly over top of potatoes.

2. Return skillet to element. Add remaining butter and leeks and cook, stirring, until leeks are softened, about 4 minutes. Add garlic, thyme, salt and pepper and cook, stirring, for 1 minute. Add flour and cook, stirring, for 1 minute. Add vegetable stock and cook, stirring, until mixture thickens, about 3 minutes. Pour over contents of stoneware.

3. Cover and cook on Low for 8 hours or on High for 4 hours, until potatoes are tender.

4. *Topping:* In a bowl, combine bread crumbs, Parmesan, if using, paprika, salt and pepper. Mix well. Add butter and stir to blend. Spread mixture evenly over leeks. Cover, leaving lid slightly ajar to prevent accumulated moisture from dripping on the topping, and cook on High for 30 minutes, until cheese is melted and mixture is hot and bubbling.

Variation

Creamy Leek, Potato and Mushroom Gratin: For a creamier version of this gratin, bring ½ to 1 cup (125 to 250 mL) of whipping (35%) cream to a boil on the stovetop or in the microwave. Pour over the cooked vegetables just before adding the topping. Proceed with Step 4.

Make ahead

This dish can be partially assembled the night before it is cooked. Complete Steps 1 and 2. Cover and refrigerate overnight. The next morning, continue cooking as directed.

NUTRITIONAL ANALYSIS PER SERVING			
Energy: 545 kcal	Carbohydrate: 93 g	Calcium: 263 mg	Folate: 180 mcg
Protein: 17 g	Fat: 16 g	Iron: 5.0 mg	Fiber: 11.0 g

**MAKES
4 SERVINGS**

This tasty and nutritious combination of sweet potatoes, carrots and pineapple, finished with a chickpea topping makes a delightfully different main course. Refrigerate any leftovers and transform them into an interesting side dish. Simply purée in a food processor fitted with a metal blade, then reheat in the microwave or over low heat on the stovetop.

Make ahead

This dish can be partially prepared the night before it is cooked. Complete Steps 1 and 2. Cover and refrigerate overnight. The next morning, continue with Step 3.

Sweet Potatoes and Carrots with Chickpea Topping

- Large (minimum 5 quart) slow cooker, greased

2	sweet potatoes, peeled and cut into ½-inch (1 cm) cubes	2
6	carrots, peeled and thinly sliced	6
1	can (14 oz/398 mL) crushed pineapple, drained, ¼ cup (50 mL) syrup set aside	1
2 tbsp	packed brown sugar	25 mL

Topping

1	can (14 to 19 oz/398 to 540 mL) chickpeas, drained and rinsed, or 2 cups (500 mL) cooked chickpeas, drained and rinsed	1
1 tbsp	minced garlic	15 mL
½ cup	vegetable stock	125 mL
	Salt and freshly ground pepper, to taste	

1. In prepared stoneware, combine sweet potato, carrots and pineapple. In a small bowl, combine brown sugar and reserved pineapple juice. Add to stoneware and stir to blend.

2. *Topping:* In a food processor fitted with a metal blade, process chickpeas, garlic and vegetable broth until mixture is well combined, but chickpeas are still a little chunky. Season with salt and pepper. Spread mixture evenly over sweet potato mixture.

3. Cover and cook on Low for 8 hours or on High for 4 hours until vegetables are tender.

NUTRITIONAL ANALYSIS PER SERVING			
Energy: 332 kcal	Carbohydrate: 70 g	Calcium: 107 mg	Folate: 170 mcg
Protein: 10 g	Fat: 3 g	Iron: 3.9 mg	Fiber: 12.0 g

Potatoes with Creamy Corn Topping

- Large (minimum 5 quart) slow cooker, greased

4 cups	corn kernels, thawed if frozen	1 L
½ cup	evaporated milk	125 mL
1 tbsp	butter	15 mL
½ tsp	freshly grated nutmeg	2 mL
	Freshly ground black pepper, to taste	
1 cup	shredded mozzarella	250 mL
1	can (28 oz/796 mL) tomatoes, including juice	1
½ cup	loosely packed parsley leaves	125 mL
1 tsp	salt	5 mL
4	medium potatoes, thinly sliced, preferably with a mandoline	4
1	red onion, halved and thinly sliced on the vertical	1

1. In a food processor, combine corn and evaporated milk. Process until combined, but corn is still a little chunky.

2. In a skillet, melt butter over medium-low heat. Add corn mixture and cook until thickened, about 5 minutes. Add nutmeg, pepper and mozzarella and stir until cheese is melted. Set aside.

3. Rinse out food processor work bowl. Add tomatoes with juice, parsley and salt and process until smooth.

4. Spread potatoes evenly over bottom of prepared slow cooker stoneware. Spread red onion over top and cover with tomato mixture.

5. Spread corn mixture evenly over top of tomato mixture. Cover and cook on Low for 8 hours or High for 4 hours, until potatoes are tender and mixture is hot and bubbling.

Excellent source of:
- Calcium

Good source of:
- Folate and fiber

Source of:
- Iron

MAKES 6 TO 8 SERVINGS

This dish reminds me of scalloped potatoes, a childhood favorite, dressed up to become a main course. It's much lighter and more nutritious than that old favorite and has an abundance of interesting flavors. Add a green salad or crisp green beans, sprinkled with toasted sesame seeds to complete the meal.

Make ahead

This dish can be partially prepared before it is cooked. Complete Steps 1 through 4. Cover and refrigerate corn mixture and stoneware separately. The next morning, continue cooking as directed in Step 5.

NUTRITIONAL ANALYSIS PER SERVING

Energy: 269 kcal	Carbohydrate: 37 g	Calcium: 336 mg	Folate: 61 mcg
Protein: 15 g	Fat: 9 g	Iron: 1.8 mg	Fiber: 4.7 g

**MAKES
6 SERVINGS**

Loaded with healthy vegetables and beans, vegetarian chili is a great dish for those of us who are trying to eat less fat and increase dietary fiber. This delicious version combines fresh green beans with dried beans and adds corn kernels and sautéed zucchini for a tasty finish.

TIPS

Substitute cranberry, romano or red kidney beans for the pinto beans, if desired.

Crush cumin seeds in a mortar with a pestle or on a cutting board, using the bottom of a measuring cup.

Two-Bean Chili with Zucchini

• Large (minimum 5 quart) slow cooker

2	dried ancho chili peppers	2
2 cups	boiling water	500 mL
1 tbsp	vegetable oil	15 mL
2	small zucchini, cut into ½-inch (1 cm) lengths and sweated	2
2	onions, finely chopped	2
2	cloves garlic, minced	2
1 tbsp	cumin seeds, coarsely crushed (see Tip, at left)	15 mL
1 tbsp	dried oregano	15 mL
1 tsp	salt	5 mL
½ tsp	cracked black peppercorns	2 mL
1	can (28 oz/796 mL) tomatoes, including juice, coarsely chopped	1
2 cups	green beans, cut into 2-inch (5 cm) lengths	500 mL
1	can (14 to 19 oz/398 to 540 mL) pinto beans, drained and rinsed, or 1 cup (250 mL) dried pinto beans, cooked and drained	1
1½ cups	corn kernels	375 mL
1 cup	shredded Monterey Jack cheese (optional)	250 mL
	Sour cream (optional)	
	Finely chopped cilantro	

1. In a heatproof bowl, soak ancho chilies in boiling water for 30 minutes. Drain, discarding soaking liquid and stems. Pat dry, chop finely and set aside.

2. In a skillet, heat oil over medium heat. Add zucchini and cook, stirring, until it begins to brown. Transfer to a bowl using a slotted spoon, cover and refrigerate.

3. In same skillet, add onions and cook, stirring, until softened, about 3 minutes. Add garlic, cumin seeds, oregano, reserved ancho chilies, salt and peppercorns and cook, stirring, for 1 minute. Add tomatoes, with juice, and green beans and bring to a boil. Transfer to slow cooker stoneware. Add beans and stir to combine.

4. Cover and cook on Low for 8 hours or on High for 4 hours, until mixture is bubbling and hot. Stir in corn and reserved zucchini. Cover and cook on High for 20 minutes, until zucchini is heated through. Ladle into bowls and top with cheese or sour cream, if using. Garnish with cilantro.

Make ahead

This chili can be partially prepared the night before it is cooked. Complete Steps 1 through 3. Cover and refrigerate overnight. The next morning, continue with Step 4.

NUTRITIONAL ANALYSIS PER SERVING			
Energy: 226 kcal	Carbohydrate: 41 g	Calcium: 133 mg	Folate: 38 mcg
Protein: 10 g	Fat: 4 g	Iron: 4.5 mg	Fiber: 10.6 mg

**MAKES
4 SERVINGS**

The tomato sauce from this recipe is so delicious, you may want to make it alone and use it over pasta, fish or vegetables. This is one recipe you will be sure to make over and over again!

Zucchini Parmesan

• Preheat oven to 300°F (150°C)
• 9-inch (2.5 L) glass baking dish

2 tbsp	vegetable oil (approx.)	25 mL
2½ lbs	zucchini (about 5), julienned	1.25 kg
2	large tomatoes, quartered, cored and seeded	2
1	small onion	1
½ cup	tomato paste	125 mL
1 tbsp	chopped fresh parley	15 mL
	Salt and freshly grated black pepper to taste	
1 cup	freshly grated Parmesan cheese	250 mL
4 oz	mozzarella cheese, thinly sliced	125 g
1	egg, beaten	1

1. In a large skillet, heat oil over medium-high heat until hot, but not smoking. Pat zucchini dry and sauté, in batches, until it begins to color, about 3 minutes. Remove with a slotted spoon to a plate lined with paper towels. Repeat, adding oil as necessary between batches.

2. In a food processor, purée tomatoes, onion, tomato paste and parsley until smooth. Season with salt and pepper.

3. Spread one-quarter of the tomato mixture over bottom of baking dish. Spread one-third of the zucchini on top, then one-third of the Parmesan, then half the mozzarella. Whisk egg into the remaining sauce and pour one-third into the pan. Repeat layers as follows: zucchini, Parmesan, mozzarella, sauce, zucchini, sauce, Parmesan.

4. Bake in preheated oven for 1 hour, until top is brown and crusty.

NUTRITIONAL ANALYSIS PER SERVING

Energy: 199 kcal	Carbohydrate: 12 g	Calcium: 432 mg	Folate: 44 mcg
Protein: 16 g	Fat: 10 g	Iron: 1.5 mg	Fiber: 3.5 g

Wild Rice with Mushrooms and Apricots

• 3½ to 6 quart slow cooker, greased

1 tbsp	vegetable oil	15 mL
1	onion, chopped	1
4	stalks celery, diced	4
2	cloves garlic, minced	2
1 cup	wild rice and brown rice mixture, rinsed (see Tip, at right)	250 mL
8 oz	portobello or cremini mushrooms stems removed and caps diced	250 g
	Salt and freshly ground black pepper, to taste	
2 cups	vegetable stock	500 mL
1 tbsp	balsamic vinegar	15 mL
¼ cup	chopped dried apricots	50 mL
	Chutney	

1. In a skillet, heat oil over medium heat. Add onion and celery and cook, stirring, until softened, about 5 minutes. Add garlic and rice and stir until coated. Stir in mushrooms and salt and pepper. Add stock and balsamic vinegar and bring to a boil. Transfer to prepared slow cooker. Stir in apricots.

2. Place two clean tea towels, each folded in half (so you will have four layers), over top of slow cooker stoneware (see Tip, at right). Cover and cook on Low for 7 to 8 hours or on High for 4 hours, until rice is tender and liquid has been absorbed. Serve hot accompanied by your favorite fruit chutney.

Good source of:
• Iron and fiber

Source of:
• Folate

MAKES 4 SERVINGS

This combination of wild and brown rice with dried apricots makes a tasty weeknight meal. Be sure to serve it with a good chutney alongside — tomato or spicy mango work very well. A grated carrot salad is a nice accompaniment.

TIPS

You can purchase wild and brown rice mixtures in many supermarkets, or you can make your own by combining ½ cup (125 mL) of each.

Accumulated moisture affects the consistency of the rice. The folded tea towels will absorb the moisture generated during cooking.

NUTRITIONAL ANALYSIS PER SERVING			
Energy: 257 kcal	Carbohydrate: 47 g	Calcium: 43 mg	Folate: 37 mcg
Protein: 7 g	Fat: 5 g	Iron: 2.7 mg	Fiber: 4.0 g

**MAKES
6 SERVINGS**

*Your family will love
this tasty one-pot dinner.
Add a green, shredded
carrot or sliced tomato
salad, if you prefer,
but if you're pressed
for time, just serve hot,
crusty rolls. This is an
ideal meal for those
evenings when everyone
is coming and going at
different times, as it
can be kept warm in the
slow cooker and people
can help themselves.*

Cheesy Rice and Mushroom Casserole with Spinach

• Large (minimum 5 quart) slow cooker

1 tbsp	cumin seeds	15 mL
1 tbsp	vegetable oil	15 mL
2	onions, finely chopped	2
4	stalks celery, peeled and thinly sliced	4
2	cloves garlic, minced	2
1 tbsp	minced gingerroot	15 mL
1 tsp	salt	5 mL
1 tsp	crushed black peppercorns	5 mL
2 cups	long-grain brown rice	500 mL
1/4 cup	oil-packed sun-dried tomatoes, finely chopped	50 mL
1	can (28 oz/796 mL) tomatoes, including juice, coarsely chopped	1
3 cups	vegetable stock	750 mL
2	large portobello mushrooms, stems removed, caps cut into 1/2-inch (1 cm) cubes	2
8 oz	fresh spinach leaves or 1 package (10 oz/300 g) spinach, washed, stems removed and chopped	250 g
2 cups	shredded Cheddar cheese	500 mL

1. In a dry skillet over medium heat, toast cumin seeds until they release their aroma and just begin to turn brown. Transfer to a mortar or a spice grinder and grind coarsely. Set aside.

2. In a skillet, heat oil over medium heat. Add onions and celery and cook, stirring, until softened, about 5 minutes. Add garlic, ginger, reserved cumin, salt, peppercorns and rice and cook, stirring, for 1 minute. Add sun-dried tomatoes, tomatoes, with juice, and vegetable stock and bring to a boil.

3. Place mushrooms in slow cooker stoneware. Pour rice mixture over mushrooms and stir to combine.

4. Place two clean tea towels, each folded in half (so you will have four layers), across the top of slow cooker stoneware. Cover and cook on Low for 7 to 8 hours or High for 4 hours, until rice is tender and has absorbed the liquid. Remove tea towels. Stir in spinach and sprinkle cheese over top of mixture. Cover and cook on High for 20 to 25 minutes, until spinach is cooked and cheese is melted. Serve piping hot.

TIP

Accumulated moisture affects the consistency of the rice. The folded tea towels will absorb the moisture generated during cooking.

Make ahead

This dish can be partially prepared the night before it is cooked. Cut mushrooms. Cover and refrigerate. Complete Steps 1 and 2. Cover and refrigerate overnight. The next day, continue cooking as directed in Step 3.

NUTRITIONAL ANALYSIS PER SERVING			
Energy: 306 kcal	Carbohydrate: 23 g	Calcium: 369 mg	Folate: 105 mcg
Protein: 14 g	Fat: 18 g	Iron: 3.0 mg	Fiber: 4.0 g

**MAKES 4 TO
6 SERVINGS**

This is a variation of spanakorizo (spinach-rice), a rustic winter staple of the eastern Mediterranean, where spinach is one of the leafy vegetables that keep growing in the cold months. The lentils are my own addition, but they are in keeping with the traditions of this kind of cuisine. They also bolster this dish into main-course status.

TIP

The lentils-rice-spinach can be served immediately, or it can wait for up to 2 hours, covered and unrefrigerated.

Lentils-Rice-Spinach

¼ cup	olive oil	50 mL
¼ tsp	salt	1 mL
¼ tsp	freshly ground black pepper	1 mL
2 cups	diced onion	500 mL
1	medium tomato, cubed	1
4 cups	chopped fresh spinach leaves, packed down	1 L
1½ cups	cooked rice (½ cup/125 mL uncooked rice)	375 mL
2 cups	cooked green lentils	500 mL
1	lemon, cut into wedges	1

1. In a pot or large skillet, heat oil over high heat for 30 seconds. Add salt and pepper and stir for 30 seconds. Add onions and stir-fry for 2 minutes, until softened. Add cubed tomato and stir-fry for 1 minute.

2. Add all the spinach at once; cook, turning over several times, until spinach has been reduced to one-third of its volume, about 1 minute.

3. Reduce heat to medium-low and add rice and lentils. Stir-cook for 3 to 4 minutes, until well mixed and everything is piping hot. Remove from heat, cover and let rest for 5 to 6 minutes as it develops flavor. Serve with lemon wedges on the side.

NUTRITIONAL ANALYSIS PER SERVING			
Energy: 232 kcal	Carbohydrate: 34 g	Calcium: 31 mg	Folate: 38 mcg
Protein: 8 g	Fat: 8 g	Iron: 1.4 mg	Fiber: 8.3 mg

Lentil Shepherd's Pie

- Large (minimum 5 quart) slow cooker

1 tbsp	vegetable oil	15 mL
2 cups	finely chopped onions	500 mL
4	stalks celery, thinly sliced	4
2	large carrots, peeled and thinly sliced	2
1 tbsp	finely chopped garlic	15 mL
1 tsp	salt	5 mL
½ tsp	dried thyme	2 mL
½ tsp	cracked black peppercorns	2 mL
1½ cups	brown or green lentils, rinsed	375 mL
1	can (28 oz/796 mL) tomatoes, including juice, coarsely chopped	1
2 cups	vegetable stock	500 mL

Topping

4 cups	mashed potatoes (see Tip, at right)	1 L
1 cup	dry bread crumbs	250 mL
½ cup	shredded Cheddar cheese (optional)	125 mL

1. In a large skillet, heat oil over medium heat. Add onions, celery and carrots and cook, stirring, for 7 minutes, until vegetables are softened. Add garlic, salt, thyme and peppercorns and cook, stirring, for 1 minute. Add lentils and tomatoes with juice and bring to boil. Transfer to slow cooker stoneware and stir in vegetable stock.

2. *Topping:* In a bowl, combine mashed potatoes and bread crumbs. Mix well. Spread mixture evenly over lentil mixture. Sprinkle cheese over top, if using. Cover and cook on Low for 7 to 8 hours or on High for 3 to 4 hours, until hot and bubbling.

Excellent source of:
- Fiber

Good source of:
- Iron and folate

Source of:
- Calcium

MAKES 6 TO 8 SERVINGS

This flavorful combination is the ultimate comfort food dish. Don't worry if you're serving fewer people — the leftovers taste great reheated.

TIP

You can use leftover mashed potatoes in this recipe or even prepared mashed potatoes from the supermarket. However, if your potatoes contain milk, don't add the topping mixture to the slow cooker until the mixture has cooked. Spread topping over the hot lentil mixture. Cover and cook on High for 30 minutes, until the potatoes are hot and the cheese has melted.

Make ahead

This recipe can be partially prepared the night before it is cooked. Complete Step 1 and refrigerate overnight. The next day, continue cooking as directed.

NUTRITIONAL ANALYSIS PER SERVING

Energy: 260 kcal	Carbohydrate: 48 g	Calcium: 113 mg	Folate: 50 mcg
Protein: 10 g	Fat: 4 g	Iron: 2.3 mg	Fiber: 6.1 mg

**MAKES
6 SERVINGS**

Shredded carrots and red pepper add a burst of color to this tasty loaf, which is also good served cold.

TIP

Use 1 can (14 to 19 oz/ 398 to 540 mL) green or brown lentils, drained and rinsed.

Make ahead

This loaf can be partially prepared before it is cooked. Complete Steps 1, 2 and 3. Refrigerate overnight. The next day, continue with Step 4.

Cashew Lentil Loaf

• Large (minimum 5 quart) slow cooker

1 tbsp	cumin seeds	15 mL
1 tbsp	vegetable oil	15 mL
1	large onion, finely chopped	1
2	stalks celery, diced	2
2 cups	shredded carrots	500 mL
2	cloves garlic, minced	2
1	red bell pepper, diced	1
½ to 1	long red or green chili pepper, diced	½ to 1
1 tsp	salt	5 mL
½ tsp	cracked black peppercorns	2 mL
2 cups	cooked green or brown lentils, drained and rinsed (see Tip, left)	500 mL
3 cups	shredded Cheddar cheese	750 mL
1 cup	coarsely chopped cashews	250 mL
3	eggs, beaten	3

1. In a large dry skillet over medium heat, toast cumin seeds until they begin to brown and release their aroma. Immediately transfer to a mortar or spice grinder and grind to a powder. Set aside.

2. Return skillet to element and heat oil. Add onion and celery and cook, stirring, until celery softens, about 5 minutes. Add carrots, garlic, red pepper, chili pepper, salt and peppercorns and cook, stirring for 2 minutes. Remove from heat and set aside.

3. In a large mixing bowl, combine lentils, cheese and cashews. Add contents of skillet and stir well. Add eggs and mix until blended. Spoon into prepared pan and cover tightly with foil, securing with a string.

4. Place in slow cooker stoneware and pour in enough boiling water to come 1 inch (2.5 cm) up the sides. Cover and cook on High for 4 to 5 hours, until loaf has set.

NUTRITIONAL ANALYSIS PER SERVING			
Energy: 523 kcal	Carbohydrate: 30 g	Calcium: 470 mg	Folate: 61 mcg
Protein: 27 g	Fat: 34 g	Iron: 3.3 mg	Fiber: 8.9 mg

Stir-Fried Vegetables with Tofu

2 tbsp	vegetable oil	25 mL
1	large onion, cut into wedges	1
3	medium carrots, sliced diagonally	3
3	celery stalks, sliced diagonally	3
¼	small cabbage, sliced thinly	¼
1 cup	snow peas, trimmed	250 mL
1 cup	sliced mushrooms	250 mL
1 cup	firm tofu, cubed	250 mL
½ cup	vegetable stock	125 mL
1 tbsp	cornstarch	15 mL
1 tsp	finely chopped gingerroot (or ½ tsp/2 mL ground ginger)	5 mL
¼ tsp	freshly ground black pepper	1 mL

MAKES 6 SERVINGS

Gingerroot adds zest to this tasty dish.

TIP

Tofu, a source of protein and some calcium, is made from soy milk, in much the same way that cheese is made from animal milk. Tofu is best stored in water in a covered container in the refrigerator. Change the water daily to keep tofu fresh for 1 week.

1. In a wok or large heavy skillet, heat oil over high heat. When oil is very hot, add onion, carrot and celery; cover and steam for 5 minutes. Add cabbage, snow peas, mushrooms and tofu; steam, covered, for 5 minutes longer.

2. Mix together chicken broth, cornstarch, ginger and pepper; pour over vegetable mixture. Stir-fry for 1 minute or until sauce thickens. Serve over hot rice.

NUTRITIONAL ANALYSIS PER SERVING			
Energy: 157 kcal	Carbohydrate: 14 g	Calcium: 357 mg	Folate: 60 mcg
Protein: 10 g	Fat: 8 g	Iron: 6.0 mg	Fiber: 3.7 g

**MAKES
4 SERVINGS**

*This recipe is great for
someone who is trying
tofu for the first time.
It's easy to prepare
and very tasty.*

TIP

Be sure to do your
preparation — washing,
chopping and dicing —
ahead of time so that
everything comes together
when you are actually at
the stove.

Teriyaki Tofu Stir-Fry

1⅓ cups	diced firm tofu	325 mL
½ cup	teriyaki sauce	125 mL
1 tsp	brown sugar	5 mL
1 tsp	cornstarch	5 mL
1 tbsp	water	15 mL
2 tsp	olive oil	10 mL
½ cup	diced onion	125 mL
1 cup	diced green bell peppers	250 mL
1 cup	diced red bell peppers	250 mL
1 tsp	minced garlic	5 mL
1 tsp	grated gingerroot	5 mL
2 cups	roughly chopped vegetables (see Variation, below, for suggestions)	500 mL
3 cups	cooked rice	750 mL
1 to 2 tbsp	chopped fresh cilantro or parsley (optional)	15 to 25 mL

1. In a medium bowl, gently toss tofu with teriyaki sauce and brown sugar until well coated. Cover and refrigerate for 10 minutes or for up to several hours.

2. In a small bowl, whisk together cornstarch and water. Set aside.

3. In a large nonstick skillet, heat oil over medium-high heat. Add onion, green peppers, red peppers, garlic and ginger; stir-fry for 3 minutes. Stir in vegetables of your choice and stir-fry for 3 to 4 minutes or until vegetables are tender-crisp.

4. Add tofu mixture and cornstarch mixture. Stir for 3 to 4 minutes or until thickened and heated through. Serve over rice. Sprinkle with cilantro, if using.

Variation

Use any vegetables you like or have on hand, such as broccoli and cauliflower, snow peas, green beans, mushrooms, tomatoes or thinly sliced carrots.

NUTRITIONAL ANALYSIS PER SERVING			
Energy: 373 kcal	Carbohydrate: 52 g	Calcium: 233 mg	Folate: 84 mcg
Protein: 21 g	Fat: 10 g	Iron: 11.6 mg	Fiber: 3.8 g

Soy-Braised Tofu, Cabbage and Ginger with Cellophane Noodles

- Preheat oven to 375°F (190°C)
- Baking sheet, greased

4 oz	bean thread noodles or 8 oz (250 g) dried angel hair pasta	125 g
1 tbsp	vegetable oil	15 mL
4 oz	medium-firm tofu, cut into ½-inch (1 cm) cubes	125 g
2 tbsp	soy sauce	25 mL
2 tbsp	minced gingerroot	25 mL
1 tbsp	minced garlic	15 mL
4 cups	vegetable stock or apple juice	1 L
2 cups	shredded green cabbage	500 mL
1 tbsp	chopped cilantro	15 mL
2 tbsp	tomato ketchup	25 mL
1 tbsp	horseradish	15 mL
1 tbsp	cornstarch, dissolved in 2 tbsp (25 mL) water	15 mL
	Salt and freshly ground black pepper to taste	

1. In a heatproof bowl or pot, cover noodles with boiling water and soak for 3 minutes. Drain. (If using pasta, prepare according to package directions, and coat with a little oil.) Set aside.

2. In a large bowl, combine tofu, oil, soy sauce, ginger and garlic. Place on a baking sheet and roast until firm and browned, about 15 minutes. Remove from oven and allow to cool slightly.

3. Meanwhile, in a saucepan over medium-high heat, combine stock, cabbage, tofu mixture, cilantro, ketchup and horseradish. Bring to a boil. Reduce heat and simmer for 5 minutes. Add dissolved cornstarch and cook until mixture begins to thicken. Add noodles and stir until heated through. Season with salt and pepper; serve immediately.

Good source of:
- Folate

Source of:
- Calcium and iron

MAKES 4 SERVINGS

Braising is a key component of Chinese cooking — it adds rich flavor to otherwise bland ingredients such as tofu. Baking also firms the tofu and allows the flavorings to penetrate.

TIPS

For added flavor, roast the cabbage along with the tofu.

Bean thread noodles are very slippery and best eaten with chopsticks.

NUTRITIONAL ANALYSIS PER SERVING

Energy: 224 kcal	Carbohydrate: 41 g	Calcium: 85 mg	Folate: 43 mcg
Protein: 6 g	Fat: 5 g	Iron: 1.7 mg	Fiber: 1.9 mg

**MAKES
4 SERVINGS**

This spicy, nutty tofu recipe has the flavor of an Asian satay dish and is guaranteed to please both vegetarians and non-vegetarians!

TIP

Freeze the tofu cubes prior to preparation; this enhances the texture of the tofu so it's more poultry-like.

Nutty Tofu and Green Vegetable Stir-Fry

1 tbsp	vegetable oil	15 mL
8 oz	firm tofu, cubed	250 g
1	green bell pepper, thinly sliced	1
1½ cups	green beans, trimmed	375 mL
½ tsp	salt	2 mL
4	cloves garlic, minced	4
1	onion, chopped	1
1	tomato, chopped	1
¼ cup	ground almonds	50 mL
½ cup	water (approx.), divided	125 mL
½ tsp	granulated sugar	2 mL
½ tsp	ground turmeric	2 mL
½ tsp	ground cumin	2 mL
½ tsp	ground coriander	2 mL

1. In a large skillet, heat oil over medium heat. Lightly brown tofu on all sides, then remove from pan and set aside.

2. Add green pepper, green beans and salt to skillet; stir-fry until tender-crisp, about 5 minutes. Add garlic, onion and tomato; stir-fry for 5 minutes. Stir in tofu pieces. Stir in almonds, ¼ cup (50 mL) of the water and sugar. Reduce heat to low and cook for 5 minutes. Stir in turmeric, cumin and coriander, then the remaining ¼ cup (50 mL) water (add more if the mixture becomes too dry and sticks to the pan).

NUTRITIONAL ANALYSIS PER SERVING			
Energy: 167 kcal	Carbohydrate: 14 g	Calcium: 127 mg	Folate: 62 mcg
Protein: 8 g	Fat: 10 g	Iron: 1.9 mg	Fiber: 4.3 mg

Tofu in Indian-Spiced Tomato Sauce

Excellent source of:
• Iron

Good source of:
• Calcium and folate

MAKES 4 TO 6 SERVINGS

This robust dish makes a lively and different meal. I like to serve it with fresh green beans and naan, an Indian bread, to soak up the sauce.

Make ahead

This dish can be partially prepared the night before it is cooked. Complete Step 1. Cover and refrigerate overnight. The next morning, continue cooking as directed.

• 3½ to 6 quart slow cooker

1 tbsp	vegetable oil	15 mL
2	onions, finely chopped	2
2	cloves garlic, minced	2
½ tsp	minced gingerroot	2 mL
1	long green chili pepper, seeded and finely chopped	1
6	whole cloves	6
4	pods white or green cardamom	4
1	2-inch (5 cm) cinnamon stick	1
1 tsp	caraway seeds	5 mL
1 tsp	salt	5 mL
½ tsp	cracked black peppercorns	2 mL
1	can (28 oz/796 mL) tomatoes, including juice	1

Tofu

¼ cup	all-purpose flour	50 mL
1 tsp	curry powder	5 mL
¼ tsp	cayenne pepper	1 mL
1 tbsp	vegetable oil	15 mL
8 oz	firm tofu, cubed	250 g

1. In a skillet, heat oil over medium heat. Add onions and cook, stirring, until softened. Add garlic, ginger, chili pepper, cloves, cardamom, cinnamon stick, caraway seeds, salt and peppercorns and cook, stirring, for 1 minute. Add tomatoes with juice and bring to a boil. Transfer to slow cooker stoneware.

2. Cover and cook on Low for 8 to 10 hours or on High for 4 to 5 hours.

3. *Tofu:* On a plate, mix together flour, curry powder and cayenne. Roll tofu in mixture until lightly coated. Discard excess flour. In a skillet, heat oil over medium-high heat. Add dredged tofu and sauté, stirring, until nicely browned. Spoon tomato mixture into a serving dish. Discard cloves, cardamom and cinnamon stick. Layer tofu on top.

NUTRITIONAL ANALYSIS PER SERVING

Energy: 250 kcal	Carbohydrate: 25 g	Calcium: 206 mg	Folate: 49 mcg
Protein: 13 g	Fat: 13 g	Iron: 8.0 mg	Fiber: 1.1 g

**MAKES
8 SERVINGS**

Unusual flavor and a kick of heat make a star out of tofu in this dish. Although the list of ingredients seems long, most of them are spices you are likely to have on hand.

TIPS

Leftover kabob vegetables make perfect pizza toppings.

The tofu can marinate overnight, covered, in the refrigerator.

Serve these kabobs with rice or pasta or on top of fresh greens.

Tofu Veggie Kabobs

- Preheat barbecue to medium
- Eight 8-inch (20 cm) wooden skewers, soaked

Spice Mixture

2 tbsp	granulated sugar	25 mL
1 tbsp	ground cinnamon	15 mL
1 tbsp	ground nutmeg	15 mL
2 tsp	salt	10 mL
2 tsp	cayenne pepper (or to taste)	10 mL
2 tsp	onion powder	10 mL
2 tsp	dried thyme	10 mL
1 tsp	freshly ground black pepper	5 mL
¼ cup	olive oil, divided	50 mL
3 tbsp	balsamic vinegar	45 mL
1 tbsp	soy sauce	15 mL
10 oz	firm tofu, cut into large cubes	300 g
1	large zucchini	1
1	large orange bell pepper	1
1	large yellow bell pepper	1
16	cherry tomatoes	16

1. *Prepare the spice mixture:* In a small bowl, combine sugar, cinnamon, nutmeg, salt, cayenne, onion powder, thyme and black pepper. Set aside.

2. In a large bowl, combine 2 tbsp (25 mL) of the olive oil, balsamic vinegar and soy sauce. Add tofu and set aside to marinate while you chop the vegetables.

3. Cut zucchini, orange pepper and yellow pepper into large pieces. In a bowl, combine zucchini, peppers and cherry tomatoes. Add spice mixture and the remaining 2 tbsp (25 mL) olive oil; toss until vegetables are evenly coated.

4. Thread zucchini, peppers, tomatoes and tofu cubes onto skewers. Place on preheated barbecue and cook, turning at least once, for about 10 minutes or until browned.

Variation

This recipe is very versatile. You can use herbed tofu or, for a non-vegetarian meal, cubes of cooked chicken or beef. You could also substitute different vegetables, such as sweet potatoes and onions, and even fresh pineapple.

NUTRITIONAL ANALYSIS PER SERVING			
Energy: 130 kcal	Carbohydrate: 11 g	Calcium: 74 mg	Folate: 38 mcg
Protein: 4 g	Fat: 9 g	Iron: 1.7 mg	Fiber: 1.7 mg

Pasta and Noodles

**MAKES 5 CUPS
(1.25 L)**

*Dinner preparation
is a cinch with a supply
of this sauce in the
refrigerator or freezer.*

Basic Red Tomato Sauce

1	can (28 oz/796 mL) diced tomatoes	1
1	can (5½ oz/156 mL) tomato paste	1
2	large onions, chopped	2
2	cloves garlic, minced	2
	Salt and freshly ground black pepper	

1. In a large saucepan, combine tomatoes, tomato paste, onions, garlic and ¾ cup (175 mL) water. Bring to a boil on medium-high heat. Reduce heat to medium-low and cook, uncovered, stirring frequently, for 1 hour or until mixture is cooked and thickened. Add additional water if sauce becomes too thick. Season with salt and pepper to taste.

2. Remove from heat. Let cool before storing in smaller containers. Freeze for longer storage or refrigerate for about 2 days.

Variations

Add any of these additions to 1 cup (250 mL) sauce.

Mushroom Sauce: 1 can (10 oz/284 mL) drained mushrooms.

Vegetable Sauce: ½ diced green or red bell pepper, ½ diced zucchini or 1 cup (250 mL) chopped broccoli and 1 stalk celery chopped.

NUTRITIONAL ANALYSIS PER SERVING			
Energy: 101 kcal	Carbohydrate: 21 g	Calcium: 33 mg	Folate: 22 mcg
Protein: 4 g	Fat: Trace	Iron: 2.1 mg	Fiber: 4.2 mg

Tuna Tomato Pasta

8 oz	penne, fusilli or spaghetti	250 g
2 cups	Basic Red Tomato Sauce (see recipe, page 260) or store-bought	500 mL
1	can (6½ oz/170 g) tuna, water-packed, drained	1
1 cup	frozen peas (see Variation, below)	250 mL
	Freshly ground black pepper	

1. In a large saucepan of boiling water, cook pasta according to package directions until al dente (tender but firm). Drain well. Return to saucepan.

2. Add sauce, tuna and peas. Cook on low for 5 minutes or until sauce is hot and peas are heated. Season with pepper to taste.

Variation

Any frozen vegetable, such as corn, mixed vegetables, carrots or green beans, works well here.

NUTRITIONAL ANALYSIS PER SERVING

| Energy: 358 kcal | Carbohydrate: 62 g | Calcium: 45 mg | Folate: 48 mcg |
| Protein: 22 g | Fat: 3 g | Iron: 2.9 mg | Fiber: 5.6 mg |

MAKES 4 SERVINGS

Basic Red Tomato Sauce, a can of tuna, some pasta and a frozen vegetable make a quick dinner. Put a salad together while the pasta is cooking.

Mac 'n' Cheese Night

2 cups	macaroni or fusilli	500 mL
3 tbsp	butter or margarine	45 mL
1½ cups	shredded Cheddar cheese	375 mL
¾ cup	sour cream	175 mL
	Salt and freshly ground black pepper	

1. In a medium saucepan of boiling water, cook macaroni according to package directions until al dente (tender but firm). Drain well. Return to saucepan.

2. Remove from heat and stir in butter until melted. Stir in cheese, adding a small amount at a time. Add sour cream and salt and pepper to taste. Stir until pasta is well coated with sauce and cheese is melted.

NUTRITIONAL ANALYSIS PER SERVING

| Energy: 412 kcal | Carbohydrate: 22 g | Calcium: 360 mg | Folate: 18 mcg |
| Protein: 15 g | Fat: 29 g | Iron: 0.7 mg | Fiber: 0.8 mg |

MAKES 4 SERVINGS

Wonder what to have for dinner tonight? This classic favorite may just be the answer.

**MAKES
4 SERVINGS**

*Timing is everything
when it comes to
cooking pasta and
preparing a stir-fry.
Before you begin
chopping the vegetables
for this recipe, put a
large pot of water on
the stove to boil. The
pasta takes just a few
minutes to cook, so
don't add it to the
boiling water until just
after you brown the
meat. This way both
pasta and stir-fry will be
ready at the same time.*

Angel Hair Pasta with Spicy Ginger Beef and Vegetables

½ cup	chicken stock	125 mL
3 tbsp	soy sauce	45 mL
1½ tsp	cornstarch	7 mL
12 oz	lean tender beef, such as sirloin, cut into very thin shreds	375 g
4 tsp	vegetable oil, divided	20 mL
2 tbsp	minced gingerroot	25 mL
2	large cloves garlic, minced	2
½ tsp	hot pepper flakes or to taste	2 mL
2 cups	snow peas, ends trimmed, halved	500 mL
1	large red bell pepper, cut into thin 2-inch (5 cm) strips	1
4	green onions, sliced	4
8 oz	angel hair pasta	250 g
⅓ cup	chopped fresh cilantro	75 mL

1. In a glass measure, combine stock, soy sauce and cornstarch. Pat meat dry with paper towels.

2. In a wok or large nonstick skillet, heat 2 tsp (10 mL) of the oil over high heat; stir-fry beef until browned. Transfer to a plate.

3. Add remaining oil to skillet; cook ginger, garlic and hot pepper flakes, stirring, for 15 seconds. Stir in snow peas, red pepper and green onions; cook, stirring, for 1 minute. Stir stock mixture and add to skillet; cook, stirring, until thickened. Return beef to skillet. Cook, stirring, for 30 seconds.

4. Meanwhile, in a large pot of boiling salted water, cook pasta until tender but firm. Drain well and return to pot. Add beef and cilantro; toss well. Serve immediately.

Variation

Use pork, chicken or firm tofu instead of the beef.

NUTRITIONAL ANALYSIS PER SERVING			
Energy: 552 kcal	Carbohydrate: 54 g	Calcium: 55 mg	Folate: 41 mcg
Protein: 37 g	Fat: 20 g	Iron: 3.9 mg	Fiber: 3.1 mg

Spaghetti with Garlic Tomato Sauce

2 tbsp	olive oil	25 mL
3	cloves garlic, thinly sliced, then coarsely chopped	3
¼ tsp	hot pepper flakes	1 mL
1	can (28 oz/796 mL) plum tomatoes, including juice, chopped	1
	Salt and freshly ground black pepper	
Pinch	granulated sugar	Pinch
12 oz	spaghetti	375 g
2 tbsp	chopped fresh parsley	25 mL
2 tbsp	chopped fresh basil or chives	25 mL

1. In a large saucepan, heat oil over medium heat; stir in garlic and hot pepper flakes. Reduce heat to low; cook, stirring, for 1 minute or until garlic is light golden. (Do not let garlic brown or sauce will be bitter.)

2. Add tomatoes with juice; season with salt, pepper and sugar to taste. Bring to a boil, reduce heat and simmer, partially covered, stirring occasionally, for 15 minutes.

3. Cook pasta in a large pot of boiling salted water until tender but firm. Drain well; return to pot. Add tomato sauce, parsley and basil; toss well. Adjust seasoning with salt and pepper. Serve immediately.

Variation

Quick Creamy Tomato Sauce: Instead of the traditional accompaniment of freshly grated Parmesan cheese, toss hot pasta with 5 oz (150 g) creamy goat cheese, soft Brie or Gorgonzola, rind removed and cut into small pieces.

Good source of:
- Iron and fiber

Source of:
- Calcium and folate

MAKES
4 SERVINGS AS
A MAIN COURSE
OR 6 SERVINGS
AS A SIDE DISH

Even when my pantry is almost empty, chances are I'll have a can of tomatoes and dried pasta on hand to whip up this easy supper dish.

TIP

Improvise if you don't have any fresh herbs by using 1 tsp (5 mL) each dried basil and dried oregano for the fresh basil and parsley.

NUTRITIONAL ANALYSIS PER SERVING			
Energy: 451 kcal	Carbohydrate: 80 g	Calcium: 86 mg	Folate: 37 mcg
Protein: 14 g	Fat: 9 g	Iron: 2.5 mg	Fiber: 4.0 mg

Spaghetti with Creamy Tomato Clam Sauce

**MAKES
4 SERVINGS**

By the time it takes to cook the pasta, a flavorful sauce using canned clams can be quickly assembled on the stovetop.

TIPS

Omit the cream if you prefer a lighter sauce.

Freeze remaining clam juice to use in other fish-based soups and sauces.

2 tbsp	olive oil	25 mL
1	onion, chopped	1
3	large cloves garlic, minced	3
¼ tsp	hot pepper flakes or to taste	1 mL
2	cans (each 5 oz/142 g) baby clams, drained, juice reserved	2
½ cup	dry white wine	125 mL
2 cups	seeded chopped fresh plum tomatoes	500 mL
½ cup	whipping (35 %) cream	125 mL
¼ cup	chopped fresh parsley	50 mL
	Salt and freshly ground black pepper	
12 oz	spaghetti, fettuccini or linguine	375 g

1. In a large skillet, heat oil over medium-high heat. Cook onion, garlic and hot pepper flakes, stirring, for 2 minutes. Add clams and cook, stirring, for 2 minutes. Add wine; cook for 1 minute or until slightly reduced.

2. Stir in tomatoes and ½ cup (125 mL) of the reserved clam juice. (Discard any juice remaining.) Reduce heat to medium and cook, stirring occasionally, for 5 minutes or until sauce-like. Add cream and parsley. Season with salt and pepper to taste. Cook for 1 minute or until heated through.

3. Meanwhile, cook pasta in a large pot of boiling salted water until tender but firm. Drain well. Return to pot and add clam sauce; toss to coat pasta in the sauce. Serve immediately.

NUTRITIONAL ANALYSIS PER SERVING			
Energy: 628 kcal	Carbohydrate: 85 g	Calcium: 149 mg	Folate: 43 mcg
Protein: 25 g	Fat: 21 g	Iron: 9.0 mg	Fiber: 3.8 mg

Fettuccine with Shrimp and Vegetables

Excellent source of:
- Iron, folate and fiber

Good source of:
- Calcium

3 tbsp	olive oil, divided	45 mL
1½ lbs	large raw shrimp, peeled and deveined, with tails left on	375 g
2	cloves garlic, finely chopped	2
½ tsp	hot pepper flakes or to taste	2 mL
⅓ cup	vodka (optional)	75 mL
2	small red bell peppers, cut into thin strips	2
1	fennel bulb, top trimmed and cut into thin strips	1
1 cup	fish or chicken stock	250 mL
1 cup	whipping (35%) cream	250 mL
1 tbsp	grated orange zest	15 mL
½ tsp	salt	2 mL
¼ tsp	freshly ground black pepper	1 mL
12 oz	fettuccine	375 g
⅓ cup	chopped fresh parsley	75 mL

MAKES 4 SERVINGS

Infusing shrimp with pungent hot peppers and garlic then flambéing with vodka as in this winning entertaining dish is sure to illicit raves from your guests.

1. In a large nonstick skillet, heat half the oil over high heat until almost smoking; add shrimp, garlic and hot pepper flakes. Cook, stirring, for 1 to 2 minutes or until shrimp are pink and almost cooked through. Add vodka, if using, and ignite with a match. Cook, shaking skillet, until flames subside. Transfer shrimp and juices to a bowl.

2. Add remaining oil to pan; cook red pepper and fennel strips, stirring, for 2 minutes or until tender-crisp. Transfer to bowl with shrimp.

3. Add stock, cream, zest, salt and pepper to pan; bring to a boil. Reduce heat to medium and boil sauce until reduced by half. Return shrimp and vegetables to skillet and heat through. Season with salt and pepper to taste.

4. In a large pot of boiling salted water, cook pasta until just tender but firm. Drain well. Return to pot. Toss with shrimp and vegetables; sprinkle with parsley.

NUTRITIONAL ANALYSIS PER SERVING			
Energy: 872 kcal	Carbohydrate: 85 g	Calcium: 198 mg	Folate: 261 mcg
Protein: 53 g	Fat: 36 g	Iron: 8.6 mg	Fiber: 6.2 mg

**MAKES
4 SERVINGS**

When I crave a rich and creamy pasta dish, this is it. Since this requires very little preparation, have all of the ingredients assembled before you start.

TIP

When to use curly versus flat-leaf parsley? While both are interchangeable in recipes, I like the more assertive taste of flat-leaf parsley, especially in recipes such as this one where it is a vital ingredient and balances nicely with the lemon and garlic.

Linguine with Seared Scallops, Lemon and Garlic

1 lb	large scallops	500 g
	Salt and freshly ground black pepper	
2 tbsp	butter	25 mL
3	cloves garlic, minced	3
½ cup	dry white wine	125 mL
1 tbsp	grated lemon zest	15 mL
1 tbsp	freshly squeezed lemon juice	15 mL
1 cup	whipping (35%) cream	250 mL
¼ cup	chopped fresh flat-leaf parsley (see Tip, at left)	50 mL
12 oz	linguine	375 g

1. Pat scallops dry with paper towels. Halve horizontally and season with salt and pepper.

2. Heat a large nonstick skillet over high heat. Add butter; heat until foamy and butter starts to brown. Add scallops and cook for 1 minute or until lightly browned. Turn and cook second side for about 30 seconds. Do not overcook. Transfer to a plate.

3. Reduce heat to medium. Add garlic and cook, stirring, for 30 seconds or until fragrant. Stir in wine and lemon zest and juice; bring to a boil. Add cream and cook, stirring, until sauce boils and is slightly reduced.

4. Add parsley and season with salt and pepper to taste. Add scallops and cook for 1 minute or just until heated in the sauce. Do not overcook.

5. Meanwhile, in a large pot of boiling salted water, cook pasta until tender but firm. Drain and return to pot.

6. Pour sauce over pasta and toss until well coated. Spoon pasta into warm bowls and serve immediately.

NUTRITIONAL ANALYSIS PER SERVING			
Energy: 712 kcal	Carbohydrate: 79 g	Calcium: 99 mg	Folate: 222 mcg
Protein: 33 g	Fat: 29 g	Iron: 3.9 mg	Fiber: 3.2 mg

Cannelloni with Tomato Eggplant Sauce

- Large (minimum 5 quart) slow cooker

Sauce

2 tbsp	olive oil	25 mL
1	medium eggplant, peeled, cut into 2-inch (5 cm) cubes and drained of excess moisture (see Tip, at right)	1
2	cloves garlic, minced	2
¼ tsp	freshly ground black pepper	1 mL
3 cups	tomato sauce	750 mL

Filling

2 cups	ricotta cheese	500 mL
½ cup	freshly grated Parmesan cheese	125 mL
1½ cups	chopped baby spinach	375 mL
1 tsp	freshly grated nutmeg	5 mL
1	egg, beaten	1
¼ tsp	salt	1 mL
¼ tsp	freshly ground black pepper	1 mL
24	oven-ready cannelloni shells	24

1. *Sauce:* In a nonstick skillet, heat oil over medium heat. Add eggplant, in batches, and cook until it begins to brown. Add garlic and black pepper and cook, stirring, for 1 minute. Add tomato sauce, stir well and bring to a boil. Remove from heat and set aside.

2. *Filling:* In a bowl, combine ricotta, Parmesan, spinach, nutmeg, egg, salt and pepper. Using your fingers, fill pasta shells with mixture and place filled shells side by side in slow cooker stoneware, then on top of each other when bottom layer is complete. Pour sauce over shells. Cover and cook on Low for 8 hours or on High for 4 hours, until hot and bubbling.

MAKES 8 SERVINGS

Here's a great recipe for cannelloni that is remarkably easy to make.

TIP

Although eggplant is delicious when properly cooked, some varieties tend to be bitter. Since the bitterness is concentrated under the skin, I peel eggplant before using. Sprinkling the pieces with salt and leaving them to "sweat" for an hour or two also draws out the bitter juice. If time is short, blanch the pieces for a minute or two in heavily salted water. In either case, rinse thoroughly in fresh cold water and, using your hands, squeeze out the excess moisture. Pat dry with paper towels and it's ready for cooking.

Make ahead

This dish can be prepared the night before it is cooked. Let tomato sauce cool before pouring over cannelloni. Refrigerate overnight in slow cooker stoneware and cook as directed.

NUTRITIONAL ANALYSIS PER SERVING			
Energy: 266 kcal	Carbohydrate: 27 g	Calcium: 268 mg	Folate: 70 mcg
Protein: 14 g	Fat: 11 g	Iron: 1.6 mg	Fiber: 3.1 mg

**MAKES
8 SERVINGS**

Everyone loves lasagna, but who has the time to make it from scratch? Try this uncomplicated version that makes even a non-cook look like a pro in the kitchen. It's also the perfect recipe for young cooks, since there's no chopping involved. Once you assemble the ingredients, it takes a mere 15 minutes to prepare and the lasagna is ready for the oven.

Make Ahead

Lasagna freezes well; cover with plastic wrap, then with foil and freeze for up to 2 months. Let defrost in the refrigerator overnight before baking.

Easy Lasagna

• Preheat oven to 350°F (180°C)
• 13-by 9-inch (3 L) baking dish, lightly greased

2 cups	ricotta cheese	500 mL
2	eggs, beaten	2
1/3 cup	freshly grated Parmesan cheese	75 mL
1/4 tsp	freshly ground black pepper	1 mL
1/4 tsp	freshly grated nutmeg	1 mL
3 cups	spaghetti sauce (homemade or store-bought)	750 mL
12	precooked lasagna noodles	12
2 cups	shredded mozzarella cheese	500 mL

1. In a bowl, combine ricotta, eggs and Parmesan cheese; season with pepper and nutmeg.

2. Depending on thickness of the spaghetti sauce, add about 3/4 cup (175 mL) water to thin sauce. (Precooked noodles absorb extra moisture while cooking.)

3. Spoon 1/2 cup (125 mL) sauce in bottom of prepared baking dish. Layer with 3 lasagna noodles. Spread with 3/4 cup (175 mL) of the sauce and then one-third of the ricotta mixture. Repeat with two more layers of noodles, sauce and ricotta cheese. Layer with rest of noodles and top with remaining sauce. Sprinkle with mozzarella cheese.

4. Bake, uncovered, in preheated oven for 45 minutes or until cheese is melted and sauce is bubbly.

NUTRITIONAL ANALYSIS PER SERVING			
Energy: 414 kcal	Carbohydrate: 40 g	Calcium: 481 mg	Folate: 87 mcg
Protein: 24 g	Fat: 18 g	Iron: 2.1 mg	Fiber: 2.4 mg

Mushroom and Artichoke Lasagna

- Large (minimum 5 quart) oval slow cooker, greased

2 tbsp	butter	25 mL
1	onion, finely chopped	1
1 lb	mushrooms, stems removed and sliced	500 g
4	cloves garlic, minced	4
3½ cups	quartered artichoke hearts, packed in water, drained, or thawed if frozen	875 mL
¾ cup	dry white wine or vegetable stock	175 mL
12	oven-ready lasagna noodles	12
2½ cups	ricotta cheese	625 mL
2 cups	baby spinach	500 mL
2½ cups	shredded mozzarella cheese	625 mL
½ cup	freshly grated Parmesan cheese	125 mL

1. In a skillet, melt butter over medium heat. Add onion and cook until softened. Add mushrooms and garlic and cook, stirring, just until mushrooms begin to release their liquid. Stir in artichokes and wine and bring to a boil. Cook, stirring, for 1 or 2 minutes, until liquid reduces slightly. Set aside.

2. Cover bottom of slow cooker stoneware with 4 noodles, breaking to fit where necessary. Spread with half of the ricotta, half of the mushroom mixture, half of the spinach, one-third each of the mozzarella and Parmesan. Repeat. Arrange final layer of noodles over cheeses. Pour any liquid remaining from mushroom mixture over noodles (see Tip, at right) and sprinkle with remaining Parmesan and mozzarella. Cover and cook on Low for 6 to 8 hours or on High for 3 to 4 hours, until hot and bubbling.

NUTRITIONAL ANALYSIS PER SERVING			
Energy: 547 kcal	Carbohydrate: 39 g	Calcium: 924 mg	Folate: 158 mcg
Protein: 40 g	Fat: 25 g	Iron: 3.8 mg	Fiber: 5.6 g

Excellent source of:
- Calcium, iron and folate

Good source of:
- Fiber

MAKES 8 SERVINGS

I love the unusual combination of flavors in this lasagna, which reminds me of a Provençal gratin. In addition to adding flavor and color, the baby spinach is a great time saver as it doesn't require precooking.

TIPS

Unlike many recipes for lasagna, this one is not terribly saucy. As a result, the noodles on the top layer tend to dry out. Leave a small amount of the cooking liquid from the mushroom mixture behind in the pan, after adding to the slow cooker. Pour that over the top layer of noodles, particularly around the edges, where they are most likely to dry out.

Use white or cremini mushrooms or a combination of the two in this recipe.

Make ahead

This dish can be prepared the night before it is cooked. Refrigerate overnight in slow cooker stoneware and cook as directed.

**MAKES
6 SERVINGS**

*Pad thai may be the
most popular dish in
Thailand, but its
addictive appeal has
spread beyond its
borders, based on the
number of restaurants
that now feature it on
their menus. Here's
how to make it in your
home kitchen.*

TIP

Fish sauce (also called
nam pla) is an important
flavoring ingredient in this
dish. You can now find it in
the Asian foods section of
most large supermarkets
or in Asian markets.

Pad Thai

8 oz	wide rice stick noodles	250 g
1/3 cup	chili sauce or ketchup	75 mL
1/4 cup	fish sauce (see Tip, at left)	50 mL
3 tbsp	freshly squeezed lime juice	45 mL
1 tbsp	packed brown sugar	15 mL
1 tsp	chili paste or to taste	5 mL
2 tbsp	vegetable oil, divided	25 mL
8 oz	medium shrimp, peeled and deveined	250 g
8 oz	boneless skinless chicken breasts, cut into thin strips	250 g
3	cloves garlic, minced	3
2	eggs, lightly beaten	2
2 cups	bean sprouts	500 mL
5	green onions, sliced	5
1/2 cup	coarsely chopped fresh cilantro	125 mL
1/3 cup	coarsely chopped roasted peanuts	75 mL
	Lime wedges	

1. Place noodles in a large bowl. Add hot water to cover. Let stand for 15 minutes or until softened. Drain.

2. In a bowl, combine chili sauce, fish sauce, lime juice, brown sugar and chili paste.

3. In a large wok or nonstick skillet, heat 1 tbsp (15 mL) of the oil over medium-high heat. Cook shrimp and chicken, stirring, for 3 minutes or until chicken is cooked through and shrimp are pink. Add to chili sauce mixture and toss.

4. Add remaining oil to the skillet. Cook garlic, stirring, for 15 seconds or until fragrant. Add eggs; cook, stirring constantly, for 30 seconds or until soft-scrambled. Add sprouts and green onions; cook, stirring, for 1 minute.

5. Add noodles and shrimp mixture; cook, stirring, for 2 minutes or until heated through. Transfer to a platter; sprinkle with cilantro and peanuts. Garnish with lime wedges.

NUTRITIONAL ANALYSIS PER SERVING			
Energy: 429 kcal	Carbohydrate: 49 g	Calcium: 90 mg	Folate: 61 mcg
Protein: 29 g	Fat: 13 g	Iron: 3.1 mg	Fiber: 2.1 mg

Thin Rice Noodles with Cauliflower and Black Bean Sauce

8 oz	thin rice vermicelli (thin rice stick noodles) or dried linguine	250 g
1 tbsp	vegetable oil, plus oil for coating noodles	15 mL
2 cups	cauliflower florets	500 mL
1 tbsp	minced garlic	15 mL
1 tbsp	minced gingerroot	15 mL
1	onion, coarsely chopped	1
1	green pepper, seeded and thinly sliced	1
2 tbsp	black bean sauce	25 mL
2 cups	water or chicken or beef stock	500 mL
1 tbsp	cornstarch, dissolved in 2 tbsp (25 mL) water	15 mL

1. In a heatproof bowl or pot, cover noodles with boiling water and soak for 3 minutes. (If using pasta, prepare according to package directions.) Drain, coat with a little oil and set aside.

2. In a colander, rinse cauliflower under cold water. Transfer to a steamer and cook for 5 minutes (or microwave in a covered container with 2 tbsp/25 mL water for 4 minutes) until tender but slightly firm. Set aside.

3. In a nonstick wok or skillet, heat oil over medium-high heat for 30 seconds. Add garlic, ginger, onion, pepper and cauliflower. Sauté for 2 minutes or until onion softens. Add black bean sauce and stir. Add water or stock and cook for another 2 minutes. Add dissolved cornstarch and stir to thicken. Add noodles, mix well and cook 1 minute to warm through. Serve immediately.

Good source of:
- Iron

Source of:
- Folate and fiber

MAKES 4 SERVINGS AS A MAIN COURSE OR 6 TO 8 SERVINGS AS A SIDE DISH

The pungent, earthy flavor of black beans makes this a hearty and satisfying vegetarian dish.

TIP

Presteaming the cauliflower gives a soft and luxurious feel. For a crunchier texture, thinly slice raw cauliflower and sauté along with the onion.

NUTRITIONAL ANALYSIS PER SERVING			
Energy: 324 kcal	Carbohydrate: 64 g	Calcium: 52 mg	Folate: 19 mcg
Protein: 7 g	Fat: 4 g	Iron: 2.6 mg	Fiber: 3.9 mg

**MAKES
4 SERVINGS AS A
MAIN COURSE OR
6 TO 8 SERVINGS
AS A SIDE DISH**

*This quick and easy
noodle dish is one of
our standbys. Add some
grilled chicken and a
big green salad, and
you can have a delicious
and nutritious dinner in
less than 20 minutes.*

Cilantro Parmesan Noodles

1 lb	fresh Shanghai noodles or fresh fettuccine	500 g
2 tbsp	whipping (35%) cream	25 mL
½ cup	freshly grated Parmesan cheese	125 mL
½ cup	chopped cilantro	125 mL
	Salt and pepper to taste	

1. In a large pot of boiling salted water, cook noodles until al dente, about 3 minutes. (If using pasta, prepare according to package instructions.) Drain.

2. Immediately return noodles to pot. Over low heat, add cream and Parmesan; mix. Add cilantro and toss thoroughly to combine. Season to taste with salt and pepper. Serve immediately.

NUTRITIONAL ANALYSIS PER SERVING			
Energy: 548 kcal	Carbohydrate: 91 g	Calcium: 194 mg	Folate: 8 mcg
Protein: 21 g	Fat: 9 g	Iron: 1.9 mg	Fiber: 2.5 mg

Side Dishes

**MAKES
6 SERVINGS**

When locally grown asparagus appears at the market, it's one of my rites of spring. I prepare them tossed with crunchy almonds and melting Parmesan — and it's every bit as pleasing as a buttery Hollandaise.

Asparagus with Parmesan and Toasted Almonds

1½ lbs	asparagus	750 g
¼ cup	sliced blanched almonds	50 mL
2 tbsp	butter	25 mL
2	cloves garlic, finely chopped	2
¼ cup	freshly grated Parmesan cheese	50 mL
	Salt and freshly ground black pepper	

1. Snap off asparagus ends; cut spears on the diagonal into 2-inch (5 cm) lengths. In a large nonstick skillet, bring ½ cup (125 mL) water to a boil; cook asparagus for 2 minutes (start timing when water returns to a boil) or until just tender-crisp. Run under cold water to chill; drain and reserve.

2. Dry the skillet and place over medium heat. Add almonds and toast, stirring often, for 2 to 3 minutes or until golden. Remove and reserve.

3. Increase heat to medium-high. Add butter to skillet; cook asparagus and garlic, stirring, for 4 minutes or until asparagus is just tender.

4. Sprinkle with Parmesan; season with salt and pepper. Transfer to serving bowl; top with almonds.

Variation

Try making this dish with green beans. Trim and cut into 1½-inch (4 cm) lengths and cook in boiling water for about 5 minutes or until tender-crisp.

NUTRITIONAL ANALYSIS PER SERVING			
Energy: 114 kcal	Carbohydrate: 7 g	Calcium: 97 mg	Folate: 147 mcg
Protein: 6 g	Fat: 8 g	Iron: 1.3 mg	Fiber: 2.4 mg

Stir-Fried Red Cabbage

5½ cups	thinly shredded red cabbage	1.4 L
1 tbsp	cider vinegar	15 mL
1 tsp	salt	5 mL
2 tbsp	vegetable oil	25 mL
¼ tsp	salt	1 mL
¼ tsp	freshly ground black pepper	1 mL
1 tsp	whole fennel seeds	5 mL
1	small green bell pepper, cut into thin strips	1
1 tbsp	cider vinegar	15 mL
	Few sprigs fresh dill, chopped	

MAKES 4 TO 6 SERVINGS

Slightly tart, startlingly red-purple cabbage adds welcome sparkle and flavor (not to mention nutrition) to any vegetarian table. The fennel seeds and fresh dill add character without drawing away any of the assertiveness of the humble cabbage.

1. In a saucepan, cover cabbage with cold water; add vinegar and salt. Place on high heat for 7 to 8 minutes, until just coming to a boil. Drain cabbage, refresh under cold water and drain again.

2. In a large frying pan, heat oil over high heat for 30 seconds. Add salt, pepper and fennel seeds and stir-fry for 1 minute or until the seeds start to pop. Add green pepper strips and stir-fry for 1 minute until pepper wilts.

3. Add drained cabbage and stir-fry for 3 to 4 minutes, until all the cabbage is shiny and warm through.

4. Remove from heat. Add cider vinegar and half of the chopped dill. Toss well to mix. Transfer to a serving dish and garnish with the remaining dill.

TIP

This dish can be served warm, or it can wait for up to 2 hours, covered and unrefrigerated, to be served at room temperature.

NUTRITIONAL ANALYSIS PER SERVING			
Energy: 64 kcal	Carbohydrate: 6 g	Calcium: 37 mg	Folate: 34 mcg
Protein: 1 g	Fat: 5 g	Iron: 0.6 mg	Fiber: 2.0 mg

Cauliflower and Red Pepper

**MAKES
6 SERVINGS**

A colorful, significantly dressed combination of lush red pepper and the oft-neglected cauliflower, this salad travels well on picnics in the summer, just as it helps to liven up a cozy dinner in winter.

1	head cauliflower, florets only	1
2	red bell peppers, roasted, skinned and cut into thick strips	2
¼ tsp	salt	1 mL
¼ tsp	freshly ground black pepper	1 mL
2 tbsp	freshly squeezed lemon juice	25 mL
1 tbsp	Dijon mustard	15 mL
1 tsp	vegetable oil	5 mL
1 tsp	black mustard seeds	5 mL
½ tsp	turmeric	2 mL
½ tsp	whole coriander seeds	2 mL
2	cloves garlic	2
2 tbsp	olive oil	25 mL

1. Blanch cauliflower florets in a large saucepan of boiling water for 5 to 6 minutes, until just cooked. Drain, refresh in iced water, drain again and transfer to a bowl. Add red peppers to cauliflower. Sprinkle with salt and pepper and toss.

2. In a small bowl, whisk together lemon juice and Dijon mustard until blended. Set aside.

3. In a small frying pan, heat vegetable oil over medium heat for 1 minute. Add mustard seeds, turmeric and coriander seeds and stir-fry for 2 to 3 minutes or until the seeds begin to pop. With a rubber spatula, scrape cooked spices from the pan into the lemon-mustard mixture. Squeeze garlic through a garlic press and add to the mixture. Add olive oil and whisk until the dressing has emulsified.

4. Add dressing to the cauliflower-red pepper mixture. Toss gently but thoroughly to dress all the pieces evenly. Transfer to a serving bowl, propping up the red pepper ribbons to properly accent the yellow-tinted cauliflower. This salad benefits greatly from a 1- or 2-hour wait, after which it should be served at room temperature.

NUTRITIONAL ANALYSIS PER SERVING			
Energy: 73 kcal	Carbohydrate: 7 g	Calcium: 21 mg	Folate: 40 mcg
Protein: 2 g	Fat: 5 g	Iron: 0.8 mg	Fiber: 2.2 mg

Fennel Mushroom Stir-Fry

1	fennel bulb (about 1 lb/500 g)	1
3 tbsp	olive oil	45 mL
¼ tsp	salt	1 mL
¼ tsp	freshly ground black pepper	1 mL
½ cup	roughly chopped red onion	125 mL
½	red bell pepper, roughly chopped	½
2½ cups	trimmed and halved mushrooms	625 mL
1 tbsp	freshly squeezed lemon juice	15 mL

1. Remove and discard any branches shooting up from the fennel bulb (they are fibrous and inedible). Cut the bulb in half and trim away triangles of hard core. Chop remaining fennel in large chunks. Set aside.

2. In a large frying pan, heat olive oil over high heat for 30 seconds. Add salt, pepper, onions and red pepper. Stir-fry for 1 minute. Add fennel and stir-fry for 3 to 4 minutes, until the vegetables are slightly charred. Add mushrooms and stir-fry actively (the pan will be crowded by now) for 3 minutes, until mushrooms are slightly browned and soft. Remove from heat and stir in lemon juice. Transfer to a presentation dish and serve.

Source of:
- Iron, folate and fiber

MAKES 4 SERVINGS

Bold, crunchy, colorful, this simple stir-fry gains its appeal from its large-chunk vegetables and its simple flavoring, which allows the subtle licorice of the fennel to shine through. It can be enjoyed hot off the pan, or at room temperature on a party buffet.

NUTRITIONAL ANALYSIS PER SERVING

Energy: 129 kcal	Carbohydrate: 9 g	Calcium: 34 mg	Folate: 31 mcg
Protein: 3 g	Fat: 11 g	Iron: 0.9 mg	Fiber: 2.9 mg

MAKES
8 SERVINGS

The cumin adds a slightly exotic note to this traditional dish, which makes a great accompaniment to many foods.

TIP

In a dry skillet, toast cumin seeds until they release their aroma. Transfer to a spice grinder or mortar, or use the bottom of a measuring cup or wine bottle to coarsely grind.

Make ahead

Peel and cut parsnips and carrots. Cover and refrigerate overnight.

Parsnip and Carrot Purée with Cumin

- 3 ½ to 6 quart slow cooker

4 cups	cubed peeled parsnips, (½-inch/1 cm cubes)	1 L
2 cups	thinly sliced carrots	500 mL
1 tsp	cumin seeds, toasted and coarsely ground (see Tip, at left)	5 mL
2 tbsp	butter or butter substitute	25 mL
1 tsp	granulated sugar	5 mL
½ tsp	salt	2 mL
¼ tsp	freshly ground black pepper	1 mL
¼ cup	water or vegetable stock	50 mL

1. In slow cooker stoneware, combine parsnips, carrots, cumin seeds, butter or butter substitute, sugar, salt, pepper and water or stock. Cover and cook on Low for 8 to 10 hours or on High for 4 to 5 hours, until vegetables are tender.

2. Using a potato masher or a food processor or blender, mash or purée mixture until smooth. Serve immediately.

Variation

Parsnip Purée with Cumin: Use 6 cups (1.5 L) cubed parsnips, instead of the parsnip-carrot combination.

NUTRITIONAL ANALYSIS PER SERVING			
Energy: 90 kcal	Carbohydrate: 15 g	Calcium: 34 mg	Folate: 45 mcg
Protein: 1 g	Fat: 3 g	Iron: 0.6 mg	Fiber: 3.0 mg

Sweet Potato French Fries

- Preheat oven to 425°F (220°C)
- Rimmed baking sheet, lightly greased

2	medium sweet potatoes, peeled	2
2 tbsp	olive oil	25 mL
2	cloves garlic, finely chopped	2
½ tsp	dried tarragon or 2 tsp (10 mL) chopped fresh	2 mL
	Salt and freshly ground black pepper	

1. Cut each potato into ½-inch (1 cm) thick slices. Cut each slice lengthwise into ½-inch (1 cm) strips. Place in a shallow bowl or plastic bag.
2. Add oil, garlic, tarragon and a dash of salt and pepper. Toss until coated.
3. Spread on prepared baking sheet. Bake in preheated oven for 15 minutes or until potatoes are tender, turning once.

Source of:
- Fiber

MAKES 4 SERVINGS

The ease of making French fries the oven way! This time, we do it with sweet potatoes, which cook even faster than the white varieties.

TIPS

Foods rich in beta-carotene are the dark orange and red vegetables and fruits such as sweet potatoes and carrots, as well as pink grapefruit.

Because of the rich flavor in sweet potatoes, they have earned a bad reputation of being high in calories. In reality, a 5-inch (12.5 cm) sweet potato contains only about 120 calories — no more than a white one of the same size.

NUTRITIONAL ANALYSIS PER SERVING			
Energy: 118 kcal	Carbohydrate: 14 g	Calcium: 24 mg	Folate: 8 mcg
Protein: 1 g	Fat: 7 g	Iron: 0.5 mg	Fiber: 2.0 mg

Herbed Potatoes

**MAKES
4 SERVINGS**

*When the palate
demands the wonderful
taste of fried potatoes,
but the waistline says
"no" to French fries,
try this zesty refry of
parboiled potato. It uses
a minimum of oil, and
delivers delightful
flavors.*

1 lb	new potatoes, unpeeled but well scrubbed (about 3)	500 g
¼ cup	olive oil	50 mL
¼ tsp	salt	1 mL
¼ tsp	freshly ground black pepper	1 mL
1 tbsp	grated lemon zest	15 mL
4	cloves garlic, finely chopped	4
	Few sprigs fresh parsley and/or rosemary, chopped	
2 tbsp	freshly squeezed lemon juice	25 mL

1. In a large saucepan, boil potatoes over high heat for 5 to 7 minutes, until they can just be pierced with a fork. Drain and refresh several times with cold water. Cut potatoes into ½-inch (1 cm) rounds.

2. In a large frying pan, heat oil over high heat for 30 seconds. Add salt and pepper and stir. Add potatoes in a single layer and fry for 2 to 3 minutes; reduce heat to medium-high, turn rounds over and fry other side for 2 to 3 minutes, then toss-fry for another 1 to 2 minutes, until golden all over. (Some of the skins will have peeled off and fried to a crisp. Don't worry: they'll add to the final appeal.)

3. Add lemon zest, garlic and most of the chopped herb(s), reserving some for the final garnish. Toss-fry for 1 to 2 minutes. Add lemon juice and toss-fry for 1 to 2 minutes, until the sizzle has stopped and the acidity of the lemon has mellowed. (Taste a piece.) Transfer potatoes to a serving bowl and garnish with the remainder of the herb(s). Serve immediately.

NUTRITIONAL ANALYSIS PER SERVING			
Energy: 207 kcal	Carbohydrate: 25 g	Calcium: 14 mg	Folate: 13 mcg
Protein: 2 g	Fat: 12 g	Iron: 0.5 mg	Fiber: 2.3 mg

Sun-Dried Tomato Quinoa

1 cup	quinoa (see Tip, at right)	250 mL
2 tbsp	chopped dry-packed sun-dried tomatoes	25 mL
2	cloves garlic, minced	2
2 cups	chicken stock	500 mL
	Salt and freshly ground black pepper	

1. Rinse quinoa under cold running water until water is clear. Set aside.

2. Soak tomatoes for 10 minutes in boiling water. Drain and chop. Set aside.

3. In a medium saucepan, combine quinoa, tomatoes, garlic and stock. Bring to a boil. Cover, reduce heat and cook for 25 minutes or until all liquid is absorbed and quinoa is tender. Season with salt and pepper to taste.

MAKES 4 SERVINGS

Quinoa is a grain from Peru that contains more protein than any other grain. In fact, it is considered to be the "supergrain of the future."

TIP

Quinoa may be fairly new to our markets, but it is actually a staple of the ancient Incas, who called it "the mother grain." It remains to this day an important food in South American cuisine. It can be found in most health food stores and in some supermarkets.

NUTRITIONAL ANALYSIS PER SERVING			
Energy: 204 kcal	Carbohydrate: 32 g	Calcium: 38 mg	Folate: 27 mcg
Protein: 12 g	Fat: 4 g	Iron: 4.6 mg	Fiber: 3.2 g

**MAKES
4 SERVINGS**

TIPS

To clean leeks: Fill sink full of lukewarm water. Split leeks in half lengthwise and submerge in water, swishing them around to remove all traces of dirt. Transfer to a colander and rinse under cold water.

In season, add some steamed yellow wax beans, tossed with butter or butter substitute, lemon juice and finely chopped fresh dill.

Make ahead

This dish can be partially prepared the night before it is cooked. Complete Step 1. Cover and refrigerate overnight. The next morning, continue with Step 2.

Leek and Barley Risotto

- 3½ to 6 quart slow cooker

1 tbsp	vegetable oil	15 mL
3	leeks, white part only, cleaned and thinly sliced (see Tip, at left)	3
1 tsp	salt	5 mL
½ tsp	cracked black peppercorns	2 mL
2 cups	pearl barley, rinsed	500 mL
1	can (28 oz/796 mL) tomatoes, including juice, coarsely chopped	1
3 cups	vegetable stock or water	750 mL
	Freshly grated Parmesan cheese (optional)	

1. In a skillet, heat oil over medium heat. Add leeks and cook, stirring, until softened. Add salt, peppercorns and barley and cook, stirring, for 1 minute. Add tomatoes, with juice, and stock and bring to a boil. Transfer to slow cooker stoneware.

2. Cover and cook on Low for 8 hours or on High for 4 hours. Stir in Parmesan, if using, and serve piping hot.

NUTRITIONAL ANALYSIS PER SERVING			
Energy: 497 kcal	Carbohydrate: 105 g	Calcium: 150 mg	Folate: 105 mcg
Protein: 13 g	Fat: 5 g	Iron: 5.5 mg	Fiber: 17.3 g

Desserts

**MAKES 6 TO
8 SERVINGS**

*I love to make this
delicious dessert in the
fall when apples and
cranberries are in
season. This version is
a little tart, which suits
my taste, but if you have
a sweet tooth, add more
sugar to the cranberry
mixture. Great on its
own, this is even better
with whipped cream or
a scoop of frozen yogurt
or vanilla ice cream.*

Delectable Apple-Cranberry Coconut Crisp

• **Large (minimum 5 quart) slow cooker, lightly greased**

4 cups	sliced peeled apples	1 L
2 cups	cranberries, thawed if frozen	500 mL
½ cup	granulated sugar	125 mL
1 tbsp	cornstarch	15 mL
½ tsp	ground cinnamon	2 mL
2 tbsp	freshly squeezed lemon juice or port wine	25 mL

Coconut Topping

½ cup	packed brown sugar	125 mL
½ cup	rolled oats	125 mL
¼ cup	flaked sweetened coconut	50 mL
¼ cup	butter	50 mL

1. In a bowl, combine apples, cranberries, sugar, cornstarch, cinnamon and lemon juice or port. Mix well and transfer to prepared stoneware.

2. *Coconut Topping:* In a separate bowl, combine brown sugar, rolled oats, coconut and butter. Using two forks or your fingers, combine until crumbly. Spread over apple mixture.

3. Place two clean tea towels, each folded in half (so you will have four layers) over top of stoneware. Cover and cook on High for 3 to 4 hours, until crisp is hot and bubbling. Serve with whipped cream or ice cream, if desired.

Variation

Apple-Coconut Crisp: Use 6 cups (1.5 L) of sliced apples, reduce sugar to ¼ cup (50 mL) and use lemon juice rather than port wine.

NUTRITIONAL ANALYSIS PER SERVING			
Energy: 228 kcal	Carbohydrate: 45 g	Calcium: 22 mg	Folate: 3 mcg
Protein: 1 g	Fat: 6 g	Iron: 0.9 mg	Fiber: 3.2 g

Sweet Potato Pecan Pie

- 7-inch (17.5 cm) springform pan, well-greased (see Tip, at right) or 7-inch (17.5 cm) 6-cup (1.5 L) soufflé dish, lined with greased heavy-duty foil
- Heavy-duty foil, if using a springform pan
- Large (minimum 5 quart) oval slow cooker

Crust

1 cup	gingersnap cookie crumbs	250 mL
3 tbsp	packed brown sugar	45 mL
½ tsp	ground ginger	2 mL
3 tbsp	melted butter	45 mL

Filling

2	medium sweet potatoes, cooked, peeled and puréed (about 2 cups/500 mL)	2
½ cup	packed brown sugar	125 mL
2	eggs, beaten	2
½ tsp	ground cinnamon	2 mL
¼ tsp	ground allspice	1 mL
Pinch	salt	Pinch

Topping

½ cup	chopped pecans	125 mL
¼ cup	packed brown sugar	50 mL
2 tbsp	melted butter	25 mL

1. *Crust:* In a bowl, combine gingersnap crumbs, brown sugar and ginger. Add butter and mix well. Press mixture into the bottom of prepared pan. Place in freezer until ready for use.

2. *Filling:* In a bowl, beat sweet potatoes, brown sugar, eggs, cinnamon, allspice and salt until smooth. Spread evenly over prepared crust.

3. *Topping:* In a bowl, combine pecans and brown sugar. Drizzle with butter and stir until combined. Sprinkle over top of pie. Place a layer of parchment or waxed paper over top of cake and cover tightly with foil.

4. Place pan in slow cooker stoneware and pour in enough boiling water to come 1 inch (2.5 cm) up the sides. Cover and cook on High for 4 hours, until filling is set. Serve warm or cold.

Good source of:
- Iron

Source of:
- Calcium, folate and fiber

MAKES 8 SERVINGS

I love everything about this mouth-watering dessert, which among its many charms makes a great alternative to pumpkin pie. The gingersnap crust, the crunchy pecan topping and the creamy sweet potato filling are a delectable combination. Serve this hot or cold, with vanilla ice cream or whipped cream flavored with vanilla or brandy.

TIP

If using a springform pan, ensure that water doesn't seep into the cake by wrapping the bottom of the pan in one large seamless piece of foil that extends up the sides and over the top. Cover the top with a single piece of foil that extends down the sides and secure with string.

NUTRITIONAL ANALYSIS PER SERVING			
Energy: 355 kcal	Carbohydrate: 53 g	Calcium: 60 mg	Folate: 32 mcg
Protein: 4 g	Fat: 15 g	Iron: 2.5 mg	Fiber: 3.1 g

MAKES 12 SERVINGS

This is an absolutely beautiful cake, full of mocha flavor. A true favorite for birthday celebrations!

Delicious Mocha Torte

• Preheat oven to 350°F (180°C)
• Two 8-inch (20 cm) round cake pans, buttered

Cake

1¾ cups	all-purpose flour	425 mL
1 tsp	baking soda	5 mL
½ tsp	salt	2 mL
1 cup	semisweet chocolate chips	250 mL
¼ cup	water	50 mL
1 cup	granulated sugar	250 mL
½ cup	unsalted butter, softened	125 mL
2	eggs, at room temperature	2
1 tsp	vanilla	5 mL
¾ cup	milk	175 mL
1 tsp	freshly squeezed lemon juice	5 mL

Mocha Cream

1 cup	semisweet chocolate chips	250 mL
¼ cup	granulated sugar	50 mL
¼ cup	strong brewed coffee	50 mL
2 cups	whipping (35%) cream	500 mL

1. *Prepare the cake:* In a bowl, combine flour, baking soda and salt; set aside.

2. In a heavy saucepan, over low heat, heat chocolate chips and water, stirring constantly, until chocolate is melted and smooth; set aside.

3. In a large bowl, using an electric mixer, cream sugar and butter until light and fluffy. Beat in eggs, one at a time. Beat in melted chocolate and vanilla.

4. In a small bowl, combine milk and lemon juice; let stand for 30 seconds.

5. Stir flour mixture into butter mixture alternately with the soured milk, making 3 additions of flour and 2 of milk, and mixing until smooth.

6. Pour batter into prepared pans. Bake in preheated oven for 25 to 30 minutes, or until a tester inserted in the center comes out clean. Let cool in pans for 15 minutes, then run a knife around edges of pans and gently invert each cake onto a wire rack to cool completely. Slice each cake horizontally into two layers.

7. *Prepare the mocha cream:* In a heavy saucepan over low heat, heat chocolate chips, sugar and coffee, stirring constantly, until chocolate is melted and smooth. Let cool.

8. In a large bowl, whip cream until it starts to thicken. Add chocolate mixture and whip until stiff peaks form.

9. Place a cake layer cut side up on a large plate and spread top with mocha cream. Add another cake layer and spread top with mocha cream. Repeat until a four-layer cake is built, placing top layer cut side down. Spread the remaining mocha cream on top. Refrigerate for at least 1 hour, until chilled, or for up to 2 days.

NUTRITIONAL ANALYSIS PER SERVING			
Energy: 498 kcal	Carbohydrate: 55 g	Calcium: 66 mg	Folate: 41 mcg
Protein: 6 g	Fat: 31 g	Iron: 1.9 mg	Fiber: 2.2 mg

**MAKES
12 SERVINGS**

This crowd-pleasing cake is as easy to make as a batch of muffins. Serve it as a dessert or enjoy it with a fresh-brewed cup of coffee or tea.

TIP

To freeze: Wrap cake in plastic wrap, then in foil. Cake freezes well for up to 1 month.

Blueberry Crumb Cake

● Preheat oven to 350°F (180°C)
● 9-inch (23 cm) springform pan, greased

Crumb Topping

½ cup	all-purpose flour	125 mL
⅓ cup	packed brown sugar	75 mL
1 tsp	ground cinnamon	5 mL
¼ cup	butter, cut into pieces	50 mL

Cake

2 cups	all-purpose flour	500 mL
1 cup	granulated sugar	250 mL
2½ tsp	baking powder	12 mL
½ tsp	baking soda	2 mL
½ tsp	salt	2 mL
2 cups	fresh or frozen blueberries	500 mL
2	eggs	2
¾ cup	plain yogurt	175 mL
⅓ cup	butter, melted	75 mL
1½ tsp	grated lemon zest	7 mL

1. *Crumb Topping:* In a bowl, combine flour, brown sugar and cinnamon. Cut in butter with a pastry blender or two knives until crumbly.

2. *Cake:* In a large mixing bowl, stir together flour, sugar, baking powder, baking soda and salt. Toss blueberries with 2 tbsp (25 mL) of the flour mixture; set aside.

3. In another bowl, beat eggs, yogurt, melted butter and lemon zest. Stir in flour mixture to make a smooth batter. Gently fold in floured blueberries. (Batter will be thick.)

4. Spoon into prepared pan. Sprinkle top with crumb mixture. Bake in preheated oven for 50 to 60 minutes or until cake tester inserted in center comes out clean. Let cool on rack. Run a knife around edge; remove side of pan, remove base and transfer cake to serving plate.

NUTRITIONAL ANALYSIS PER SERVING			
Energy: 305 kcal	Carbohydrate: 49 g	Calcium: 69 mg	Folate: 58 mcg
Protein: 5 g	Fat: 10 g	Iron: 1.7 mg	Fiber: 1.5 mg

Sour Cream Raspberry Coffee Cake

- Preheat oven to 350°F (180°C)
- 9-inch (23 cm) springform pan, greased

1½ cups	all-purpose flour	375 mL
¾ cup	granulated sugar	175 mL
½ cup	shredded sweetened coconut	125 mL
2 tsp	baking powder	10 mL
½ tsp	baking soda	2 mL
Pinch	salt	Pinch
2	eggs	2
1 cup	sour cream	250 mL
1 tsp	vanilla	5 mL
1 cup	fresh or frozen raspberries or blueberries	250 mL

Crumb Topping

⅓ cup	packed brown sugar	75 mL
¼ cup	quick-cooking rolled oats	50 mL
¼ cup	all-purpose flour	50 mL
¼ cup	shredded sweetened coconut	50 mL
½ tsp	ground cinnamon	2 mL
¼ cup	butter, cut into pieces	50 mL

1. In a bowl, combine flour, sugar, coconut, baking powder, baking soda and salt. In another bowl, beat eggs with sour cream and vanilla. Stir in flour mixture; mix well. Gently fold in raspberries; spread batter in prepared pan.

2. *Crumb Topping:* In a bowl, combine brown sugar, oats, flour, coconut and cinnamon. Cut in butter using a pastry blender or two knives to make coarse crumbs. Sprinkle evenly over top.

3. Bake on middle rack in preheated oven for 40 to 45 minutes or until tester inserted in center comes out clean. Set cake on rack to cool. Serve warm or at room temperature.

MAKES 8 SERVINGS

I keep individual quick-frozen berries stocked in my freezer to make this delectable cake year-round.

TIP

If using frozen berries, individual quick-frozen berries do not need to be defrosted before adding to batter.

NUTRITIONAL ANALYSIS PER SERVING			
Energy: 384 kcal	Carbohydrate: 59 g	Calcium: 85 mg	Folate: 61 mcg
Protein: 6 g	Fat: 14 g	Iron: 2.1 mg	Fiber: 1.9 mg

**MAKES
6 SERVINGS**

This is a delicious old-fashioned dessert. As it cooks, the batter separates into a light soufflé-like layer on top, with a rich, creamy custard on the bottom. Serve hot or warm, accompanied by a light cookie, with whipped cream on the side, if desired.

TIP

I make this in a 7-inch (17.5 cm) square baking dish. The cooking times will vary in a differently proportioned dish.

Raspberry Custard Cake

- 6-cup (1.5 L) baking or soufflé dish, lightly greased
- Large (minimum 5 quart) oval slow cooker

1 cup	granulated sugar, divided	250 mL
2 tbsp	butter, softened	25 mL
4	eggs, separated	4
	Grated zest and juice of 1 lemon	
Pinch	salt	Pinch
¼ cup	all-purpose flour	50 mL
1 cup	milk	250 mL
1½ cups	raspberries, thawed if frozen	375 mL
	Confectioner's (icing) sugar	

1. In a bowl, beat ¾ cup (175 mL) sugar with butter until light and fluffy. Beat in egg yolks until incorporated. Stir in lemon zest and juice. Add salt, then flour and mix until blended. Gradually add milk, beating to make a smooth batter.

2. In a separate bowl, with clean beaters, beat egg whites until soft peaks form. Add remaining ¼ cup (50 mL) sugar and beat until stiff peaks form. Fold into lemon mixture, then fold in raspberries.

3. Pour mixture into prepared dish. Cover with foil and tie tightly with a string. Place dish in slow cooker stoneware and add boiling water to come 1 inch (2.5 cm) up the sides. Cover and cook on High for 3 hours, until the cake springs back when touched lightly in the center. Dust lightly with confectioner's sugar and serve.

Variation

Blueberry Custard Cake: Substitute blueberries for the raspberries.

NUTRITIONAL ANALYSIS PER SERVING			
Energy: 323 kcal	Carbohydrate: 58 g	Calcium: 84 mg	Folate: 42 mcg
Protein: 6 g	Fat: 8 g	Iron: 1.3 mg	Fiber: 3.1 g

Prune Cake

- Preheat oven to 350°F (180°C)
- 9-inch (23 cm) springform pan, buttered

Cake

1¾ cups	pitted prunes	425 mL
1 tbsp	freshly squeezed lemon juice	15 mL
¾ cup	all-purpose flour	175 mL
1 tsp	baking powder	5 mL
Pinch	salt	Pinch
1 cup	granulated sugar	250 mL
½ cup	unsalted butter, softened	125 mL
2	eggs	2

Topping

1 tbsp	granulated sugar	15 mL
¼ tsp	ground cinnamon	1 mL
	Whipped cream (optional)	

1. *Prepare the cake:* In a small bowl, toss prunes with lemon juice; set aside.

2. In a bowl, combine flour, baking powder and salt; set aside.

3. In a large bowl, using an electric mixer, cream sugar and butter until light and fluffy. Beat in eggs, one at a time. Add flour mixture and mix on low speed until well combined.

4. Spread batter evenly in prepared pan. Arrange prunes in concentric circles on top of the batter.

5. *Prepare the topping:* In a small bowl, combine sugar and cinnamon; sprinkle over prunes.

6. Bake in preheated oven for 50 to 60 minutes or until cake is golden and a tester inserted in the center comes out clean. Serve warm, each slice topped with a dollop of whipped cream, if desired.

Source of:
- Iron

MAKES 8 SERVINGS

Prunes never tasted so good. This cake is not too sweet and has the added bonus of fiber and iron.

NUTRITIONAL ANALYSIS PER SERVING

Energy: 242 kcal	Carbohydrate: 35 g	Calcium: 37 mg	Folate: 10 mcg
Protein: 3 g	Fat: 11 g	Iron: 1.7 mg	Fiber: 1.0 g

MAKES 6 TO 8 SERVINGS

This is a delicious light cake. It makes a perfect finish to a great meal and is excellent to have on hand for snacking.

TIPS

Although the orange glaze is a nice finish to this cake, it is also very tasty without a glaze. Allow cake to cool, unmold and dust lightly with confectioner's sugar.

If using a springform pan, ensure that water doesn't seep into the cake by wrapping the bottom of the pan in one large seamless piece of foil that extends up the sides and over the top. Cover the top with a single piece of foil that extends down the sides and secure with string.

Italian-Style Cornmeal Cake with Orange

- 7-inch (17.5 cm) springform pan, well-greased, or 7-inch (17.5 cm) 6-cup (1.5 L) soufflé or baking dish, lined with greased heavy-duty foil
- Large (minimum 5 quart) oval slow cooker

1 cup	fine cornmeal	250 mL
1/4 cup	finely chopped walnuts or pecans	50 mL
2 tsp	baking powder	10 mL
1/2 tsp	salt	2 mL
3/4 cup	granulated sugar	175 mL
1/2 cup	butter, softened	125 mL
2	eggs	2
1 tsp	vanilla	5 mL
1 tbsp	grated orange zest	15 mL
1/4 cup	plain yogurt	50 mL

Orange Glaze (optional)

1/2 cup	confectioner's (icing) sugar, sifted	125 mL
1/4 cup	orange juice	50 mL
1 tbsp	orange-flavored liqueur (optional)	15 mL

1. In a bowl, mix together cornmeal, walnuts, baking powder and salt.

2. In another bowl, beat sugar and butter until light and fluffy. Beat in eggs until incorporated. Stir in vanilla and orange zest. Add dry ingredients in 2 additions alternately with yogurt, mixing until blended. Spoon batter into prepared pan. Wrap securely in foil (see Tips, at left) and place in slow cooker. Cook on High for 4 hours, until cake is puffed and pulling away from side of pan. Glaze cake, if desired.

3. *Orange Glaze:* In a bowl, combine confectioner's sugar, orange juice and orange-flavored liqueur, if using. With a skewer, poke several holes in the cake. Spread glaze over hot cake.

4. Let cake cool in pan for 30 minutes, then unmold.

NUTRITIONAL ANALYSIS PER SERVING			
Energy: 326 kcal	Carbohydrate: 43 g	Calcium: 36 mg	Folate: 18 mcg
Protein: 4 g	Fat: 16 g	Iron: 0.6 mg	Fiber: 0.2 g

Best Cupcakes

- Preheat oven to 350°F (180°C)
- 12-cup muffin tin, buttered

Cupcakes

1½ cups	all-purpose flour	375 mL
1 tsp	baking powder	5 mL
Pinch	salt	Pinch
½ cup	milk	125 mL
1 tsp	vanilla	5 mL
1 cup	granulated sugar	250 mL
½ cup	unsalted butter, softened	125 mL
2	eggs, at room temperature	2

Chocolate Icing

2 cups	confectioner's (icing) sugar	500 mL
¼ cup	unsalted butter, softened	50 mL
3 tbsp	unsweetened cocoa powder, sifted	45 mL
3 tbsp	milk	45 mL
½ tsp	vanilla	2 mL

1. *Prepare the cupcakes:* In a bowl, combine flour, baking powder and salt; set aside.

2. In a small bowl, combine milk and vanilla; set aside.

3. In a large bowl, using an electric mixer, cream sugar and butter until light and fluffy. Beat in eggs, one at a time. Stir in flour mixture alternately with milk mixture, making 3 additions of flour and 2 of milk, and mixing until smooth.

4. Divide batter evenly among muffin cups and bake in preheated oven for 15 to 20 minutes or until tops are slightly browned and a tester inserted in the center of a cupcake comes out clean. Let cool in pan on a rack for 10 minutes.

5. *Prepare the icing:* In a bowl, beat confectioner's sugar, butter, cocoa, milk and vanilla. Ice cupcakes while still warm. Serve immediately.

Source of:
- Iron

MAKES
12 CUPCAKES

These cupcakes freeze well for up to 1 month. I recommend freezing them without the icing. When ready to eat, thaw and top with icing before serving.

NUTRITIONAL ANALYSIS PER SERVING (1 CUPCAKE)

Energy: 335 kcal	Carbohydrate: 53 g	Calcium: 34 mg	Folate: 10 mcg
Protein: 4 g	Fat: 13 g	Iron: 1.1 mg	Fiber: 1.5 g

**MAKES
16 SQUARES**

These classy lemon treats with a shortbread crust are always appreciated when friends are invited for a fresh-brewed cup of tea or coffee.

Luscious Lemon Squares

● Preheat oven to 350°F (180°C)
● 8-inch (2 L) square baking pan

1 cup	all-purpose flour	250 mL
1/4 cup	granulated sugar	50 mL
1/2 cup	butter, cut into pieces	125 mL

Filling

2	eggs	2
1 cup	granulated sugar	250 mL
2 tbsp	all-purpose flour	25 mL
1/2 tsp	baking powder	2 mL
Pinch	salt	Pinch
1 tbsp	grated lemon zest	15 mL
1/4 cup	freshly squeezed lemon juice	50 mL
	Confectioner's (icing) sugar	

1. In a bowl, combine flour and sugar; cut in butter with a pastry blender to make coarse crumbs. Press into bottom of baking pan. Bake in preheated oven for 18 to 20 minutes or until light golden. Let cool on rack.

2. *Filling:* In a bowl, beat eggs with sugar, flour, baking powder, salt, lemon zest and juice. Pour over base.

3. Bake for 25 to 30 minutes or until filling is set and light golden. Place pan on rack to cool. Dust with confectioner's sugar; cut into squares.

NUTRITIONAL ANALYSIS PER SERVING (1 SQUARE)			
Energy: 151 kcal	Carbohydrate: 23 g	Calcium: 9 mg	Folate: 20 mcg
Protein: 2 g	Fat: 7 g	Iron: 0.5 mg	Fiber: 0.2 mg

Fabulous Date Squares

- Preheat oven to 350°F (180°C)
- 8-inch (2 L) square baking pan

Filling

3 cups	chopped pitted dates (about 12 oz/375 g)	750 mL
1 cup	water	250 mL
¼ cup	packed brown sugar	50 mL
1 tsp	grated lemon zest	5 mL

Crumb Layer

1½ cups	quick-cooking rolled oats	375 mL
1 cup	all-purpose flour	250 mL
¾ cup	packed brown sugar	175 mL
½ tsp	baking powder	2 mL
¼ tsp	salt	1 mL
¾ cup	cold butter, cut into pieces	175 mL

1. *Filling:* In a saucepan, combine dates, water, brown sugar and lemon zest. Place over medium heat; cook, stirring, for 8 to 10 minutes or until dates form a smooth paste. Let cool.

2. *Crumb Layer:* In a bowl, combine rolled oats, flour, brown sugar, baking powder and salt. Cut in butter with a pastry cutter or fork to make coarse crumbs.

3. Press two-thirds of crumb mixture in bottom of baking pan. Spread evenly with date filling. Sprinkle with remaining crumb mixture, pressing down lightly.

4. Bake in preheated oven for 30 minutes or until golden. Let cool on a rack; cut into squares.

Source of:
- Iron, folate and fiber

MAKES 16 SQUARES

Here's a heritage recipe that never grows old. My version of date squares has a burst of lemon in the filling, which only enhances its traditional appeal.

TIP

Rather than using a knife to cut sticky dried fruits like dates and apricots, you'll find that kitchen scissors do a better job.

NUTRITIONAL ANALYSIS PER SERVING (1 SQUARE)

Energy: 257 kcal	Carbohydrate: 44 g	Calcium: 37 mg	Folate: 15 mcg
Protein: 3 g	Fat: 9 g	Iron: 1.4 mg	Fiber: 2.8 mg

**MAKES
60 COOKIES**

A favorite since my university days, these spice cookies would provide fuel for cram sessions before exams. Now, continuing the tradition, my kids bake a batch when they have to hit the books.

TIP

Be sure to use fresh baking soda as it makes these cookies crisp and light. Like baking powder, an open box of baking soda has a shelf life of only 6 months, so make sure to replenish both regularly. As a reminder, write the date when they need to be replaced on the container.

Gingersnaps

- Cookie sheets, lightly greased

1/2 cup	shortening	125 mL
1/2 cup	butter, softened	125 mL
3/4 cup	packed brown sugar	175 mL
1/4 cup	fancy molasses	50 mL
1	egg	1
2 1/4 cups	all-purpose flour	550 mL
1 1/2 tsp	baking soda	7 mL
1 1/2 tsp	ground ginger	7 mL
1 tsp	ground cinnamon	5 mL
1 tsp	ground cloves	5 mL
1/4 tsp	salt	1 mL
	Granulated sugar	

1. In a large bowl, cream shortening and butter with brown sugar until light and fluffy; beat in molasses and egg until creamy.

2. In another bowl, sift together flour, baking soda, ginger, cinnamon, ground cloves and salt. Stir into creamed mixture to make a soft dough. Refrigerate for 1 hour or until firm.

3. Preheat oven to 350°F (180°C). Shape dough into 1-inch (2.5 cm) balls; roll in bowl of granulated sugar. Arrange 2 inches (5 cm) apart on prepared cookie sheets. Flatten to 1/4-inch (0.5 cm) thickness using bottom of large glass dipped in sugar.

4. Bake in preheated oven for 12 to 14 minutes or until golden. Cool 2 minutes on baking sheets; transfer to rack and let cool.

NUTRITIONAL ANALYSIS PER SERVING (2 COOKIES)

Energy: 124 kcal	Carbohydrate: 14 g	Calcium: 14 mg	Folate: 18 mcg
Protein: 2 g	Fat: 8 g	Iron: 0.8 mg	Fiber: 0.2 g

Crunchy Almond Biscotti

- Preheat oven to 325°F (160°C)
- Baking sheets, lined with parchment paper

½ cup	butter, softened	125 mL
1¼ cups	granulated sugar	300 mL
3	eggs	3
1 tbsp	finely grated lemon zest	15 mL
1 tsp	almond extract	5 mL
3 cups	all-purpose flour	750 mL
2½ tsp	baking powder	12 mL
¼ tsp	salt	1 mL
1 cup	whole unblanched almonds, coarsely chopped	250 mL

1. In a bowl, using an electric mixer, cream butter with sugar until light and fluffy; beat in eggs, lemon zest and almond extract until incorporated.

2. In another bowl, combine flour, baking powder and salt; stir into butter mixture until combined. Stir in almonds.

3. Turn dough out onto lightly floured surface. With floured hands, shape into a ball and divide in two. Pat into 2 logs, each about 2 inches (5 cm) wide and 14 inches (35 cm) long. Place on prepared baking sheet, about 2 inches (5 cm) apart.

4. Bake on middle rack of preheated oven for 25 minutes or until firm to the touch. Let cool for 10 minutes. Using a long spatula, transfer to a cutting board. With a serrated knife, cut diagonally into ½-inch (1 cm) slices.

5. Place cookies upright on sheet ½-inch (1 cm) apart, using 2 sheets, if necessary. Return to oven and bake for 20 minutes or until dry and lightly browned. Transfer cookies to a rack to cool.

Source of:
- Iron and folate

MAKES 60 COOKIES

Biscotti are much easier to bake than delicate cookies like shortbread and they're also less rich. A double whammy — perfect for these twice-baked Italian specialties.

TIP

Store cookies in covered container, separating layers with waxed paper, for 1 week, or freeze for up to 1 month.

NUTRITIONAL ANALYSIS PER SERVING (2 COOKIES)

Energy: 140 kcal	Carbohydrate: 20 g	Calcium: 28 g	Folate: 26 mcg
Protein: 2 g	Fat: 6 g	Iron: 0.8 mg	Fiber: 1.0 mg

**MAKES
48 COOKIES**

*These crunchy morsels
make wonderful gifts
for friends and family.
Pack biscotti in fancy
containers or tins, or
wrap in clear cellophane
and add a bright ribbon.*

TIP

To toast and skin hazelnuts:
Place nuts on a rimmed
baking sheet in preheated
350°F (180°C) oven for
8 to 10 minutes or until
lightly browned. Place in
a clean, dry towel and rub
off most of the skins.

Hazelnut and Dried Cranberry Biscotti

• Preheat oven to 325°F (160°C)
• Baking sheets, lined with parchment paper

½ cup	butter, softened	125 mL
1 cup	packed brown sugar	250 mL
2	eggs	2
2⅓ cups	all-purpose flour	575 mL
1½ tsp	baking powder	7 mL
1½ tsp	ground cinnamon	7 mL
¼ tsp	ground cloves	1 mL
¼ tsp	ground allspice	1 mL
¼ tsp	salt	1 mL
½ cup	dried cranberries	125 mL
¾ cup	hazelnuts, toasted, skinned and coarsely chopped (see Tip, at left)	175 mL

1. In a bowl, using an electric mixer, cream butter with brown sugar until light and fluffy; beat in eggs until incorporated.

2. In another bowl, combine flour, baking powder, cinnamon, cloves, allspice and salt; stir into butter mixture until combined. Fold in dried cranberries and hazelnuts.

3. Turn dough out onto lightly floured surface. With floured hands, shape into a ball and divide in two. Pat into 2 logs, each about 2 inches (5 cm) wide and 12 inches (30 cm) long. Place on prepared baking sheet, about 2 inches (5 cm) apart.

4. Bake on middle rack of preheated oven for 20 to 25 minutes or until firm to the touch. Let cool for 10 minutes. Using a long spatula, transfer to a cutting board. With a serrated knife, cut diagonally into ½-inch (1 cm) slices.

5. Place cookies upright on sheet ½-inch (1 cm) apart, using 2 sheets, if necessary. Return to oven and bake for 15 to 20 minutes or until dry and lightly browned. Transfer cookies to a rack to cool.

Variation

Dried cranberries add a sweet-tart flavor; substitute golden raisins or chopped dried apricots, if desired.

NUTRITIONAL ANALYSIS PER SERVING (2 COOKIES)			
Energy: 148 kcal	Carbohydrate: 22 g	Calcium: 26 mg	Folate: 28 mcg
Protein: 2 g	Fat: 6 g	Iron: 1.0 mg	Fiber: 0.8 mg

✳ Acknowledgments

THE WRITING OF A BOOK can be quite a challenge, but if the subject is one that has significant meaning to the author, then that challenge becomes a welcome one. I feel most fortunate to have been given yet another opportunity to write about a subject that is dear to my heart — nutrition and the well-being of children and their families. I sincerely believe that the information presented in this book will benefit many and that the benefits of new knowledge received will be lifelong for many.

It would not have been possible to prepare *Better Breastfeeding* without the help of so many important individuals, to whom I am so very grateful:

A very sincere thanks to Debbie O'Connor, for all her ongoing support over the years and for sharing her knowledge on folic acid and nutrition. Thank you so much, Debbie.

I feel so fortunate to work with a great team of dietitians at Sick Kids. Your advice and reviews of the material are most appreciated. Thank you to my RD colleagues, for whom I have the greatest respect — Alisa BarDayan, Jennifer Buccino, Megan Carricato, Cristina Cicco, Gloria Green, Lorrie Hagen, Brenda Hartman Craven, Joann Herridge, Jaimie Kennedy, Joanne Njhuis, Vanita Pais, Anna Tedesco-Bruce and Kellie Welch. Thanks for all your enthusiasm and support, Aneta Plaga. Thanks to Andrea Nash, Joanne Saab, Lisa Houghton and Myla Moretti for your comments and reviews. We wish to gratefully acknowledge the following lactation consultants for reviewing Strategies for Healthy Breastfeeding: Tammy McBride, Kathy Buller, Joan Turnbull and Jennifer Vaughan.

To my colleagues at Sick Kids, who shared their knowledge in their respective specialty areas, thank you so very much — Dr. Sharon Dell, Dr. David Farkouh, Dr. Charlotte Miller, Dr. Paul Pencharz and Dr. Stan Zlotkin. I have learned and continue to learn so much from all of you. A special thanks to Dr. Kirsten Smith for your help.

Thank you, Linda Chow, for completing the recipe analysis. You are, as always, such a pleasure to work with. You continue to show great enthusiasm for your work. Thanks also to Len Piche and Kimberley Zammit.

Thank you, Heidi Falkch. You are a great listener, always supportive and encouraging. Your enthusiasm throughout made it an exciting project from the very beginning.

Thank you to Bob Dees and Marian Jarkovich — I feel truly fortunate to have your team behind this work.

Thank you, Bob Hilderley and Sue Sumeraj. Once again, your expertise really shaped this book and brought out the important messages.

We wish to acknowledge Donna Weissinger, Leon Mitoulas, Amy Spangler and Jules Robinson at Childbirth Graphics®, www.ChildbirthGraphics.com, 1-800-299-3366, ext. 287, for their generous support in giving permission to adapt their illustrations for this book.

Joyce and Debbie, it was so wonderful working with you on this book. Thank you for providing such an important contribution to the project, and for all your wise words and knowledge. I am sure that many will succeed with breastfeeding because of your experiences put in words.

Maureen B, you are such a dear dear friend — thank you for providing some great recipes and for your support and constant encouragement. (And welcome back to the world of nutrition!) Nicole Inch, thanks for your friendship and never-ending kindness (I know who I can go to when I am out of flour).

Joanne S, I missed working with you on this book. I so appreciate your friendship. Thank you for all your support, always.

To my mother, Ilze, paldies, paldies, paldies. You are always so encouraging and thoughtful. You are my role model.

And finally, to Blair, Natali and Matis. You are the world to me. Thank you for understating when I had those late nights and when I just could not be there to do what you wanted while I was buried in the papers all around the house. Natali and Matt, I am so proud of who you are, and how considerate and thoughtful you always try to be. I love you so so much. Blair, you support me always. I am so lucky. Es tev mil.

✷ Contributing Authors

Byron Ayanoglu
125 Best Vegetarian Recipes
Recipes from this book can be found on pages 250, 275–77 and 280.

Johanna Burkhard
400 Best Comfort Food Recipes
Recipes from this book can be found on pages 147–48, 153, 178–79, 181–82, 185, 188, 262–66, 268, 270, 274, 288–89 and 294–98.

Dietitians of Canada
Cook Great Food
Recipes from this book can be found on pages 140–43, 145–46, 149, 151–52, 154, 169, 191–94, 196–99, 202, 204–5, 209, 218, 221–23, 226, 233, 238 and 253–54.

Simply Great Food
Recipes from this book can be found on pages 156, 161, 183–84, 200, 239, 256 and 258.

Judith Finlayson
125 Best Vegetarian Slow Cooker Recipes
Recipes from this book can be found on

pages 174, 240, 242–44, 247–48, 251–52, 257, 267, 269, 278, 282, 284–85, 290 and 292.

Margaret Howard
The 250 Best 4-Ingredient Recipes
Recipes from this book can be found on pages 219–20, 224–25, 236, 260, 261, 279 and 281.

Bill Jones and Stephen Wong
New World Chinese Cooking
Recipes from this book can be found on pages 230–31.

New World Noodles
Recipes from this book can be found on pages 176, 186, 210, 212, 229, 232, 234, 255 and 271–72.

Lynn Roblin, RD, Nutrition Editor
500 Best Healthy Recipes
Recipes from this book can be found on pages 157–59, 160, 162 (top), 163, 166, 168, 171–73, 175, 195, 203, 206–8 and 213–16.

✳ Resources

General Information

Hospital for Sick Children
(About Kids Health and Motherisk)
555 University Avenue
Toronto, ON M5G 1X8
Tel: 416-813-7500
www.sickkids.ca

Canadian Health Network
Public Health Agency of Canada
10th Floor, Jeanne Mance Building
Tunney's Pasture, A.L. 1910B
Ottawa, ON K1A 0K9
www.canadian-health-network.ca

Institute of Medicine of the National Academies
Food and Nutrition Board
Tel: 202-334-1732
Fax: 202-334-2316
E-mail: fnb@nas.edu
www.iom.edu
For information on Dietary Reference Intakes (DRIs), go to the home page, select Food and Nutrition, and then select DRIs

Dietitians of Canada
480 University Avenue, Suite 604
Toronto, ON M5G 1V2
Tel: 416-596-0857
Fax: 416-596-0603
www.dietitians.ca

American Dietetic Association
120 South Riverside Plaza, Suite 2000
Chicago, IL 60606-6995
Tel: 800-877-1600
www.eatright.org

Health Canada
Address Locator 0900C2
Ottawa, ON K1A 0K9
Tel: 619-957-2991 or 866-225-0709

www.hc-sc.gc.ca
See sections on Nutrition for a Healthy Pregnancy — National Guidelines for the Childbearing Years; Food and Nutrition — Canada's Food Guide; Nutrition and Healthy Eating; Advisories, Warnings and Recalls.

World Health Organization (WHO)
The WHO Child Growth Standards
www.who.int/childgrowth/en

Canadian Paediatric Society
2305 St. Laurent Boulevard
Ottawa, ON K1G 4J8
Tel: 613-526-9397
Fax: 613-526-3332
www.cps.ca

American Academy of Pediatrics
3400 Research Forest Drive, Suite B7
The Woodlands, TX 77381
Tel: 281-419-0052
Fax: 281-419-0082
Email: info@aps-spr.org
www.aps-spr.org

Allergy Information

American Academy of Allergy Asthma and Immunology
555 East Wells Street, Suite 1100
Milwaukee, WI 53202-3823
Tel: 414-272-6071
Patient Information and Physician Referral Line: 800-822-2762
E-mail: info@aaaai.org
www.aaaai.org

Food Allergy and Anaphylaxis Network
11781 Lee Jackson Highway, Suite 160
Fairfax, VA 22033-3309
Tel: 800-929-4040
Fax: 703-691-2713
www.foodallergy.org

Breast-Feeding Information

The Academy of Breastfeeding Medicine
140 Huguenot Street, Third Floor
New Rochelle, NY 10801
Tel: 800-990-4ABM
Fax: 914-740-2101
E-mail: abm@bfmed.org
www.bfmed.org

Canadian Lactation Consultants Association
www.clca-accl.ca

HMBANA (Human Milk Banking Association of North America)
www.hmbana.org

International Lactation Consultants Association
1500 Sunday Drive, Suite 102
Raleigh, NC 27607
Tel: 919-861-5577
Fax: 919-787-4916
E-mail info@ilca.org
http://ilca.org

La Leche League International
1400 N. Meacham Road
Schaumburg, IL 60173-4808
Tel: 847-519-7730
www.lalecheleague.org

Dental Health Information

The Canadian Dental Association
1815 Alta Vista Drive
Ottawa, ON K1G 3Y6
Tel: 613-523-1770
www.cda-adc.ca

American Dental Association
211 East Chicago Avenue
Chicago, IL 60611-2678
Tel: 312-440-2500
www.ada.org

Diabetes Information

Canadian Diabetes Association
National Life Building
1400-522 University Avenue
Toronto, ON M5G 2R5

Tel: 800 BANTING (226-8464)
E-mail: info@diabetes.ca
www.diabetes.ca

American Diabetes Association
1701 North Beauregard Street
Alexandria, VA 22311
Tel: 800-DIABETES (800-342-2383)
www.diabetes.org

Food Safety Information

Canada Organic Office
Agri-Food Division
Tel: 613-221-7165
Fax: 613-221-7296

Canadian Food Inspection Agency
159 Cleopatra Drive
Ottawa, ON K1A 0Y9
www.inspection.gc.ca

Health Canada Food and Nutrition
Advisories, Warnings and Recalls
Health Canada
Address Locator 0900C2
Ottawa, ON K1A 0K9
Tel: 613-957-2991 or 866-225-0709
Fax: 613-941-5366
E-mail: Info@hc-sc.gc.ca
www.hc-sc.gc.ca/fn-an/advisories-avis/index_e.html

Environmental Protection Agency
Ariel Rios Building
1200 Pennsylvania Averue, N.W.
Washington, DC 20460
Tel: 202-272-0167
www.epa.gov

United States Department of Agriculture
Food Safety and Inspection Service
USDA Meat & Poultry Hotline
Tel: 888-MPHotline (888-674-6854) or
800-256-7072 (TTY)
mphotline.fsis@usda.gov

United States Food and Drug Administration
Center for Food Safety and Applied Nutrition
5600 Fishers Lane
Rockville, MD20857
Tel: 888-INFO-FDA (1-888-463-6332) or
888-SAFEFOOD
www.cfsan.fda.gov

Pregnancy Information

American College of Obstetricians and Gynecologists
409 12th Street, S.W., PO Box 96920
Washington, DC 20090-6920
Tel: 202-638-5577 or 800-762-2264
www.acog.org

The Society of Obstetricians and Gynaecologists of Canada
780 Echo Drive
Ottawa, ON K1S 5R7
Tel: 613-730-4192 or 800-561-2416
Fax: 613-730-4314
E-mail: helpdesk@sogc.com
http://sogc.medical.org

March of Dimes
Pregnancy and Newborn Health Education Center
1275 Mamaroneck Avenue
White Plains, NY 10605
www.marchofdimes.com

Motherisk
Hospital for Sick Children
555 University Avenue
Toronto, ON M5G 1X8
Tel: 416-813-6780
www.motherisk.org

Other Motherisk Services:
Nausea and Vomiting in Pregnancy:
800-436-8477
   (Telephone counseling service for pregnant women suffering from nausea and vomiting)

Motherisk HIV Healthline and Network:
888-246-5840
   (Information on the effects of HIV and HIV medication in pregnancy and breastfeeding)

Motherisk Alcohol and Substance Use Line:
877-FAS-INFO (327-4636)
   (Information on alcohol and other substances of abuse in pregnancy)

U.S. Department of Health and Human Services
The National Women's Health Information Center
Pregnancy and a Healthy Diet
Tel: 800-994-9662
www.womenshealth.gov

✳ References

Books on Breastfeeding

Kerkhoff Gromada K. Mothering Multiples: Breastfeeding and Caring for Twins. Franklin Park: La Leche League International, 1993.

Lang S. Breastfeeding Special Care Babies. London: Bailliere Tindall, 1997.

Lawrence R. Breastfeeding: A Guide for the Medical Profession, 5th ed. Philadelphia: Mosby, 2005.

Ludington S, Golant S. Kangaroo Care: The Best You Can Do to Help Your Preterm Infant. New York: Bantam Books, 1993.

Morbacher M, Stock J. The Breastfeeding Answer Book, 3rd ed. Schaumberg, IL: La Leche League International, 2003.

Newman J, Pitman T. Dr. Jack Newman's Guide to Breastfeeding. New York: HarperCollins, 2000.

Renfrew M, Fisher C, Arms S. Bestfeeding: Getting Breastfeeding Right for You. Berkeley: Celestial Arts, 2004.

Riordan J. Breastfeeding and Human Lactation, 3rd ed. Sudbury, UK: Jones and Bartlett, 2005.

Walker M. Breastfeeding Management for the Clinician Using the Evidence. Mississauga, ON: Jones and Bartlett, 2006.

———. Core Curriculum for Lactation Consultant Practice. Mississauga, ON: Jones and Bartlett, 2002.

General Pregnancy and Breastfeeding

Bazzano LA. The high cost of not consuming fruits and vegetables. J Am Diet Assoc 2006;106(9):1364–68.

Bell KI, Tepper BJ. Short-term vegetable intake by young children classified by 6-n-propylthoiuracil bitter-taste phenotype. Am J Clin Nutr 2006;84(1):245–51.

Blumberg S. Infant feeding: Can we spice it up a bit? J Am Diet Assoc 2006;106(4):504–5.

Breast cancer and breastfeeding: Collaborative reanalysis of individual data from 47 epidemiological studies in 30 countries, including 50,302 women with breast cancer and 96,973 women without the disease. Lancet 2002;360(9328):187–95.

Butte NF, et al. Energy requirements during pregnancy based on total energy expenditure and energy deposition. Am J Clin Nutr 2004;79(6):1078–87.

de Onis M, Onyango AW. The Centers for Disease Control and Prevention 2000 growth charts and the growth of breastfed infants. Acta Paediatr 2003;92(4):413–19.

Dewey KG. Impact of breastfeeding on maternal nutritional status. Adv Exp Med Biol 2004;554:91–100.

———. Nutrition, growth, and complementary feeding of the breastfed infant. Pediatr Clin North Am 2001;48(1):87–104.

Eberhardt MV, et al. Antioxidant activity of fresh apples. Nature 2000;405(6789):903–4.

Ekstrom A, Nissen E. A mother's feelings for her infant are strengthened by excellent breastfeeding counseling and continuity of care. Pediatrics 2006;118(2):e309–14.

Fiocchi A, et al. Food allergy and the introduction of solid foods to infants: A consensus document. Adverse Reactions to Foods Committee, American College of Allergy, Asthma and Immunology. Ann Allergy Asthma Immunol 2006;97(1):10–20; quiz 1, 77.

Fox MK, et al. Sources of energy and nutrients in the diets of infants and toddlers. J Am Diet Assoc 2006;106(1 Suppl 1):S28–42.

Gale CR, et al. Critical periods of brain growth and cognitive function in children. Brain 2004;127(Pt 2):321–29.

Godfrey KM, Barker DJ. Fetal nutrition and adult disease. Am J Clin Nutr 2000;71(5 Suppl):1344S–52S.

Guenther PM, et al. Most Americans eat much less than recommended amounts of fruits and vegetables. J Am Diet Assoc 2006;106(9):1371–79.

Heyman MB. Lactose intolerance in infants, children, and adolescents. Pediatrics 2006;118(3):1279–86.

Hibbeln JR, et al. Maternal seafood consumption in pregnancy and neurodevelopmental outcomes in childhood (ALSPAC study): An observational cohort study. Lancet 2007;369(9561):578–85.

Jones CA. Maternal transmission of infectious pathogens in breast milk. J Paediatr Child Health 2001;37(6):576–82.

Kaiser LL, Allen L. Position of the American Dietetic Association: Nutrition and lifestyle for a healthy pregnancy outcome. J Am Diet Assoc 2002;102(10):1479–90.

Kent JC, et al. Volume and frequency of breastfeedings and fat content of breast milk throughout the day. Pediatrics 2006;117(3):e387–95.

King JC. Physiology of pregnancy and nutrient metabolism. Am J Clin Nutr 2000;71(5 Suppl):1218S–25S.

Krebs NF, Hambidge KM. Complementary feeding: Clinically relevant factors affecting timing and composition. Am J Clin Nutr 2007;85(2):639S–45S.

Labbok MH. Effects of breastfeeding on the mother. Pediatr Clin North Am 2001;48(1):143–58.

Li R, et al. Changes in public attitudes toward breastfeeding in the United States, 1999–2003. J Am Diet Assoc 2007;107(1):122–27.

Mandel D, et al. Fat and energy contents of expressed human breast milk in prolonged lactation. Pediatrics 2005;116(3):e432–5.

Martin R, et al. Human milk is a source of lactic acid bacteria for the infant gut. J Pediatr 2003;143(6):754–58.

McCrory MA. Does dieting during lactation put infant growth at risk? Nutr Rev 2001;59(1 Pt 1):18–21.

Mennella JA, et al. Flavor programming during infancy. Pediatrics 2004;113(4):840–45.

———. Prenatal and postnatal flavor learning by human infants. Pediatrics 2001;107(6):e88.

Penders J, et al. Factors influencing the composition of the intestinal microbiota in early infancy. Pediatrics 2006;118(2):511–21.

Position of the American Dietetic Association and Dietitians of Canada: Nutrition and Women's Health. JADA 2004;104:984–1001.

Scott JA, et al. Predictors of breastfeeding duration: Evidence from a cohort study. Pediatrics 2006;117(4):e646–55.

Shroff R, et al. Life-threatening hypernatraemic dehydration in breastfed babies. Arch Dis Child 2006;91(12):1025–26.

Stricker T, Braegger CP. Cholesterol intake, biosynthesis of cholesterol and plasma lipids in infants. Effects of early cholesterol intake on cholesterol biosynthesis and plasma lipids among infants until 18 months of age. J Pediatr Gastroenterol Nutr 2006;42(5):591.

Transfer of drugs and other chemicals into human milk. Pediatrics 2001;108(3):776–89.

Win NN, et al. Breastfeeding duration in mothers who express breast milk: A cohort study. Int Breastfeed J 2006;1:28.

Allergy/Eczema

Boyle RJ, Tang ML. Can allergic diseases be prevented prenatally? Allergy 2006;61(12):1423–31.

Dell S, To T. Breastfeeding and asthma in young children: Findings from a population-based study. Arch Pediatr Adolesc Med 2001;155(11):1261–65.

Friedman NJ, Zeiger RS. The role of breast-feeding in the development of allergies and asthma. J Allergy Clin Immunol 2005;115(6):1238–48.

Khakoo A, Lack G. Preventing food allergy. Curr Allergy Asthma Rep 2004;4(1):36–42.

Kramer MS, Kakuma R. Maternal dietary antigen avoidance during pregnancy or lactation, or both, for preventing or treating atopic disease in the child. Cochrane Database Syst Rev 2006;3:CD000133.

Lawrence RM, Pane CA. Human breast milk: current concepts of immunology and infectious diseases. Curr Probl Pediatr Adolesc Health Care 2007;37(1):7–36.

Muraro A, et al. Dietary prevention of allergic diseases in infants and small children. Part I: Immunologic background and criteria for hypoallergenicity. Pediatr Allergy Immunol 2004;15(2):103–11.

Oddy WH, et al. Atopy, eczema and breast milk fatty acids in a high-risk cohort of children followed from birth to 5 yr. Pediatr Allergy Immunol 2006;17(1):4–10.

Saarinen KM, et al. Breast-feeding and the development of cows' milk protein allergy. Adv Exp Med Biol 2000;478:121–30.

Sausenthaler S, et al. Maternal diet during pregnancy in relation to eczema and allergic sensitization in the offspring at 2 y of age. Am J Clin Nutr 2007;85(2):530–37.

Schoetzau A, et al. Effect of exclusive breast-feeding and early solid food avoidance on the incidence of atopic dermatitis in high-risk infants at 1 year of age. Pediatr Allergy Immunol 2002;13(4):234–42.

Semic-Jusufagic A, et al. Environmental exposures, genetic predisposition and allergic diseases: One size never fits all. Allergy 2006;61(4):397–99.

Snijders BE, et al. Breastfeeding and infant eczema in the first year of life in the KOALA birth cohort study: A risk period–specific analysis. Pediatrics 2007;119(1):e137–41.

Vadas P, et al. Detection of peanut allergens in breast milk of lactating women. Jama 2001;285(13):1746–48.

Wegienka G, et al. Breastfeeding history and childhood allergic status in a prospective birth cohort. Ann Allergy Asthma Immunol 2006;97(1):78–83.

Zeiger RS. Food allergen avoidance in the prevention of food allergy in infants and children. Pediatrics 2003;111(6 Pt 3):1662–71.

Zutavern A, et al. The introduction of solids in relation to asthma and eczema. Arch Dis Child 2004;89(4):303–8.

———. Timing of solid food introduction in relation to atopic dermatitis and atopic sensitization: results from a prospective birth cohort study. Pediatrics 2006;117(2):401–11.

Anatomy of the Breast

Ramsay D, et al. Anatomy of the lactating breast redefined with ultrasound imaging. J. Anat 2005;206: 525–34.

Benefits of Breastfeeding for Mom and Child

Bachrach VR, et al. Breastfeeding and the risk of hospitalization for respiratory disease in infancy: A meta-analysis. Arch Pediatr Adolesc Med 2003;157(3):237–43.

Barone JG, et al. Breastfeeding during infancy may protect against bed-wetting during childhood. Pediatrics 2006;118(1):254–59.

Chantry CJ, et al. Full breastfeeding duration and associated decrease in respiratory tract infection in US children. Pediatrics 2006;117(2):425–32.

Chen A, Rogan WJ. Breastfeeding and the risk of postneonatal death in the United States. Pediatrics 2004;113(5):e435–39.

Hanson LA. Breastfeeding provides passive and likely long-lasting active immunity. Ann Allergy Asthma Immunol 1998;81(6):523–33; quiz 33–34, 37.

Helewa M, et al. Breast cancer, pregnancy, and breastfeeding. J Obstet Gynaecol Can 2002;24(2):164–80; quiz 81–84.

Lopez-Alarcon M, et al. Breast-feeding lowers the frequency and duration of acute respiratory infection and diarrhea in infants under six months of age. J Nutr 1997;127(3):436–43.

Martin RM, et al. Breast-feeding and childhood cancer: A systematic review with metaanalysis. Int J Cancer 2005;117(6):1020–31.

McVea KL, et al. The role of breastfeeding in sudden infant death syndrome. J Hum Lact 2000;16(1):13–20.

Morrow AL, et al. Human milk oligosaccharides are associated with protection against diarrhea in breast-fed infants. J Pediatr 2004;145(3):297–303.

Oddy WH. Breastfeeding protects against illness and infection in infants and children: A review of the evidence. Breastfeed Rev 2001;9(2):11–18.

Paricio Talayero JM, et al. Full breastfeeding and hospitalization as a result of infections in the first year of life. Pediatrics 2006;118(1):e92–99.

Quigley MA, et al. Breastfeeding and hospitalization for diarrheal and respiratory infection in the United Kingdom Millennium Cohort Study. Pediatrics 2007;119(4):e837–42.

Breastfeeding Twins

Leonard LG. Breastfeeding twins: Maternal-infant nutrition. JOGN Nurs 1982;11(3):148–53.

Saint L, et al. Yield and nutrient content of milk in eight women breast-feeding twins and one woman breast-feeding triplets. Br J Nutr 1986;56(1):49–58.

Caffeine

Frary CD, et al. Food sources and intakes of caffeine in the diets of persons in the United States. J Am Diet Assoc 2005;105(1):110–13.

James JE. Critical review of dietary caffeine and blood pressure: A relationship that should be taken more seriously. Psychosom Med 2004;66(1):63–71.

Calcium and Vitamin D

Cantorna MT, Mahon BD. Mounting evidence for vitamin D as an environmental factor affecting autoimmune disease prevalence. Exp Biol Med (Maywood) 2004;229(11):1136–42.

Hashim N, Norliza ZA. Calcium status among pregnant women. Asia Pac J Clin Nutr 2004;13(Suppl):S97.

Hollis BW, Wagner CL. Assessment of dietary vitamin D requirements during pregnancy and lactation. Am J Clin Nutr 2004;79(5):717–26.

Reichrath J, Querings K. Vitamin D deficiency during pregnancy: A risk factor not only for fetal growth and bone metabolism but also for correct development of the fetal immune system? Am J Clin Nutr 2005;81(5):1177; author reply, 8.

Specker B. Vitamin D requirements during pregnancy. Am J Clin Nutr 2004;80(6 Suppl):1740S–47S.

Colic

Garrison MM, Christakis DA. A systematic review of treatments for infant colic. Pediatrics 2000;106(1 Pt 2):184–90.

Woolridge MW, Fisher C. Colic, "overfeeding," and symptoms of lactose malabsorption in the breast-fed baby: A possible artifact of feed management? Lancet 1988;2(8607):382–84.

Contraception and Breastfeeding

Black A, et al. Canadian contraception consensus. J Obstet Gynaecol Can 2004;26(4):347–87, 389–436.

Truitt ST, et al. Hormonal contraception during lactation: Systematic review of randomized controlled trials. Contraception 2003;68(4):233–38.

Dental Health and Fluoride

Loesche WJ. Nutrition and dental decay in infants. Am J Clin Nutr 1985;41(2 Suppl):423–35.

Nainar SM, Mohummed S. Diet counseling during the infant oral health visit. Pediatr Dent 2004;26(5):459–62.

Essential Fatty Acids

Helland IB, et al. Maternal supplementation with very-long-chain n-3 fatty acids during pregnancy and lactation augments children's IQ at 4 years of age. Pediatrics 2003;111(1):e39–44.

Jensen CL. Effects of n-3 fatty acids during pregnancy and lactation. Am J Clin Nutr 2006;83(6 Suppl):1452S–57S.

Exercise and Weight

Davies GA, et al. Joint SOGC/CSEP clinical practice guideline: Exercise in pregnancy and the postpartum period. Can J Appl Physiol 2003;28(3):330–41.

Dewey KG, McCrory MA. Effects of dieting and physical activity on pregnancy and lactation. Am J Clin Nutr 1994;59(2 Suppl):446S–52S; discussion 52S–53S.

O'Toole ML, et al. Structured diet and physical activity prevent postpartum weight retention. J Women's Health (Larchmt) 2003;12(10):991–98.

Stotland NE, et al. Body mass index, provider advice, and target gestational weight gain. Obstet Gynecol 2005;105(3):633–38.

Wright KS, et al. Infant acceptance of breast milk after maternal exercise. Pediatrics 2002;109(4):585–89.

Fiber

Marlett JA, et al. Position of the American Dietetic Association: Health implications of dietary fiber. J Am Diet Assoc 2002;102(7):993–1000.

Folic Acid

Robbins JM, et al. Hospitalizations of newborns with folate-sensitive birth defects before and after fortification of foods with folic acid. Pediatrics 2006;118(3):906–15.

Scholl TO, Johnson WG. Folic acid: Influence on the outcome of pregnancy. Am J Clin Nutr 2000;71(5 Suppl):1295S–303S.

Sherwood KL, et al. One-third of pregnant and lactating women may not be meeting their folate requirements from diet alone based on mandated levels of folic acid fortification. J Nutr 2006;136(11):2820–26.

Food Safety/Drugs and Breast Milk

Ho E, et al. Alcohol and breast feeding: Calculation of time to zero level in milk. Biol Neonate 2001;80(3):219–22.

Noakes PS, et al. Maternal smoking is associated with impaired neonatal toll-like-receptor-mediated immune responses. Eur Respir J 2006;28(4):721–29.

Qutaishat SS, et al. Transmission of Salmonella enterica serotype typhimurium DT104 to infants through mother's breast milk. Pediatrics 2003;111(6 Pt 1):1442–46.

Yagev Y, Koren G. Eating fish during pregnancy: Risk of exposure to toxic levels of methylmercury. Can Fam Physician 2002;48:1619–21.

Herbs

Tesch BJ. Herbs commonly used by women: An evidence-based review. Am J Obstet Gynecol 2003;188(5 Suppl):S44–S55.

Iron

Domellof M, et al. Iron absorption in breast-fed infants: Effects of age, iron status, iron supplements, and complementary foods. Am J Clin Nutr 2002;76(1):198–204.

Duncan B, et al. Iron and the exclusively breast-fed infant from birth to six months. J Pediatr Gastroenterol Nutr 1985;4(3):421–25.

Griffin IJ, Abrams SA. Iron and breastfeeding. Pediatr Clin North Am 2001;48(2):401–13.

Halvorsen S. Iron balance between mother and infant during pregnancy and breastfeeding. Acta Paediatr 2000;89(6):625–27.

Scholl TO. Iron status during pregnancy: Setting the stage for mother and infant. Am J Clin Nutr 2005;81(5):1218S–22S.

Zhou SJ, et al. Effect of iron supplementation in pregnancy on IQ of children at 4 years of age. Asia Pac J Clin Nutr 2004;13(Suppl):S39.

Mastitis/Engorgement/ Insufficient Milk/ Breast Surgery

Cotterman K. Reverse pressure softening: A simple tool to prepare areola for easier latching during engorgement. J Human Lactation 2004;20(2):227–37.

Williams N. Supporting the women coming to terms with persistent insufficient milk supply: The role of the lactation consultant. J Human Lactation 2002;18(3):262–63.

Pacifier Use

Canadian Paediatric Society. Recommendations for the use of pacifiers. Canadian Paediatric Society 2007.

Jones H, et al. Pacifier use, early weaning, and cry/fuss behavior. JAMA 2001;286(3):322–26.

Positioning and Latching/ Sore Nipples

Albright LM. Sore nipples in breastfeeding mothers: Causes and treatments. Intl J Pharm Compounding 2003;7(6):426–35.

Blair A. The relationship between positioning, the breastfeeding dynamic, the latching process and pain in breastfeeding mothers with sore nipples. Breastfeeding Rev 2003;11(2):5–10.

Canadian Paediatric Society. Position statements: Ankyloglossia and breastfeeding. Canadian Paediatric Society 2007.

Centuori S, et al. Nipple care, sore nipples, and breastfeeding: A randomized trial. J Human Lactation 1999;15(2):125–30.

Chertok I, et al. A pilot study of maternal and term infant outcomes associated with ultrathin nipple shield use. J Obstet, Gynecol, and Neonatal Nursing 2006;35(2):265–72.

Colson S. Maternal breastfeeding position: Have we got it right? Practicing Midwife 2005;8(11):29–32.

Dias de Oliveira L, et al. Effect of an intervention to improve breastfeeding technique on the frequency of exclusive breastfeeding and lactation-related problems. J Human Lactation 2006;22(3):315–21.

Harper M. Latching on. Practicing Midwife 1998;1(7–8):46–48.

Henderson RM, et al. Postpartum positioning and attachment education for increasing breastfeeding: A randomized trial. Birth 2001:28(4):236–41.

Kassing D. Bottle feeding as a tool to reinforce breastfeeding. J Human Lactation 2002;18(1):56–60.

Livingstone V, Stringer J. The treatment of staphylococcus aureus infected sore nipples: A randomized comparative study. J Human Lactation 1999;15(3):241–46.

Neifert MR. Breast transfer: Positioning, latch-on and screening for problems in milk transfer. Clin Obstet and Gynecol 2004;47(3):656–75.

Porter J. Treating sore, possibly infected nipples. J Human Lactation 2006:20(2):221–22.

Thorley V. Latch and the fear response: Overcoming an obstacle to successful breastfeeding. Breastfeeding Rev 2005:13(1):9–11.

Weigert EML, et al. The influence of breastfeeding technique on the frequencies of exclusive breastfeeding and nipple trauma in the first month of lactation. J de Pediatria 2006:81(4):310–16.

Weissinger D. Insights in practice: A breastfeeding teaching tool using a sandwich analogy for latch-on. J Human Lactation 1998;14(1):51–56.

Postpartum Depression

Beard JL, et al. Maternal iron deficiency anemia affects postpartum emotions and cognition. J Nutr 2005;135(2):267–72.

Carter AS, et al. Body mass index, eating attitudes, and symptoms of depression and anxiety in pregnancy and the postpartum period. Psychosom Med 2000;62(2):264–70.

Chen TH, et al. Postpartum mood disorders may be related to a decreased insulin level after delivery. Med Hypotheses 2005.

Corwin EJ, et al. Low hemoglobin level is a risk factor for postpartum depression. J Nutr 2003;133(12):4139–42.

Freeman MP, et al. Randomized dose-ranging pilot trial of omega-3 fatty acids for postpartum depression. Acta Psychiatr Scand 2006;113(1):31–35.

Prebiotics/Probiotics

Boyle RJ, et al. Probiotic use in clinical practice: What are the risks? Am J Clin Nutr 2006;83(6):1256–64; quiz 446–47.

Rinne M, et al. Effect of probiotics and breastfeeding on the bifidobacterium and lactobacillus/enterococcus microbiota and humoral immune responses. J Pediatr 2005;147(2):186–91.

Salminen S, Isolauri E. Intestinal colonization, microbiota, and probiotics. J Pediatr 2006;149(5 Suppl):S115–20.

Premature Infants

Kangaroo Care: A Practical Guide. Geneva: World Health Organization. 2003.

Meier P. Breastfeeding in the special care nursery: Prematures and infants with medical problems. Pediatr Clinics of N Am 2001;48(2).

———. Nipple shield for preterm infants: Effect on milk transfer and duration of breastfeeding. J Human Lactation 2000;16(2):106–13.

———. Supporting lactation in mothers with very low birth weight infants. Pediatr Ann 2003;32(5).

Pinelli J, Symington A. Non-nutritive sucking for promoting physiological stability and nutrition in preterm infants (Review). The Cochrane Library 2005;1.

Pumping and Milk Storage

The Academy of Breastfeeding Medicine. Protocol #8: Human Milk Storage for Home Use for Healthy Full-Term Infants. The Academy of Breastfeeding Resources Inc. 2004.

Rechtman D, et al. Effect of environmental conditions on pasteurized donor human milk. Breastfeeding Med 2006;1(1):24–26.

Trans Fats

Mojska H. Influence of trans fatty acids on infant and fetus development. Acta Microbiol Pol 2003;52 Suppl:S67–S74.

Mozaffarian D, et al. Trans fatty acids and cardiovascular disease. N Engl J Med 2006;354(15):1601–13.

Vegetarian

Finley DA, et al. Breast milk composition: Fat content and fatty acid composition in vegetarians and non-vegetarians. Am J Clin Nutr 1985;41(4):787–800.

Position of the American Dietetic Association and Dietitians of Canada: Vegetarian diets. Can J Diet Pract Res 2003;64(2):62–81.

Weiss R, et al. Severe vitamin B12 deficiency in an infant associated with a maternal deficiency and a strict vegetarian diet. J Pediatr Hematol Oncol 2004;26(4):270–71.

Library and Archives Canada Cataloguing in Publication

Kalnins, Daina

    Better breastfeeding : a mother's guide to feeding and nutrition /
Daina Kalnins, Debbie Stone, Joyce Touw.

Includes index.
ISBN 978-0-7788-0164-1 (pbk.)

    1. Breastfeeding. 2. Mothers–Nutrition. 3. Cookery. I. Stone, Debbie
II. Touw, Joyce III. Title.

RJ216.K335 2007   649'.33   C2007-903023-8

* Index